ULTRASOUND IMAGING

Edited by **Masayuki Tanabe**

Ultrasound Imaging
Edited by Masayuki Tanabe

Published by InTech
Janeza Trdine 9, 51000 Rijeka, Croatia

Publishing Process Manager Katarina Lovrecic

Technical Editor Teodora Smiljanic

Cover Designer InTech Design Team

Additional hard copies can be obtained from orders@intechopen.com

Ultrasound Imaging, Edited by Masayuki Tanabe
p. cm.
ISBN 978-953-307-239-5

For EU product safety concerns:
IN TECH d.o.o., Prolaz Marije Krucifikse Kozulić 3, 51000 Rijeka, Croatia,
info@intechopen.com or visit our website at intechopen.com.

Meet the editor

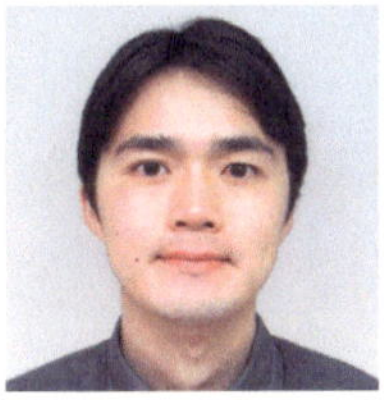

Masayuki Tanabe was born in Japan in 1983. He received both his B.Sc. Degree in 2006 and his M.Sc. Degree in 2008 from the Tokyo Metropolitan University in Japan. He is currently a Ph.D student under guidance of Norio Tagawa at the Tokyo Metropolitan University. He is also a JSPS Research Fellow since 2009. He teaches digital image processing at the Tokyo University of Technology, and is a lecturer since 2008. His current research interests include coded excitation in medical ultrasound imaging and ultrasound motor.

Contents

Preface

Ultrasound is one of the most useful sources for visualizing the inside of materials and has been used in many applications such as NDT (non destructive testing) and medical ultrasound imaging. Specifically, medical ultrasound imaging has been actively applied to abdominal, breast, heart, blood vessel, and fetus imaging. Nowadays, not only visualization of the inside of the body but also the measurements of tissue motion, blood flow and elasticity can be realized.

In this book, we present a dozen state of the art developments for ultrasound imaging, for example, hardware implementation, transducer, beamforming, signal processing, measurement of elasticity and diagnosis. The editors would like to thank all the chapter authors, who focused on the publication of this book.

Masayuki Tanabe
Tokyo Metropolitan University
Japan

1

Hardware-Software Partitioning of Digital Signal Processing in Ultrasound Medical Devices a Case Study

Marcin Lewandowski
Institute of Fundamental Technological Research, Polish Academy of Sciences
Pawinskiego 5B, 02-106 Warsaw,
Poland

1. Introduction

The development of ultrasound devices and diagnostic methods is closely related with the development of microelectronics and digital signal processing. In most of the state of the art electronic devices, the signal is digitally processed. These devices may be generally categorized based on the number of parallel processing channels. Imaging devices with multi-element linear or phased arrays usually have 16-256 transmission/reception channels. Single channel processing is usually performed in imaging devices with mechanically moved single element sector heads, the so-called "wobbler" and in dedicated Doppler devices. The methods of signal processing are much the same in all device categories.

The paper presents a general overview of ultrasound signal processing and its digital implementation with emphasis on hardware-software partitioning. The available state of the art methods and systems of digital signal processing using both hardware and software are presented as well as the issues pertaining to algorithm implementation methodology. The state of the art system solutions are presented based on the descriptions of representative ultrasound devices, found in literature. The similarities between the presented devices and radio signal processing systems used in telecommunication are also discussed in the paper. Based on device description, the authors present the architecture of processing and communication as well as specific design solutions. The discussed issues and system solutions are analyzed based on two ultrasound medical devices, namely:

- ***uScan*** - high frequency ultrasonograph with coded transmission (Lewandowski & Nowicki, 2008),
- ***digiTDS*** - transcranial Doppler system (Lewandowski et al., 2009).

Both devices have been designed and built by the author and co-workers at the Institute of Fundamental Technological Research, Polish Academy of Sciences. They have been designed for commercial purposes, in conformity with medical standards and economic limitations.

The analysis of the presented solution comprises:

- description of the presented systems architecture and of the processing algorithm implementation,
- decisions concerning the design and hardware-software partitioning.

2. Digital signal processing of the ultrasound echoes

Diagnostic medical ultrasound devices utilize ultrasound waves at the frequency of 1-15 MHz. The transmitted ultrasound wave, mainly in the form of a train of short pulses, propagates in the tissue where the structures are reflected and returned to the head as echoes. The signal of echoes is initially amplified and filtered in an analogue chain and next, digitally processed using ADC (Analog-Digital Converter) with 8-14 bit of resolution (Thomenius, 2006). The received high frequency signal (called RF – radio frequency) of the echoes is amplitude- and phase modulated carrier frequency signal. The signal is demodulated in the device to obtain baseband frequency. The demodulated echo signal is further processed, depending on the application (Ali et al., 2008).

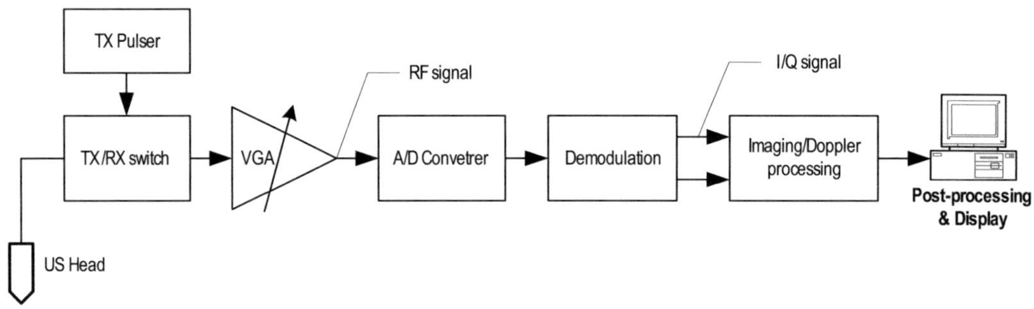

Fig. 1. Simplified block diagram of an ultrasound diagnostic device

The chain of ultrasound signal processing (Fig. 1) is much the same as the chain used in digital telecommunication. Therefore, in both cases, similar system solutions and processing methods are applied. For adaptation to quickly changing processing algorithms used in telecommunication, the Software-Defined Radio (SDR) was developed, in which RF signals are processed using software (Reed, 2002).

The generic architecture of SDR systems composed of GPP (General Purpose Processor), DSP (Digital Signal Processor), FPGA (Field Programmable Gate Array) and high frequency front-end blocks was proposed by (Bassam et al., 2009). According to the authors, universal systems of RF signal processing can be implemented based on this architecture.

The most popular example of an SDR platform is the GNU Radio project, and the compatible Universal Software Radio Peripheral (USRP) module, designed by a group of enthusiasts, later used in multiple designs and studies. The USRP module consists of a set of broadband ADC and DAC connected to the FPGA, which in turn communicates with the PC via USB interface. The board is prepared to host analogue transmitter and receiver modules, which tailor the solution to specific applications. The FPGA is responsible for signal modulation and demodulation and stream data to and from PC. The developed digital signal processing in C language with interface to Python script language enables quick and easy prototyping of radio signal processing algorithms. With its universal design and availability of a relatively cheap hardware module, the system is quite popular. The project website (http://gnuradio.org) contains information on the application of the project, as well as protocols and telecommunication standards including WiFi, RFID, DVB, DAB, GSM and DECT.

The newer and more advanced version of SDR platform named SORA was developed by Microsoft® Research. It has a significantly larger FPGA (Xilinx Virtex 5) chip and a faster

PCI-e x8 interface. Moreover, a software stack for multicore processors containing drivers and processing libraries, optimized for efficiency and latency minimization was developed (Tan et al., 2009). The authors also presented a demonstrative implementation of SoftWiFi supporting the 802.11a/b/g communication protocol.
The reader will probably notice a very high similarity between the USRP solution and coder-digitizer module of the ***uScan*** system described later in the paper. It definitely indicates a similarity between the system solutions and the architecture of SDR and ultrasound devices. Interestingly, the author has not found any report on using SDR solutions for ultrasound RF signal processing.

3. Digital signal processing systems

Nowadays, there is a vast number and diversity of digital signal processing systems and methods. Therefore, it is extremely difficult to select an optimal system solution for signal processing of suitable processing power, data throughput and power consumption at a reasonable price. If we limit our choice to the solutions commonly applied in ultrasonography, these will include:

- hardware processing - programmable logic systems (FPGA) and ASIC (Application Specific Integrated Circuits),
- software processing - general purpose processors (GPP), digital signal processors (DSP) and graphic processors (GPU).

Recently there is a tendency to increase software processing because of the development of processor systems and significantly easier implementation process and algorithm debugging as compared to hardware implementations. This tendency has resulted in the development of ultrasound medical devices, requiring a more efficient digital processing and working in a real time regime.
The main advantage of software solutions is easy code modification and simpler testing and debugging methods. Implementations in high level languages (e.g. C language) can be easily simulated and verified on different platforms before being implemented on the target platform. Nowadays, the majority of DSP are programmed in C language and have more advanced tools for development. Thanks to their computing power, easy high-level code development, DSP are the core of processing chain in modern devices. There is an alternative trend in software processing, namely general purpose processors (GPP). Modern PC processors have high computing power and special parallel executive units for multimedia processing. These units are in fact separate vector processors, optimized for digital signal processing. Adequate use of parallel processing and multimedia units can replace several DSP working at the same time. As PCs are frequently part of these devices and are used both as controller and user interface, the implementation of processing algorithms using PC seems natural. Real time application of operational systems, such as Microsoft® Windows is problematic as these are not real time systems and therefore they do not guarantee adequate time precision and the required operations being performed in the required time period.
Recently, graphic processor units (GPU) are used for signal processing; they are traditionally used for 3D graphics rendering in PCs. The quick development of computer graphics resulted in the development of graphic processors with new capabilities. From specialized 3D processors, GPU have been developed into versatile programmable vector processors. Thanks to its massive parallel internal architecture and advanced memory

interfaces, the floating point processing power of GPUs can be even 100 times higher than the power of the fastest PC processors. The new tools for graphic processor programming allow to utilize new computing power, not only for graphic purposes, but also in other, more general applications (Owens et al., 2005).
Hardware implementation of digital signal processing is presently dominated by programmable logic systems (FPGA). Thanks to the availability of cheap FPGA versions, they are used not only in small scale production, but also in products released onto the consumer market. The possibility of reprogramming within the system (also during operation), a very wide range of system density (from thousands to millions of gates) and increasingly advanced design tools (McDonald, 2009) contribute to the growing popularity of FPGA systems. Hardware methods offer the highest potential processing speed (Sirowy & Forin, 2008), however the implementation costs are also high, probably the highest. Therefore, hardware and software methods are frequently applied as complementary methods to achieve the required efficiency and versatility at minimal costs.
The discussion presented above indicates that digital processing algorithms can be implemented in different ways, based on different solutions. The optimal use of various computational tools and system architecture providing development opportunities is a complex problem from the point of view of science and engineering.

4. Ultrasound devices - state of the art

The combined architecture of hardware-software processing devices is currently the main feature of various digital signal processing devices, requiring high processing speed and characterized by a high bandwidth of input data stream. The combined architecture incorporates hardware systems (FPGA/ASIC), responsible for initial processing and aggregation and/or distribution and further software processing systems (DSP, GPP, GPU processors). We can see a clear tendency to extend the scope of software processing and minimize hardware solutions. The popularity of software solutions results not only from easier implementation, testing and debugging, but also from the possibility of adaptation of these devices to quickly changing market requirements and new algorithms.
On the other hand, the state of the art FPGA systems should be now more frequently treated as programmable SOC (System on Chip) systems rather than simple gate arrays. The availability of new tools for algorithm implementation in FPGA (e.g. Xilinx® AccelDSP, Altera® DSP Builder) significantly facilitates the design and transfer of complex computational algorithms without the need to encode them in hardware description languages. The available IP (Intellectual Property) processor blocks (e.g. Xilinx® Microblaze, Altera® NIOS, Actel® Cortex-M) enable the creation of single- and multiprocessor systems directly in FPGA structures. The processor blocks support the implementation of extended instruction sets using hardware solutions built from the surrounding logic (the so called instruction accelerators). Alter® C2H tool is an example of such solution that compiles selected code fragments in C language directly for hardware implementation, warranting 15-73-fold speedup for selected functions (Altera, 2006). Integrated systems based on the reprogrammable FPGA were described by (Garcia et al., 2006).
The model example of combined ultrasound system architecture is a Doppler device developed by (Ricci et al., 2008). The construction of this system is much the same as that of ***digiTDS*** system presented below. The module designed by Ricci et al. is composed of FPGA (Altera® Stratix) executing hardware processing functions, and DSP (Texas Instruments®

TMS320C67). The module communicates with a PC and is responsible for the control and display functions through the USB interface. The FPGA has implemented a quadrature demodulator, a set of digital filters and a decimator. The initially demodulated and decimated data stream is transferred to the DSP, executing standard Doppler algorithms. Although the reported system is not a commercial solution, its construction is similar to that of the devices offered on the market.

Another device, an ultrasonograph platform ULA-OP, was designed by the same group (Tortoli et al., 2009). Although it is a 64-channel system, it is based on the same general concept. The basic difference is that this system utilizes multiple FPGA chips connected to multichannel ADC and a central hub FPGA, responsible for data aggregation (in total: 5 FPGA Altera® Stratix systems, each having its own 512 MB of DDR memory). The efficient DSP (Texas Instruments® TMS320C6455) is responsible for software processing. The system is connected to PC via USB port and the PC controls the system and displays the results. As we can see, although it has many channels, the general scheme of device design does not differ from that of a dual channel Doppler system.

The next system described in literature is a hand-held 32-channel ultrasonograph, developed by (Lee et al., 2009). Its architecture resembles the ULA-OP system. The main differences are that the ultrasonograph uses a single large FPGA (Xilinx® Virtex 4) and an additional application processor (Intel® XScale PXA270), executing the user interface and display on the integrated LCD panel. The system is completely independent (does not require connection to PC) and optimized for the size and power consumption. The distribution of processing tasks between the hardware and software is in conformity with previous solutions.

1024-channel SARUS (Jensen et al., 2007) system is a unique ultrasound research platform. Unlike the previously described solutions, the system is mainly based on the on-line hardware and off-line software processing. It consists of 64 identical DAUP (Digital Acquisition and Ultrasound Processing) boards, each operating 16 transmitting-receiving channels and an external computer cluster with a disk array. Each of the DAUP boards contains 4 FPGA (Xilinx® Virtex XC4VFX100) with a dedicated 1-4 GB DDR2 memory and one control FPGA (Xilinx® Virtex XC4VFX12). Technical solutions and the potential of SARUS system are overwhelming, however, this is only a research system and its architecture does not allow it to be directly adapted to commercial systems.

The hardware only processing chain for ultrasound system was presented by (Chang et al., 2009). A single-channel acquisition and processing system consists of ADC (Analogue Devices® AD9430) connected to FPGA (Altera® Stratix EP1S60F1020C6), executing the entire processing. Due to the planned application of the above system in studies on mice whose heart rate reaches 13 beats per second, the authors made an attempt to perform imaging with the speed of 400 images per second. The application of simplified and optimized processing algorithms (including envelope detector) allowed to obtain the designed processing speed. The reconstructed images were next transmitted to PC via PCI interface and displayed using a graphics card with the implemented scan-converter. The presented solution indicates how high processing speed can be obtained in systems using hardware processing.

A completely different solution is a C-scan imaging system presented by (Fuller et al., 2009). It has a custom built ultrasonic array transducer, composed of 3600 elements with an integrated transmission-reception electronics. The echoes received from selected depth are then transmitted to a DSP (Analog Devices® Blackfin BF561) which executes the entire digital signal processing and display on the built-in LCD monitor screen. The obtained display speed of 43 images per second for the C-scan indicates that in some applications, pure software processing is sufficient to obtain a practical outcome.

Interestingly, ready-to-use solutions for commercial ultrasound scanners are offered by Texas Instruments® company, the leading manufacturer of DSP. Texas Instruments® has developed an optimized function library for applications in ultrasonography using the offered TMS320C64 series DSPs (Thomas, 2010). Moreover, (Pailoor & Pradhan, 2008) present specific architectures and solutions for portable medical ultrasonography systems. These are systems with combined hardware-software processing. As in the previous presented systems, the first processing stage (beamforming and demodulation) is executed by hardware, while the subsequent stages are executed by DSP. The TI offers a complete development environment and integrated circuits portfolio to build almost the complete systems (TI doesn't offer FPGA).

The final solution presented in this paper is a cheap ultrasonograph with a single processing channel in the form of an integrated head connected to PC via USB port (Richard et al., 2008). The entire simplified electronics is integrated on a miniature board, placed directly in the ultrasound head. The RF echo signal undergoes analogue demodulation and it is digitally processed and transmitted to PC via USB interface. An analogue demodulation of RF signals is no longer used in the devices; in the presented case its application results from construction simplification. Due to low power consumption, the head is supplied directly from PC via USB. The whole processing and visualization were implemented as software for PC. The quality of an ultrasound image fails to meet contemporary standards, however, on the other hand, its price is unmatched. The concept of system solution, minimization of electronics and total PC processing is similar to that of the ***uScan*** described further in the paper.

5. Case study

Both systems are based on a mixed model of hardware-software signal processing. The systems of RF echo signal acquisition are based on a fast A/D converter and FPGA, being an interface to the further part of the system. The application of FPGA at the beginning of the digital chains is now a standard solution. Apart from signal acquisition, the FPGA most often executes hardware processing of a digital signal, whose goal is to reduce the data stream for further processing. Next, the processing is executed by DSP, GPP, GPU or combinations of these processors.

5.1 High frequency ultrasound scanner - *uScan*

High frequency ultrasonography is an imaging method using ultrasound waves of more than 20 MHz frequency. Due to the obtained high resolution and low penetration depth of imaging, this method is applied in dermatology, ophthalmology, cosmetology and for examining small animals.

uScan system is a high frequency ultrasound scanner (20-40 MHz) with the implemented coded transmission/excitation function. The coded transmission method involves transmission of long series of impulses and subsequent time compression of the received echoes to restore resolution. With the long bursts, it is possible to obtain a better signal-to-noise ratio, and the resulting image contrast improvement. Unfortunately, the echo time compression algorithm, which is in fact, matched filter to the transmitted signal, requires a very high computing power.

The device is based on the concept of absolute minimization of electronics and computation based solely on CPU and GPU. The electronic module of coder-digitizer (Fig. 2) executing all the transmission and reception functions is 90 mm × 90 mm in size and is based on a single low-cost FPGA chip (Xilinx® Spartan 3 XC3S200). The transmission involves the use of an arbitrary waveform generator with a 14-bit DAC (Analogue Devices® AD9744) operating at 200 MSPS speed. The acquisition is performed using a 12-bit DAC (Maxim® MAX1214) also working at a speed of 200 MSPS. The digital RF echo signal is transmitted to PC via USB 2.0 interface (Cypress Semiconductor® CY7C68013A). The processing software executes the function of time compression on a CPU processor. The sector geometry conversion function (scan-converter) required to obtain a correct display of an image generated by the sector head is executed by a graphics processor.

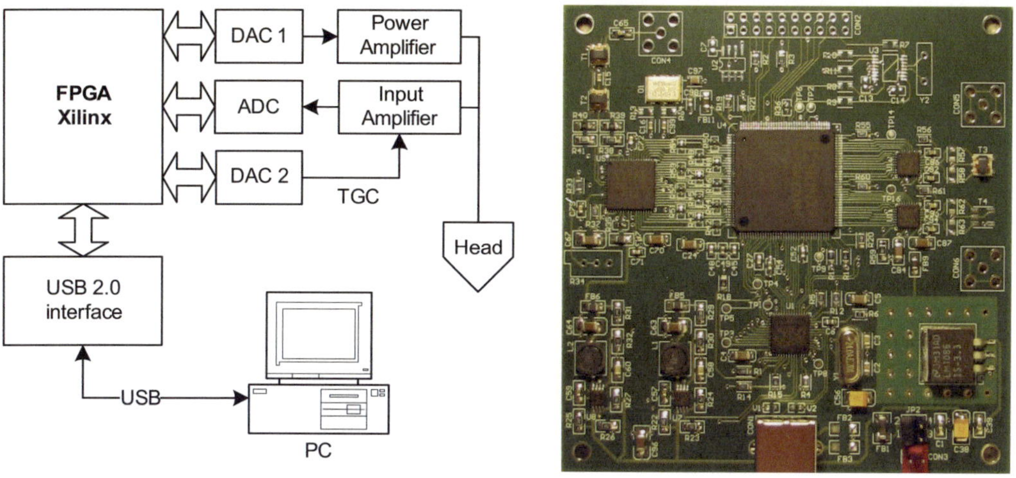

Fig. 2. Block diagram of the coder-digitizer module (left), and the board photo of size 90 mm x 90 mm (right)

The module was designed for stream data transmission; therefore it contains only a buffer in FPGA for a single RF signal line. The line data have to leave the buffer before the next acquisition, i.e. they have to be sent to the USB controller system. The USB system contains 4 buffers 512 bytes each, which are used for communication in the ping-pong mode. A typical length of a RF line is 2048 samples, which gives 4096 bytes of data (two bytes per sample). On an *ACER TravelMate 4650* notebook (Intel® Pentium M processor with a clock 1.7 GHz, 512 MB of RAM), the USB transmission throughput obtained in the test mode was close to 40 MB/s. However, in real conditions, when signal line acquisition was released periodically by ultrasound head movements, buffer overflow errors were observed. This indicates minor transmission interruption, i.e. changes in instantaneous data reception speed by PC. It was concluded that the "interruptions" occurred at system driver level. Microsoft® Windows does not guarantee the time limit of event and interruptions handling from the input/output devices. The overflow errors result in image loss and entail the necessity of subsequent image acquisition synchronization with the extreme position of the head movement. As the coder-digitizer module featured no larger data buffer, it was necessary to limit the head movement speed (and thus image display) to 10 images per second, which is still a sufficient speed for still structure imaging. An alternative solution would be to number the transmitted lines and an additional image filling algorithm with the obtained complete lines. Incomplete or deleted lines of the image would be filled by the fragments of previous lines or by interline interpolation.

The digital RF signal processing functions were implemented as a whole in the software domain and distributed between the CPU of the PC and graphic card processor depending on their specificity (Fig. 3). The code compression and detection algorithm is executed on CPU, while the scan-converter and additional post-processing functions are executed on GPU. Such architecture enables execution of more demanding processing systems without the need to employ specialized and expensive multiprocessor systems.

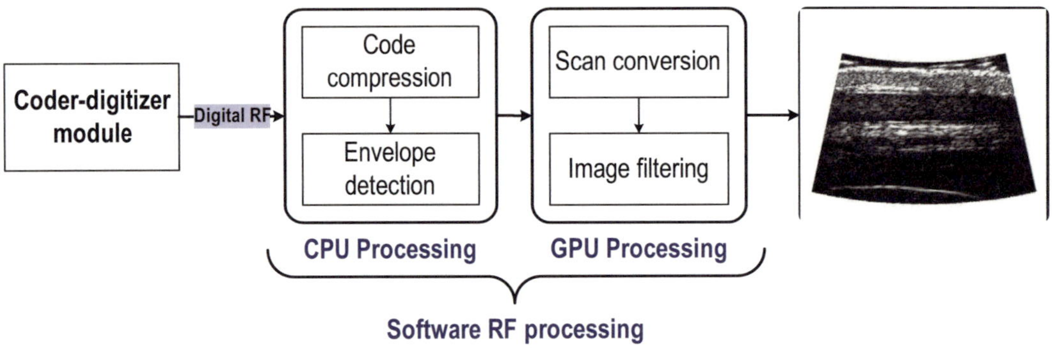

Fig. 3. Data flow of the software RF digital signal processing

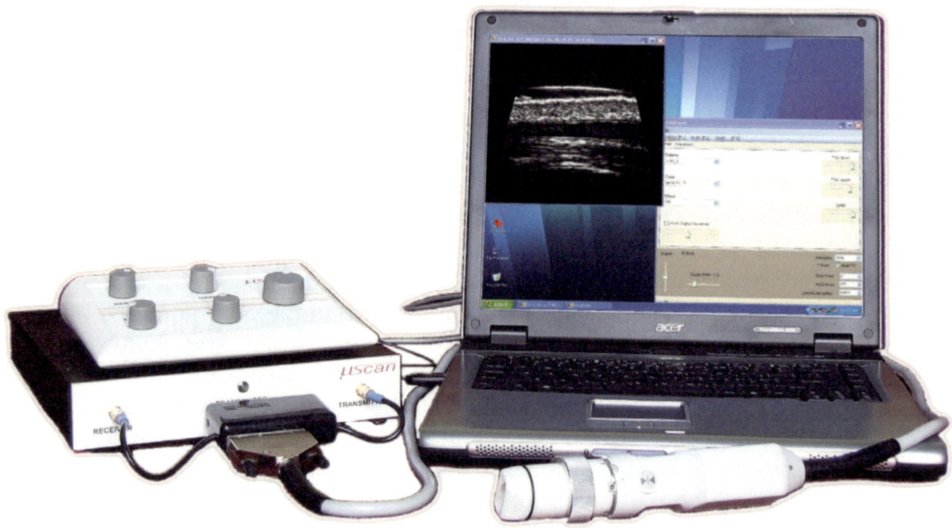

Fig. 4. Photo of the complete ***uScan*** system

Software efficiency tests for processing and visualization were performed on *ACER TravelMate 4650* notebook in configuration: Intel® Pentium M processor with 1.7 GHz clock, 2 MB second level cache, 512 MB RAM, graphic processor Nvidia GeForce Go 6600 with

64 MB of video memory. For an ultrasound head scanning with the speed of 7 images/s, the CPU load was 37%. When extrapolating the processing time, the system was found to be able to run at the speed up to 25 images/s in this configuration.

The obtained solution meets the presented requirements for processing speed and image display in a real time regime (up to 10 frames per second). The applied balanced architecture of digital processing with task distribution between CPU and GPU ensures very high processing efficiency with simultaneous limitation of electronic systems and hardware processing. The limitation of this system is the speed of data transfer via USB interface, as the computing power would allow for significantly faster display. The quick development and increase of CPU/GPU system efficiency ensures the possibility of increasingly complex processing algorithms without the need of hardware replacement.

5.2 Transcranial Doppler System - *digiTDS*

The pulse wave Doppler method is applied as a standard for intracranial diagnosing allowing to measure the flow at selected depth. The state of the art diagnostic solutions are mainly focused on complex assessment and monitoring of cerebrovascular flow in different pathological conditions, especially those potentially affecting normal function of the central nervous system.

The ***digiTDS*** device is a multigate transcranial Doppler system. This system is composed of two electronic modules of 130 mm × 82 mm dimensions (Fig. 5), responsible for high frequency signal transmission, acquisition and demodulation, and the PC responsible for Doppler signal processing after demodulation and data presentation. Fig. 6 presents the

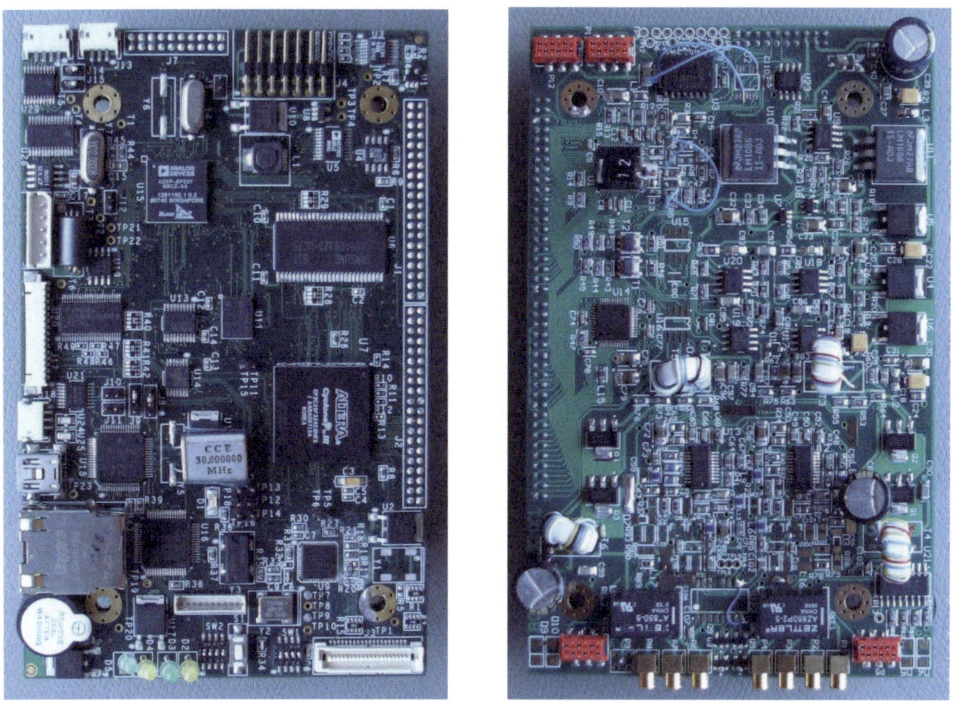

Fig. 5. Photos of the ***digiTDS***'s electronic modules: digital module (left), mixed-signal module (right)

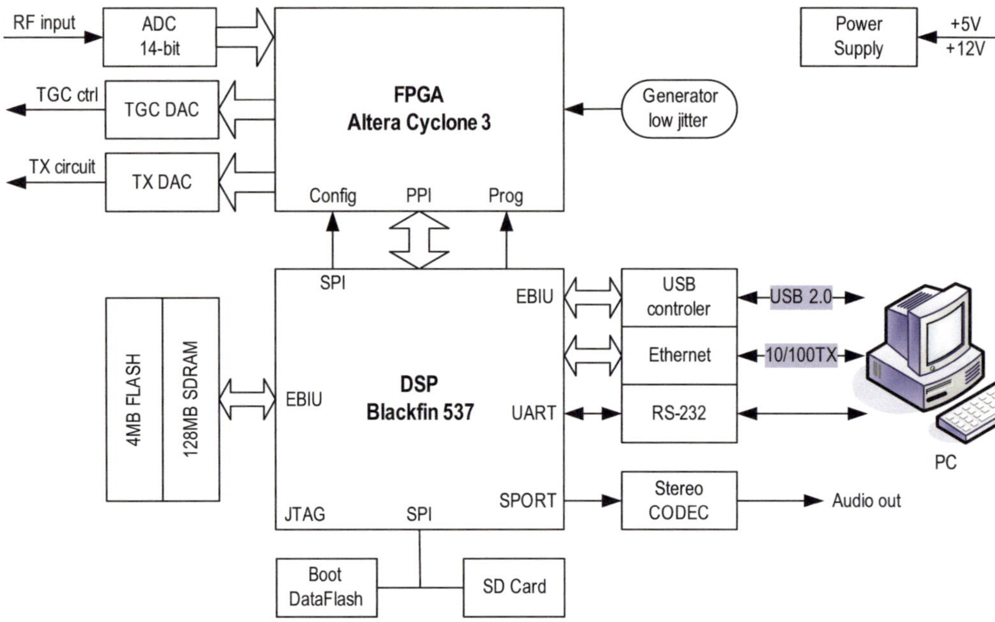

Fig. 6. Simplified block diagram of the ***digiTDS*** system

system block scheme. On an analogue-digital module board, there are two independent transmission-reception channels (the device supports two heads operation, the so called bilateral operation). A 10-bit DAC (Texas Instruments® DAC5652A) operating at a speed of 64 MSPS is used to generate the transmitted signal. The reception track contains amplifiers with the function of time gain compensation (Analogue Devices® AD8331) and a dual 14-bit ADC (Analogue Devices® AD9640) with sampling frequency of 64 MHz. The digital signals from/to converters are connected to FPGA on the digital module board via intermodule connector. The digital module consists of FPGA (Altera® Cyclone 3 EP3C25), DSP (Analog Devices® Blackfin BF537) as well as USB device controller (PLX® NET2272) and an Ethernet interface.

Unlike the ***uScan***, ***digiTDS*** may run independently of PC, thanks to its own control resources - DSP processor. The system communicates with PC via USB 2.0 interface. The digital processing chain consists of hardware processing in the FPGA and software processing using DSP and PC's CPU. The application of hardware resources during early processing stage allowed to significantly decrease the required data throughput and computing load of PC. It also allowed to use a low-power single-board PC with Intel® ATOM processor and to extend the operating time on batteries. The distribution and implementation of processing tasks were performed on a constructed device prototype. Especially moving the realization of filtration in multiple gates from the software to FPGA enabled significant processor time saving.

Fig. 7 presents the Doppler digital signal processing track on ***digiTDS*** device with task distribution between the FPGA system and software.

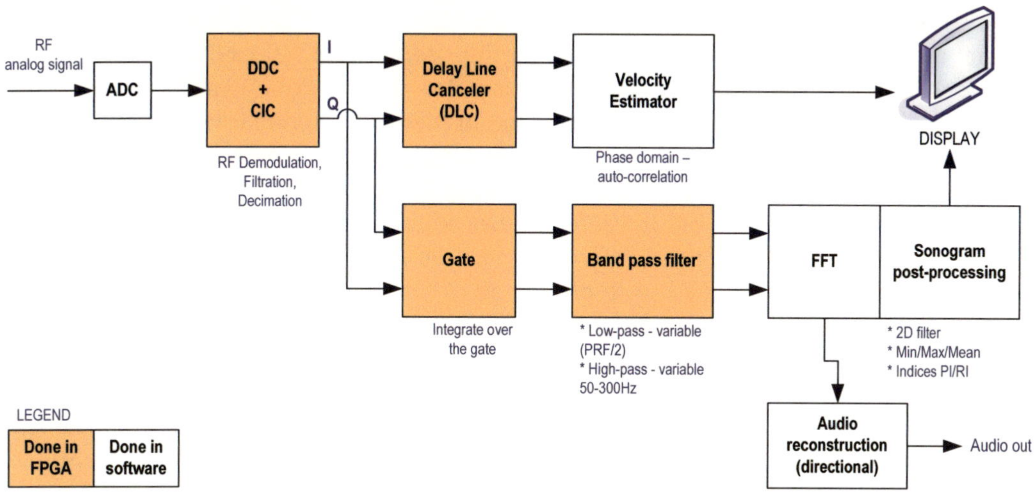

Fig. 7. Doppler digital signal processing chain

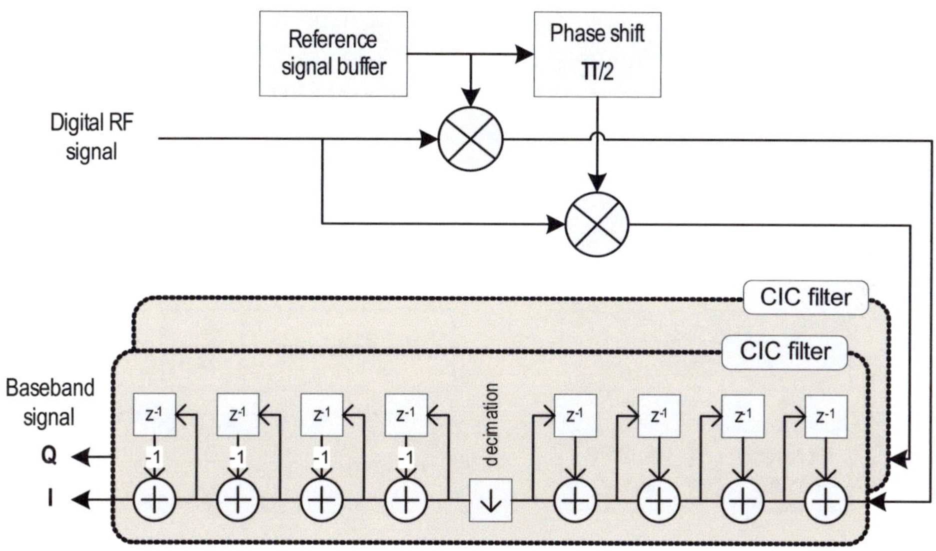

Fig. 8. Block diagram of the digital quadrature demodulator with CIC filter implemented in the FPGA

The received RF echo signal, after the amplification and digital conversion, is sent to the quadrature demodulator (DDC – Digital Down Converter) and CIC (Cascaded Integrator Comb) filter, implemented in the FPGA (Fig. 8). The demodulator is composed of two multipliers, memory containing reference signal samples with the frequency of 1-16 MHz and two low-pass filters. The samples of high frequency echo signal are mixed with 14-bit samples of reference sine and cosine signals. As a result, two signals are formed, namely in-phase (I) and quadrature (Q) signals, which are next subjected to low-pass filtration and decimation so that only baseband frequency components were retained in the signal. The low pass filters and the decimator were implemented in the FPGA as a CIC filter (Harris, 2004). The 4th order CIC filter enables regulation of the Doppler gate size and the degree of filtration and decimation.

The subsequent processing component of the FPGA system is a set of constant echo filters. In a multigate system, the signal in each gate has to be filtered in order to eliminate slow changing signals from still or slowly moving structures. In the FPGA, 200 parallel FIR filters are implemented, each with the length of 64 coefficients; they provide filtration in real time in 100 Doppler gates (independently I & Q signals are filtered in each gate). The cumulative utilization of logical resources of the applied FPGA (Altera® EP3C25) amounted to 5% of logic cells, 39% of internal block RAM and 3% of dedicated 18-bit multipliers. Time closure was obtained for the frequency of 64 MHz, and thus the processing speed matched the speed of input data stream (RF signal sampling). It is of note that the software execution of such a task on Intel® ATOM processor would be impractical.

The processed signal is next sent to PC where it is processed specifically for a given application. Recently, standard Doppler processing methods have been implemented, namely Color and Spectrum. Digital signal processing software algorithms have been implemented using Intel® IPP libraries (Taylor, 2004), which use SSE (Streaming SIMD Extensions) vector extensions of x86 family processors. SSE extensions enable execution of floating point operations on multiple data at the same time, which ensures a very high efficiency of multimedia applications (Martinez-Nieto et al., 2009).

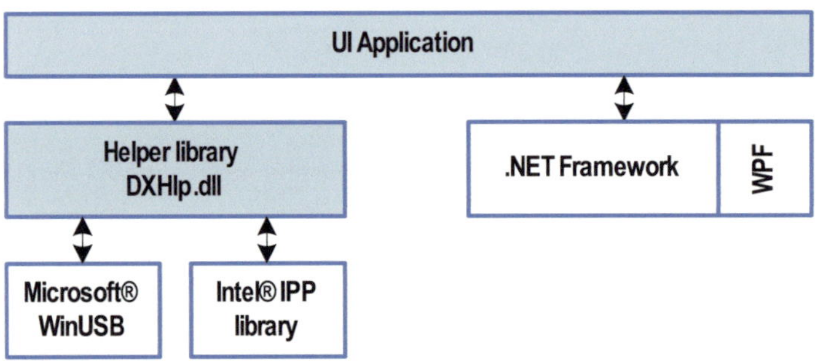

Fig. 9. PC software stack of the ***digiTDS*** system

The control and user software (Fig. 9) was implemented in Microsoft® Windows Embedded Standard 2009 environment, based on NET 3.5 framework. For communication with the digital module via USB interface, Microsoft® WinUSB drivers were applied. User interface was created based on on .NET WPF (Windows Presentation Foundation). Obtaining short delay of Doppler signal transmission, processing and visualization required optimal data buffering, processing optimization and multithreaded implementation.

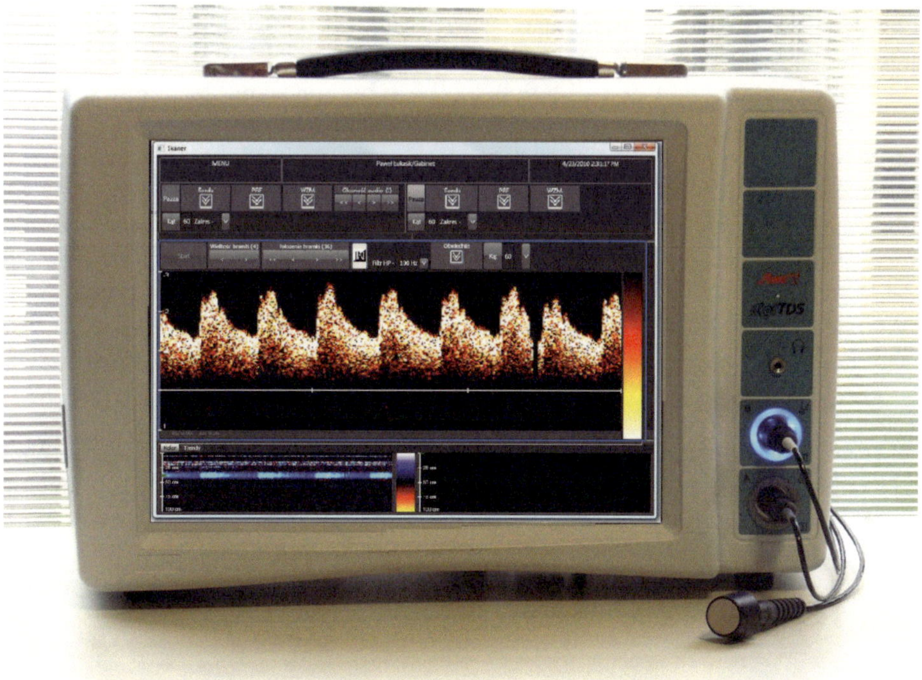

Fig. 10. Photo of the complete ***digiTDS*** system

6. Conclusions

The paper presents technical issues pertaining to the architecture of digital signal processing and task distribution between software and hardware in ultrasound diagnostic devices. The solutions reported in literature were reviewed and the similarities between the presented solutions and SDR systems used in digital telecommunication were discussed.

The two presented examples of combined hardware-software processing architecture in the ultrasound devices represent current state of the art.

The experience gained during designing and implementation of digital processing algorithms on these platforms show their unquestionable advantages, namely:

- possibility of algorithm migration between hardware and software solutions,
- possibility of equalization of load distribution in all system elements and data transfer between sub-systems,
- possibility of optimization of the selected system parameter (time delay, data transfer, power consumption, etc.) by changing the method/place of processing execution.

It is also of note that the problems can be encountered during system development requiring advanced real time processing, namely:

- difficulty in defining the required efficiency and throughput of each system component at the design stage,

- problems with operating the system in real time with minimal time delay of result presentation (image, audio),
- time synchronization of hardware and software subsystems (particularly those controlled by not real-time operating system),
- complicated verification & validation of the whole system, as required for medical device.

The future development of ultrasound medical systems will be interrelated with the development of electronics and digital signal processing systems. The present trend of extending the scope of software processing will be probably continued with the next generation of multicore GPP, DSP and GPU. Rapid development of portable devices can be expected, due to the availability of increasingly fast, integrated and low-power System on Chip integrated circuits.

7. Acknowledgements

Acknowledgements to my co-workers from the Institute of Fundamental Technological Research, Polish Academy of Sciences who cooperated with me in the project development: Andrzej Nowicki, Bogusław Zienkiewicz, Mateusz Walczak, Paweł Karłowicz, Ryszard Tymkiewicz, Piotr Karwat, and Beata Witek.

Funding: The European Regional Development Fund under the Innovative Economy Operational Programme & Ministry of Science and Higher Education, Poland.

8. References

Ali M., Magee D., Dasgupta U. (2008). Signal Processing Overview of Ultrasound Systems for Medical Imaging, Texas Instruments, White Paper SPRAB12

Altera (2006). *Automated Generation of Hardware Accelerators With Direct Memory Access from ANSI/ISO Standard C Functions*, ALTERA White Paper, WP-AGHRDWR-1.0

Bassam S. A., Ebrahimi M. M., Kwan A., Helaoui M., Aflaki M. P., Hammi O., Fattouche M., Ghannouchi F. M. (2009). A Generic architecture for smart multi-standard software defined radio systems, SDR'09 Technical Conference and Product Exposition, 1-4 December 2009, Washington, DC, USA

Chang J. H., Sun L., Yen J.T., Shung K. K. (2009). Low-cost, high-speed back-end processing system for high-frequency ultrasound B-mode imaging, *IEEE Transactions on Ultrasounds, Ferroelectrics, and Frequency Control*, Vol. 56, No. 7

Fuller M. I., Owen K., Blalock T. N., Hossack J. A., Walker W. F. (2009). Real Time Imaging with the Sonic Window: A Pocket-Sized, C-Scan, Medical Ultrasound Device, *Proceedings of IEEE International Ultrasounds Symposium*, pp. 196-199, Roma, Italy, 20-23 September 2009, IEEE

Garcia P., Compton K., Schulte M., Blem E., Fu W. (2006). An Overview of Reconfigurable Hardware in Embedded Systems , *EURASIP Journal on Embedded Systems*, Volume 2006, Article ID 56320

Harris F. J. (2004). *Multirate Signal Processing for Communication Systems*, Prentice Hall PTR, ISBN 978-0131465114

Jensen J. A., Hansen M., Tomov B. G., Nikolov S. I., Holten-Lund H. (2007). System Architecture of an Experimental Synthetic Aperture Real-Time Ultrasound System, *Proceedings of IEEE International Ultrasounds Symposium*, pp. 636-640, New York, USA, 28-31 October 2007, IEEE

Lee H., Sohn H., Yoon Ch., Mo Yoo Y., Song T. (2009). Software-based Hand-Held Ultrasound Color Doppler Imaging System, *Proceedings of IEEE International Ultrasounds Symposium*, pp. 1844-1847, Roma, Italy, 20-23 September 2009, IEEE

Lewandowski M., Nowicki A. (2008). High Frequency Coded Imaging System with RF Software Signal Processing, *IEEE Transactions on Ultrasounds, Ferroelectrics, and Frequency Control*, 55(8):1878-82

Lewandowski M., Walczak M., Nowicki A. (2009). Compact Modular Doppler System with Digital RF Processing, *Proceedings of IEEE International Ultrasounds Symposium*, pp. 1848-1851, Roma, Italy, 20-23 September 2009, IEEE

Martinez-Nieto D., McDonnell M., Carlston P., Reynolds K., Santos V. (2009). Digital Signal Processing on Intel® Architecture, Intel® Technology Journal, Vol. 13, No. 1

McDonald J., (2009). Insiders' Guide: FPGAs, Tools, and Boards, http://www.eg3.com

Owens J. D., Luebke D., Govindaraju N., Harris M., Krüger J., Lefohn A.E., Purcell T.J. (2005). A Survey of General-Purpose Computation on Graphics Hardware, *Eurographics 2005 State of the Art Reports*, August 2005, pp. 21-51.

Reed J. H. (2002). *Software Radio: A Modern Approach to Radio Engineering*, Prentice Hall, ISBN 978-0130811585

Ricci S., Dallai A., Boni E., Bassi L., Guidi F., Cellai A., Tortoli P. (2008). Embedded System for Real-Time Digital Processing of Medical Ultrasound Doppler Signals, *EURASIP Journal on Advances in Signal Processing*, Volume 2008, Article ID 418235

Richard W. D., Zar D. M., Solek R. (2008). A low-cost B-mode USB ultrasound probe, *Ultrason Imaging*, Vol. 30, No. 1, pp. 21-8

Pailoor R, Pradhan D. (2008). Digital Signal Processor (DSP) for Portable Ultrasound, Texas Instruments , Application Report SPRAB18A

Sirowy S., Forin A. (2008). Where's the Beef? Why FPGAs Are So Fast, Microsoft Research, Technical Report MSR-TR-2008-130

Tan T., Zhang J., Fang J., Liu H., Ye Y., Wang S., Zhang Y., Wu H., Wang W., Voelker G. M. (2009). Sora: High Performance Software Radio Using General Purpose Multi-core Processors, Proceedings of the 6th USENIX Symposium on Networked Systems Design and Implementation, April 22–24, 2009, Boston, MA, USA

Taylor S. (2004). *Intel Integrated Performance Primitives*, Intel Press, ISBN 978-0971786134

Thomas D. (2010). Using TI's Embedded Processor Software Toolkit for Medical Imaging (STK-MED), Texas Instruments, Application Report SPRABB8

Thomenius K. E. (2006). Instrumentation Design For Ultrasound Imaging, In: *Biomedical Engineering And Design Handbook Vol. 2: Applications*, Myer Kutz, (Ed.), 249-256, McGraw-Hill, ISBN 978-0-07-170474-8

Tortoli P., Bassi L., Boni E., Dallai A., Guidi F., Ricci S. (2009). ULA-OP: An Advanced Open Platform for Ultrasound Research. *IEEE Transactions on Ultrasounds, Ferroelectrics, and Frequency Control*, Vol. 56, No. 10

2

Design of Curvilinear Array Apertures for 3D Ultrasonic Imaging

Oscar Martínez-Graullera[1], Luis Gomez-Ullate[2], David Romero[3], Carlos J. Martín[4] and Gregorio Godoy[5]

[1,2,3,4]*Centro de Acústica Aplicada y Evaluación No Destructiva. UPM-CSIC. Ctra. Campo Real KM 0,200 28500 Arganda del Rey (Madrid)*

[5]*Dpto. Ing Electrónica. Universidad de Jaen*

Spain

1. Introduction

The development of ultrasonic volumetric imaging is closely linked to the development of systems that are able to operate bidimensional array transducers. These arrays are useful for ultrasonic volumetric imaging, because they produce steered and focused beams throughout a volume of interest. Typical 2-D arrays are based on a Squared Matrix (SM) configuration, where the array elements are the matrix cells. Their performance is determined by their width in terms of wavelenght. Resolution and the dynamic range are determined by wavelenght/aperture diameter ratio and number of elements and the wavelenght/interelement distance ratio respectively (Smith et al. (1991)).

In SM apertures, since element distribution is uniform, the composition of the secondary lobes is determined by interelement distance. All elements contribute to its formation. These lobes are known as grating lobes and produce image artifacts that can reduce the signal-to-noise ratio. Nowadays avoiding image artifacts is key to array design. For matrix and linear arrays the composition of these lobes can only be avoided by limiting the interelement distance to $\lambda/2$. In practice, it means that for 1° of lateral resolution a 60λ diameter aperture with 14400 elements is needed. Then, several problems can be identified:

- Thousands of electronic channels are needed, which increases the cost and complexity of the imaging system.
- Thousands of elements are needed, which increases the complexity of the transducer manufacture.
- The small size of the elements is associated to low signal-to-noise ratios.
- Considerable difficulties in making the electrical connections.

These problems pose a technological challenge which is the basis for the main research lines in array design. To meet these challenges and reduce the cost and complexity of 3-D systems, the main design strategy is to break the periodicity in the aperture, using different thinning strategies to reduce the number of active elements and maintaining good field characteristics at the same time(Smith et al. (1991); Schwartz & Steinberg (1998)).

Traditionally, the design strategy for matrix distribution has been based on undersampling the 2-D array by connecting only some of the available elements (Hendricks (1991)). Array designers then try to select those elements that produce the most appropriate beam pattern or image for a given set of constraints (Smith et al. (1991); Hendricks (1991); Schwartz & Steinberg (1998); Lockwood & Foster (1996)). Most thinning solutions are based on random distribution but over the last decades some solutions that use the multiplicative nature of the pulse-echo process have been presented (Schwartz & Steinberg (1998); Lockwood & Foster (1996); Austeng & Holm (2002); Nikolov & Jensen (2000)). It has been proposed that an imaging system can be composed by two different apertures in emission and reception, where the grating lobes in emission and the grating lobes in reception appear at different positions and thus they are partly suppressed in the two-way response. However, these solutions are mainly aimed at reducing the number of elements; elements are still very small. For such solutions the SNR can become too low and in general the image contrast achieved is only limited.

Alternatively apertures with curvilinear deployment have been proposed (Schwartz & Steinberg (1998); Mendelsohn & Wiener-Avnear (2002); Ullate et al. (2006); Bavaro et al. (2008); Sumanaweera et al (1999)). Unlike matrix distributions, curvilinear apertures have no privileged direction. Therefore only some and not all elements generate grating lobes and thus curvilinear apertures outperform rectilinear designs. Furthermore, curvilinear arrays can be designed so that grating lobes are distributed in wide areas, significantly reducing their impact. Therefore, layouts with inter-element distance beyond $\lambda/2$ can be considered. In this sense, in curvilinear arrays the number of elements is reduced while element size can be increased which improves the signal-to-noise ratio associated with element impedance and the array active area (Ullate et al. (2006); Martínez-Graullera et al (2010)).

In this paper, two curvilinear designs are analysed. On the one hand, array designs based on the Fermat Spiral (FS), an alternative that provides both curvilinear deployment and reduction in the number of elements. On the other hand, Segmented Annular Apertures or Circular Apertures (CA) which is a curvilinear array composed of a set of concentric rings that are divided into sectors. Grating lobes are not eliminated, but they are spread over a large region generating a pedestal sidelobe. It is shown that the formation of grating lobes can be modelled with a reduced number of parameters. The design parameters of both apertures are studied, and specific thinning strategies are presented.

Some issues have been considered for greater focus on specific problems:

1. Taking into account the technology nowadays available, the number of elements in the aperture is limited to 128.
2. The configuration considered is composed by different apertures in emission and reception.
3. The apertures have a diameter of 60λ, providing a lateral resolution of 1°.
4. The minimum inter-element distance is λ so that element area can be increased up to that size.

2. Analysis tools

Three different mathematical models are used for analysis and design strategies.

- Narrowband analysis. It models the response at a given frequency, producing the worst case of interference. Therefore, it can be used as a reference for performance asessment.

This model allows to identify which elements determine the formation of grating lobes. The knowledge adquired from this analysis can be used to develop a desing strategy. From the computational point of view, it is the fastest simulation model, adequate for intensive computation operations.

- Wideband analysis. It is based on point elements and the spatial impulse response computational model. Its computational cost is higher than that of the narrowband, but it provides a good estimate of aperture behaviour without interference from elements response. A design strategy, based on the parameters identified in the narrowband analysis, can be developed using optimization algorithms.
- Wideband acoustic field modelling. The model presented here is based on the spatial impulse response and the Piwackovski solution (Piwakowsky & Sbai (1999)). It is used to validate the best solution obtained .

Each model can be used at different design stages. It is a three-part process: learning (Narrowband and Wideband analysys), searching (Wideband analysys), and evaluating (Wideband acoustic field modelling). All three stages compose the general procedure for array design.

2.1 Narrowband analysis tool

The first stage of the design process (Learning), in which an array model of punctual elements, narrowband excitation and far field approximation are used, is based on the Array Factor response (AF). The Array Factor is a very fast computational model that explains or shows how the difraction pattern is developed for different aperture parameters. In this way, it helps us identify which are the key parameters and design the most appropriated strategy to improve the array performance.

$$|AF(\theta,\phi)| = \left| \sum_{i=1}^{N_e} \exp^{-jk((x_i \cos\phi + y_i \sin\phi)\sin\theta - \xi_i(\theta_o,\phi_o))} \right| \tag{1}$$

Where (x_i, y_i) are the cartesian coordinates of the ith element and $\xi_i(\theta_o, \phi_o)$ is the corresponding phase delay value to focus on (θ_o, α_o).

$$\xi_i(\theta_o,\phi_o) = (x_i \cos\phi_o + y_i \sin\phi_o)\sin\theta_o \tag{2}$$

The Array Factor response in pulse-echo can be evaluated using:

$$|AF_{er}(\theta,\phi)| = |AF_e(\theta,\phi)AF_r(\theta,\phi)| \tag{3}$$

Where $AF_e(\theta,\phi)$ and $AF_r(\theta,\phi)$ are respectively the array factor on emission and reception of aperture, which are computed by equation 1.

2.2 Wideband analysis tool

A wideband model is based on the spatial impulse response. Punctual elements are used. Echo-pulse response can be modelled by Nikolov & Jensen (2000):

$$s(\vec{x},t) = \frac{1}{c^2}\frac{\partial^2 v(t)}{\partial t^2} * \{h_T(\vec{x},t) * h_R(\vec{x},t)\} \tag{4}$$

Where $h_T(\vec{x},t)$ and $h_R(\vec{x},t)$ are the emitting and the receiving spatial impulse response of the array, and $v(t)$ is the excitation signal. To reduce the computational cost and suppress the element diffraction response, each one is reduced to a pointwise located at the center of the element. Then, the spatial impulse response of the array is computed as:

$$h(\vec{x},t) = \sum_{i=1}^{N_e} \frac{\delta(t - \frac{r_i}{c} - T_i)}{2\pi r_i} \tag{5}$$

Where r_i is the distance from the center of the ith element to the field point $\vec{x}$, and T_i is the corresponding focussing delay. Then, using equation 5 to model emission and reception arrays in equation 4, the presure wave obtained is mainly determined by excitation pulse and element distribution in the aperture.
The Point Spread Function (PSF) in wide-band in a $\vec{x}$ position can be calculated by the maximum value of the modulus of $s(\vec{x},t)$. The PSF is evaluated in a hemisphere as follows:

$$PSF(\theta,\phi) = \max_t \left(\left| s\left((R = \tfrac{D^2}{(4\lambda)}, \theta, \phi), t \right) \right| \right) \tag{6}$$

Futhermore, the equation 4 is used to obtain the general expression of the acoustic pressure generated by an array working in emission-reception. Where h_E and h_R are, respectively, the impulse responses in emission and reception of the array obtained by the sum of the spatial impulse response of each element:

$$h_E(\vec{x},t) = \sum_{i=1}^{N_e} a_i^E h_i(\vec{x}, t - T_i^E) \tag{7}$$

$$h_R(\vec{x},t) = \sum_{i=1}^{N_e} a_i^R h_i(\vec{x}, t - T_i^R) \tag{8}$$

Where T_i^E and T_i^R are, respectively, the focusing delays in emission and reception, a_i is its gain, and h_i is the impulse response of the ith array element computed by the Rayleigh integral.

$$h_i(\vec{x},t) = \int\int_{A_i} \frac{\delta(t - \frac{r_i}{c} - T_i)}{2\pi r_i} \delta s \tag{9}$$

Where A_i is the area of the emitting/receiving transducer. The Piwakowsky method was used to calculate this equation. This method makes a direct computation of the Rayleigh integral by means of transducer surface discretization into squared cells of elemental area ΔS, and time sampling with intervals of Δt. Hence, the contribution of every element to the array impulse response at a given instant t_S is obtained by adding the contributions of the cells contained between two concentric spherical waves, which are separated by the discretization interval $c\Delta t$ (Piwakowsky & Sbai (1999)). Thus, the contribution of the ith array element at the instant $t = t_s$ is given by:

$$h_i(t = t_S) = \frac{1}{\Delta t} \sum_j b_j, \quad t_S - \frac{\Delta t}{2} \leq t_j \leq t_S + \frac{\Delta t}{2} \tag{10}$$

$$b_j = \frac{a_i \Delta S}{2\pi(R_j - T_i)} \quad \text{and} \quad R_j = ct_j \tag{11}$$

Where T_i denotes the focusing delay in emission or reception and R_j is the distance from each cell to the field point $P(\vec{x})$.

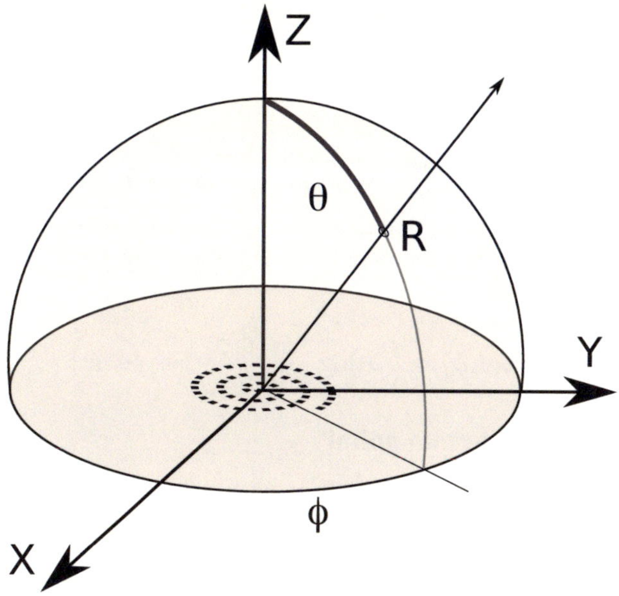

Fig. 1. Coordinate system used to compute de array beampattern. The array is located in the XY plane ($\theta = 0$) and the field is computed in a hemisphere, defined for narrowband by (θ, ϕ) and for wideband by (R, θ, ϕ).

2.3 Nomenclature

A generalized nomenclature is used for the apetures in the design:

$$F(N_t, N_r) \tag{12}$$

Where F is the main geometry organization in the element distribution. SP stands for spiral configuration, CA for Circular Apertures and M for Matrix configuration. N_t and N_r are the number of elements in the emision and reception aperture respectively. When the apertures in emission and in reception are the same the notation is F(N_e).

2.4 Evaluation parameters

In figure 1 the coordinate system used to evaluate the diffraction response in the hemisphere is presented. For simplicity, the hemisphere is presented as a disk by its projection over the XY plane. Several examples can be seen in figure 3.

To evaluate the apertures , the acoustic field (narrowband and wideband) is computed in a far field hemisphere ($R = \frac{D^2}{(4\lambda)}, \theta = 0^o : 1^o : 90^o, \phi = 0^o : 1^o : 360^o$), focusing on ($R = \frac{D^2}{(4\lambda)}, \theta = 0^o, \phi = 0^o$) in emision and reception. Also, lateral profiles in wideband are employed to show the aperture performance. Maximum, mean and minimum sidelobes at each elevation angle ($\theta = 0^o : 1 : 90^0$) are shown. See figure 6 for examples.

With this results, a number of parameters was considered to assess apertures in wideband:

- The lateral resolution at two levels of -6dB and -40dB, in order to analyse the main lobe sharpness
- The grating lobe maximum level, which is determined by analysing the PSF for 60% signal bandwidths:

- The mainlobe-to-sidelobe energy ratio (MSR).

This last parameter MSR was proposed in Nikolov & Jensen (2000) as a measurement of how energy is spread in the field, and can be computed by:

$$MSR = 20\log\frac{\sum\sum|PSF(\theta,\phi)|^2 ML(\theta,\phi)}{\sum\sum|PSF(\theta,\phi)|^2(1-ML(\theta,\phi))} \tag{13}$$

Where $ML(\theta,\phi)$ is a logical function that delimits the main lobe region. Here, due to the nature of the results, we considered that the main lobe is defined by those points having pressure amplitude higher than -40dB:

$$ML(\theta,\phi) = \left(20\log\frac{PSF(\theta,\phi)}{PSF(0,0)} > -40dB\right) \tag{14}$$

3. Arrays desing based on fermat spiral

In the search of a pattern for element distribution with reduced periodicity, we also worked on the Fermat Spiral. Although previous studies looked into the spiral layout (Sumanaweera et al (1999)), the Fermat spiral has not been studied yet. Fermat spiral is defined by the divergence angle α that determines the angular distance between two consecutive elements. The radial position of each element is determined by the square root of its angular position.

$$x_n = (R_n, \alpha_i) = \left(R_0\sqrt{n\alpha}, n\alpha\right), n = 0, ...(N_e - 1) \tag{15}$$

Where the element centre x_n is defined by its polar coordinates and N_e is the number of elements. R_0 is a constant value which is needed to obtain a particular aperture size. It is defined as:

$$R_0 = \frac{D}{2\sqrt{(N_e-1)\alpha}} \tag{16}$$

Where D is the aperture diameter.
In Figure 2 different spiral arrangements with N_e=128 and divergence angles (α= 9°, 174°, 116°, 92°) are shown. It can be seen that although only one line is drawn for the divergence angle, each spiral seems to be configured by different number of branches, or inner spirals, which grow from the centre of the array. We named the configurations of Figure 2 as SPx, where x is the number of branches.
Figure 3 shows the Array Factor in the plane ($\theta = 0^o : 30^o, \phi = 0^o : 360^o$) for $\xi_{\theta_o,\phi_o} = 0$ for the apertures shown. The figure shows how grating lobes are organized in branches, generating different diffraction patterns for each divergence angle.
In our opinion, the Fermat spiral is interesting for array design because of a number of issues.

1. Only the divergence angle and the number of elements are needed to define the layout.
2. It is a biological pattern, which in fact it is used by Phyllotaxis as a reference to model several leaves arrangements (Jean (1983); Ridley (1982)).
3. The outer elements show a more compact distribution than other spiral layouts, like Archimedean, Hyperbolic, Lituus or Logarithmic. This compactness leads to the element shadowing effect described in Schwartz & Steinberg (1998) and Ullate et al. (2006).

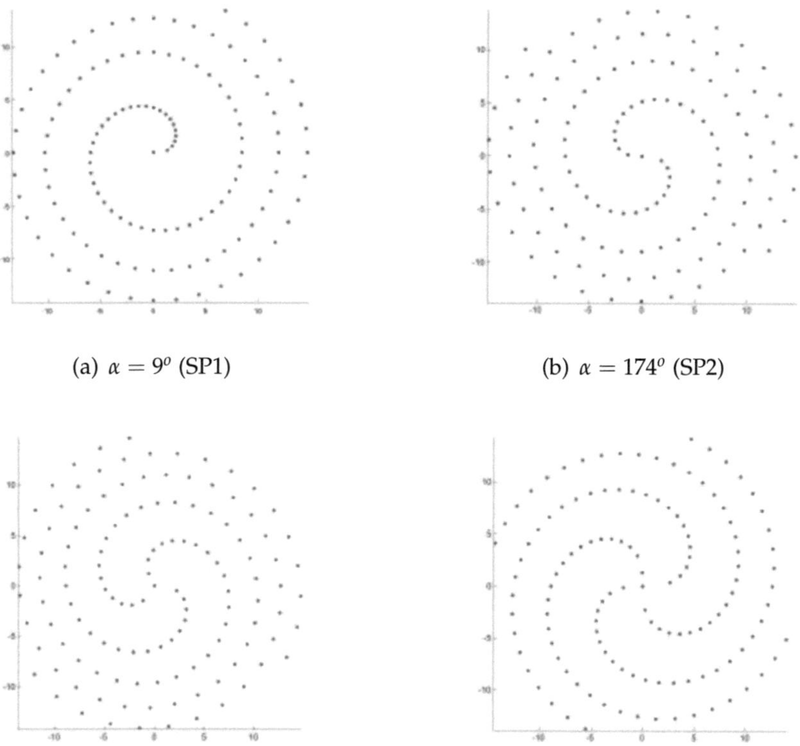

(a) $\alpha = 9^o$ (SP1) (b) $\alpha = 174^o$ (SP2)

(c) $\alpha = 116^o$ (SP3) (d) $\alpha = 92^o$ (SP4)

Fig. 2. Aperture distribution with different spiral arrangements. We have classified them in SP1, SP2, SP3 and SP4, according to the formation of branches.

4. Although elements are organised following a determined line, they compose other spiral structures in the layout. This particular arrangement distributes elements contribution to grating lobes, which are extended over wide but well located areas. Its general level is reduced.

3.1 Design strategie

In our project, taking into account the limitations described at the begining of the chapter, we propose a global array composed by two spirals of 128 elements, one for emission and another for reception, composing a configuration SP(128,128). The design strategy is based on the multiplicative nature of the pulse-echo process, and it tries to locate tgrating lobes in emission and grating lobes in reception at different positions. Hence, they are partly suppressed in the two-way response.

This principle can be applied to Fermat layouts where grating lobes are located in well defined positions. Rather than searching different complementary apertures, we use the same aperture for emission and reception and apply a phase displacement $\Delta\alpha$ between them in order to locate emission and reception grating lobes in complementary angular positions. Then the arrays that compose the SP(128,128) configuration can be determined by the equations:

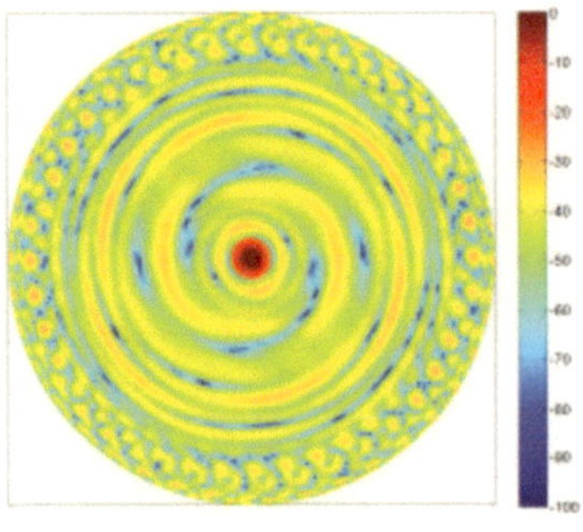

(a) $\alpha = 9^o$ (SP1)

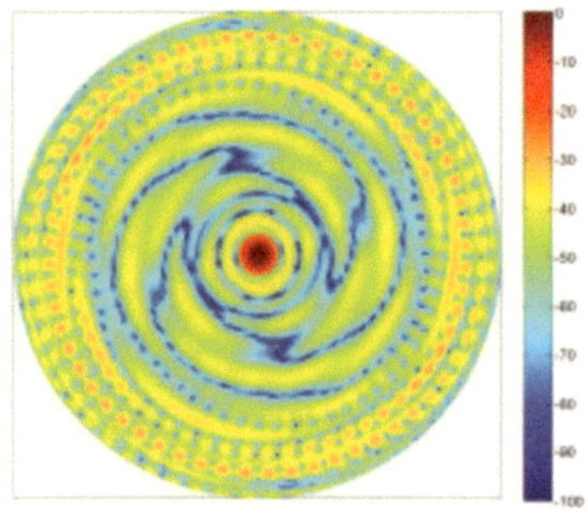

(b) $\alpha = 174^o$ (SP2)

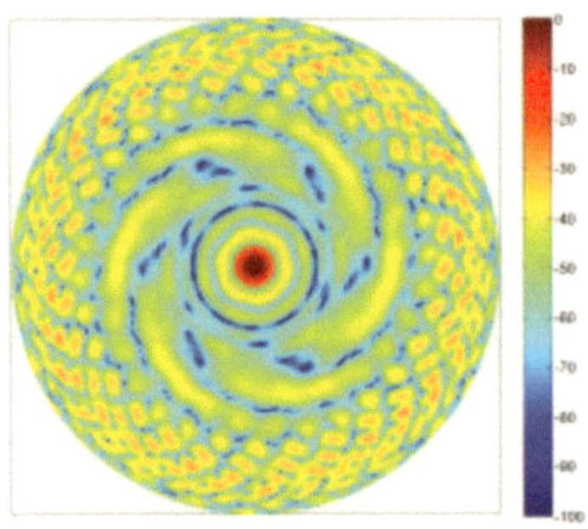

(c) $\alpha = 116^o$ (SP3)

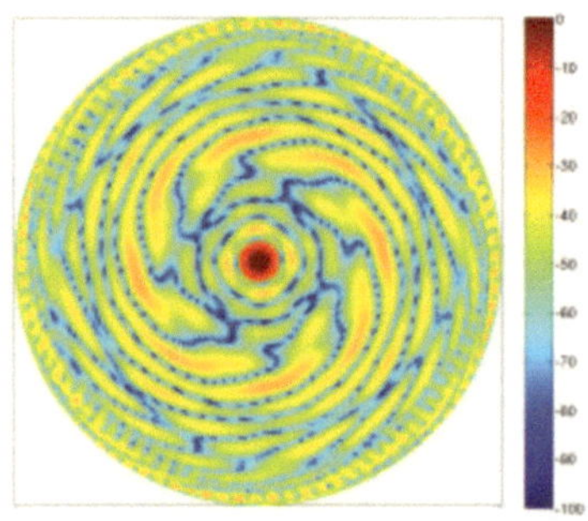

(d) $\alpha = 92^o$ (SP4)

Fig. 3. Narrowband Array Factor $\theta = 0^o : 30^o$ for different spiral arragements.

$$x_{En} = (R_n, \alpha_n) = (R_0\sqrt{n\alpha}, n\alpha), n = 0, ...127 \tag{17}$$

$$x_{Rn} = (R_n, \alpha_n) = (R_0\sqrt{n\alpha}, n\alpha + \Delta\alpha), n = 0, ...127 \tag{18}$$

Where, x_{En} and x_{Rn} are the element centres of the emission and reception apertures.
In narrowband, the highly efficient computational model allows an exhaustive analysis. We analysed 18,000 spiral apertures that were obtained varying the divergence angle. For each viable solution with spiral apertures, the two way array factor response of all possible complementary apertures ($\Delta\alpha = 0^o : 0.1^o : 180^o$) was evaluated.
The grating lobe peak values for all apertures are summarised in figure 4 and table 1, where the most representative solutions are shown. Although the results for the case $\Delta\alpha = 0^o$ are in the -15dB to -25.6dB range, the combination of two complementary apertures produces a general improvement of the results. The best results are obtained at -31dB.
Our best outcome in narrowband shows a grating lobe level of -43.6dB in wideband. In spite of the promising results for narrowband signal, the transferal to wideband (table 1) does not guarantee similar best results.

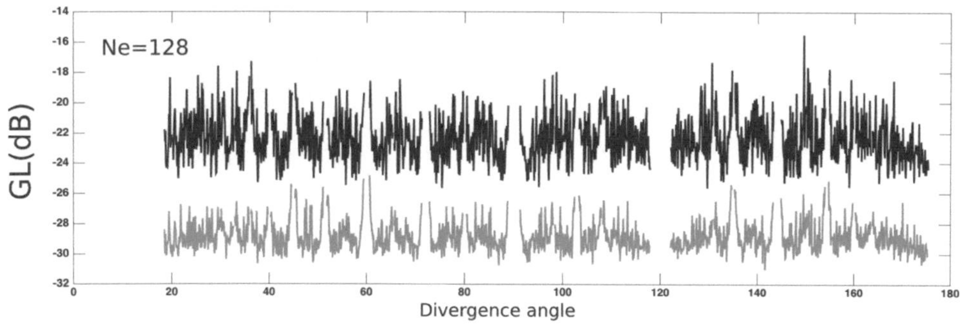

Fig. 4. Narrowband Grating lobe distribution per divergence angle. Black line represents the echo-pulse response if $\Delta\alpha = 0^0$; the gray line represents the echo-pulse response of the better case obtained when $\Delta\alpha > 0^0$.

	Narrow-band		Wide-band	
α	$\Delta\alpha = 0^o$	$\Delta\alpha > 0^o$	$\Delta\alpha = 0^o$	$\Delta\alpha > 0^o$
141.6	-23.7dB	**-31dB**	-40.27dB	-43.61dB
75.4	**-25.6dB**	-30dB	-37.5dB	-39.9dB

Table 1. Grating lobe levels for SP(128,128) apertures with best results in narrowband ($\Delta\alpha = 0^o$ and $\Delta\alpha > 0^o$); and its corresponding grating lobe levels in wideband. Results for Golden angle are also presented.

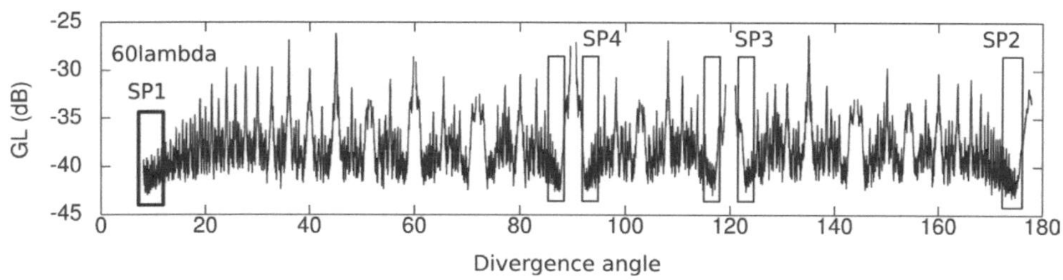

Fig. 5. Grating lobe levels vs the divergence angle, for wideband response (two ways, $\Delta\alpha = 0^o$, λ=0.5mm, BW=60%). Rectangles show the location of the best apertures.

3.1.1 Wideband analysys

The computational cost of the wideband model is higher than that of the narrowband model. As a consequence it is difficult to produce an exhaustive study. However, from the analysis of narrowband results a reduction in the number of cases can be obtained.

Our First objective is to find the best solution, then with the aim of obtaining the best apertures, an exhaustive search based on the divergence angle is subsequently carried out. Fortunately, the aperture design conditions reduce the total amount of cases under study. Furthermore, the diameter normalisation $R_{N_e} = R_0$ generates symmetries in the aperture layout that can be used to reduce the total number of apertures and consequently the set of apertures can be reduced to viable solutions of α in (0°: 0.005^o: 180°).

When $\Delta\alpha = 0^o$ is evaluated for each aperture, it is possible to obtain a general overview of the grating lobe level distribution and thus reduce the set of possible solutions. Results are shown in Figure 5. The three aperture diameters show similar grating lobes distributions but the widest aperture shows more cases, specially for low values of α.

After examining the results, the -42.5dB value was chosen as a grating lobe threshold to limit the set of apertures to be evaluated in the complementary configuration (figure 5). For D=60λ, 42 cases were identified and they could improve the result obtained in the narrowband analysis.
The set of possible solutions is divided in four groups according to element organisation (figure 5) . Figure 2 shows the most representative cases.

- SP1: Aperture defined by one branch. Range of divergence angles 8.5^o : 9.5^o.
- SP2: Aperture defined by two branches. Range of divergence angles 172.8^o : 175.5^o.
- SP3: Aperture defined by three branches. Range of divergence angles 116.5^o : 123.5^o.
- SP3: Aperture defined by three branches. Range of divergence angles 116.5^o : 123.5^o.
- SP4: Aperture defined by four branches. Range of divergence angles 87.5^o : 93.5^o.

3.1.2 Best solution

Table 2 shows the best apertures. A viable solution is given in three regions. The number of cases with a grating lobe peak value lower than -45.5dB (N_a), the lateral resolution, the MSR and the grating lobe for 60% are also shown. No representative cases were found in SP4 region.

					GL Level (60%)		Lat. Res.		MSR
Region	N_a	best α	$\Delta\alpha$	D	$\Delta\alpha > 0^o$	$\Delta\alpha = 0^o$	-6dB	-40dB	-40dB
SP1	7	9.3050^o	66.6^o	60λ	-46.1dB	-42.5dB	1.0^o	3.2^o	17.9dB
SP2	18	174.525^o	46.6^o	60λ	-46.4dB	-42.5dB	1.0^o	3.2^o	18.0dB
SP3	3	116.64^o	29.82^o	60λ	-45.6dB	-42.5dB	1.0^o	4.8^o	17.8dB

Table 2. Performance of the best F(128,128) configurations for each region and diameter. Lateral resolution at -6dB and -40dB and grating lobe level. Grating lobe peak levels for pulse bandwidth of 70% and 80%.

Figure 13 shows the best case ($\alpha = 174.525^o$) beampatterns. Lateral profiles show maximum, mean and minimum grating peak lobe level for each elevation angle. Optimised apertures have almost flat profiles with elevation.

4. Circular aperture

The Circular aperture, also known as Segmented Annular Aperture, is composed by a set of concentric rings that are divided in several elements. This aperture introduces several design factors that are useful to reduce distribution regularity. For instance, it is possible to use non equal spacing between rings or to use different interelement distance in each ring. Therefore the analysis could be very complex. To reduce the number of variables, this study is focused on what we have called Regular Distribution. This set of apertures is defined by one condition: all elements are the same size and the interelement distance is uniform. With this simple condition two consequences can be formulated:

- The distance between rings is constant.
- The number of elements in each ring is increased with the radius maintaning a similar distance between elements in all rings.

Figure 7 shows an example composed by four rings and the principal design paramenters:

- The radial distance (d_R).

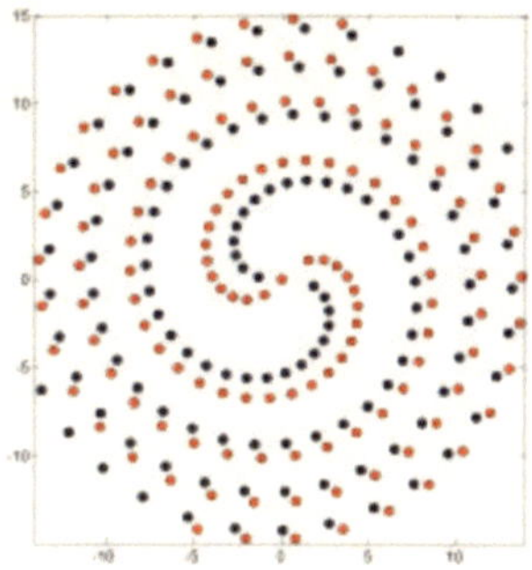

(a) Element distribution: in black emission aperture; in red reception aperture

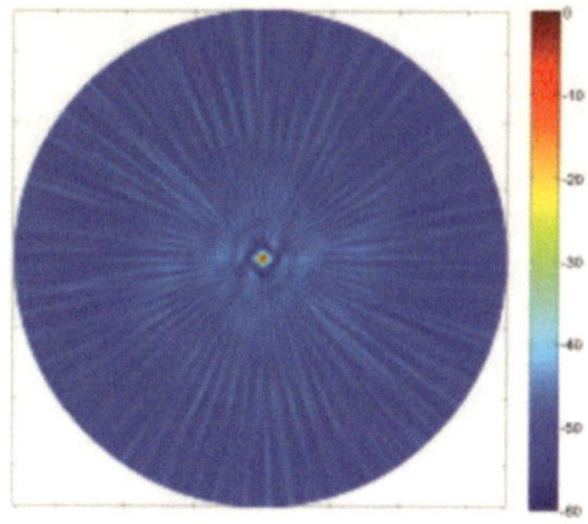

(b) Beampattern in the semisphere

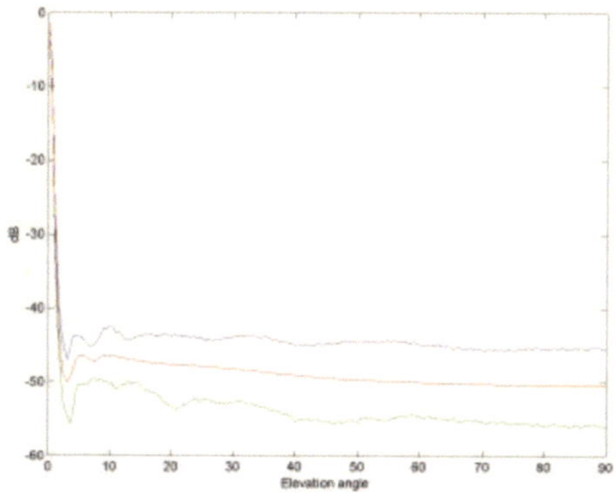

(c) Lateral profile. Maximum, mean and minimum side lobes in elevation are presented

Fig. 6. Best result for SP(28,128) is presented, $\alpha = 174.525^o$.

- The angular distance (d_A).
- The phase alignment per ring (ϕ_i).
- The aperture size (D).

4.1 Grating lobes distribution

It is well known that the factor which determines the generation of grating lobes for any array is the distance between elements. The same applies to annular segmented apertures. In this sense the most relevant distances in the aperture are angular and radial distances.
Two apertures were developed to evaluate how these distances determine the grating lobe formation. The aperture shown in figure 8 (a), was designed to garantee that d_A is lower than $\lambda/2$ and $d_R = 2\lambda$. The aperture shown in figure 8 (b), was designed to garantee that d_R is lower than $\lambda/2$ and $d_A = 2\lambda$.
By manipulating these distances we conclude that two different kinds of grating lobes can be easily distinguished:

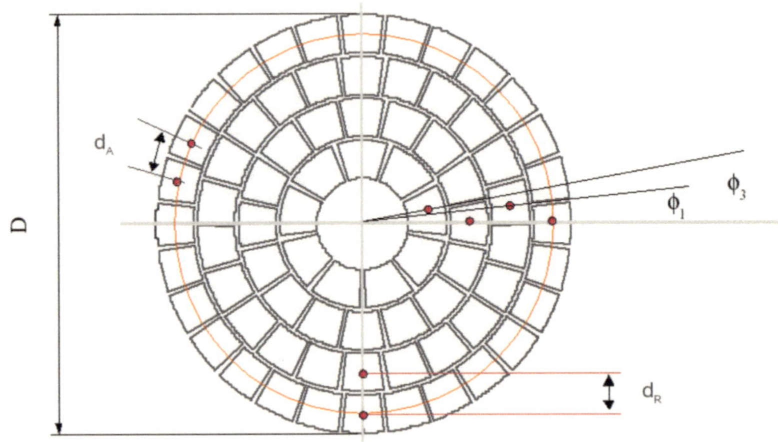

Fig. 7. Annular segmented array.

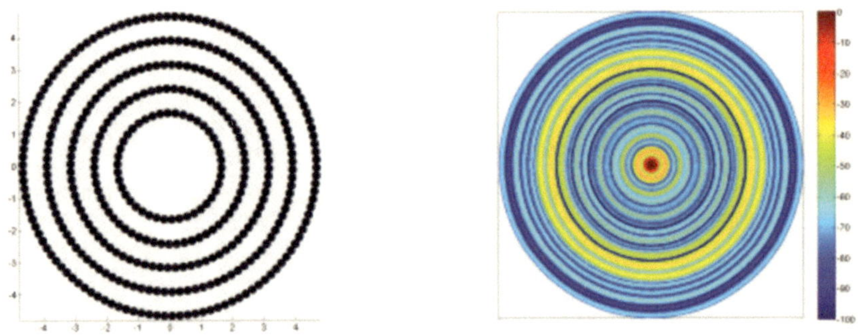

(a) Grating lobes generated by radial distance. Aperture with d_A is lower than $\lambda/2$ and $d_R = 2\lambda$.

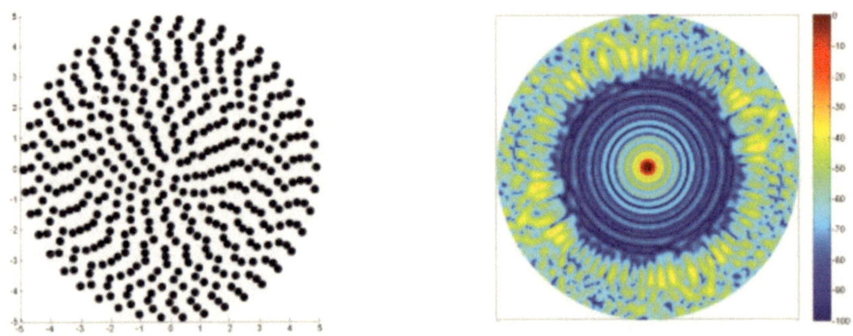

(b) Grating lobes generated by angular distance. Aperture with d_R is lower than $\lambda/2$ and $d_A = 2\lambda$.

Fig. 8. Grating Lobe generation in Circular Apertures and main distances between elements.

- The Radial Lobe (R_L) that has a narrow circular shape and shows continuity for any azimuth direction (figure 8 (a)). Its position is determined by d_R.
- The Angular Lobes (A_L), beam shaped, are distributed in different elevation positions for each azimuth direction (figure 8 (b)). The nearest lobes are determined by d_A distance and the rest are determined by the projection of d_A in the linear equivalent array, which depends on the azimuth angle.

Then, the position of this grating lobes can be determined in elevation by the equations:

$$R_L = \arcsin\left(\frac{\lambda}{d_r}\right) \tag{19}$$

$$A_L = \arcsin\left(\frac{\lambda}{d_a}\right) \tag{20}$$

Nevertheless, for a given azimuth direction, the lobes amplitude is linked with the number of coincident elements for that direction, which is not always the same. In the equivalent linear array, our first option to reduce the number of coincidences is changing the element Aspect Ratio (AR), which is the ratio between angular distance d_A and radial distance d_R. The objective of this technique is to avoid the grating lobe reinforcement that occurs when both dimensions are equal.

Figure 9 presents the array factor for three different cases, Aspect Ratio: 0.5, 1.0 and 1.5. All the arrays were designed as demonstrators, with $d_R = 2\lambda$ and $D = 20\lambda$, and AF was computed to show how grating lobes can be combined.

- For AR = 0.5, both lobes are completely uncoupled and it is easy to remark its properties (figure 9(a)). The Radial Lobe has a narrow circular shape; Angular Lobes have a straight shape and are distributed in different azimuth directions.
- For AR = 1, both lobes coincide in the same position and there is a reinforcement, specially for those directions with higher angular lobes (figure 9(b)).
- For AR = 1.5, due to the fact that Angular Lobes spread their influence over a wide region there is still a coincidence in position with the Radial Lobes, but with lower intensity than in the AR = 1 case (figure 9(c)).

Aspect Ratio and phases alignment are both design elements. Phases alligment allows to distribute angular grating lobes by generating an interference pattern between them that can be used to decrease its presence. Phase alignment is implemented by shifting elements from one ring to another in order to avoid privileged directions in the aperture. Phases alignment introduces a random factor in the array design. Figure 10 shows the histogram of the maximum grating lobe obtained in pulse-echo wideband response (60%). One thousand random phase-alignment cases for the same aperture with different aspect ratio were computed. The worst results are obtained for AR=0.5 where the coincidences in grating lobe position are higher. For AR=1 grating lobes values vary between -29dB and -36dB, and for AR=1.5 the results are quite similar (-30dB and -37dB). In short, the figure shows that small corrections in elements positions can improve results by 5dB, which should be taken into account in the design process.

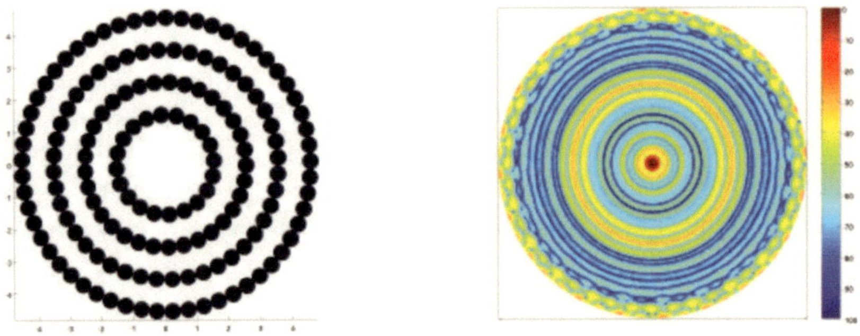

(a) AR = .5

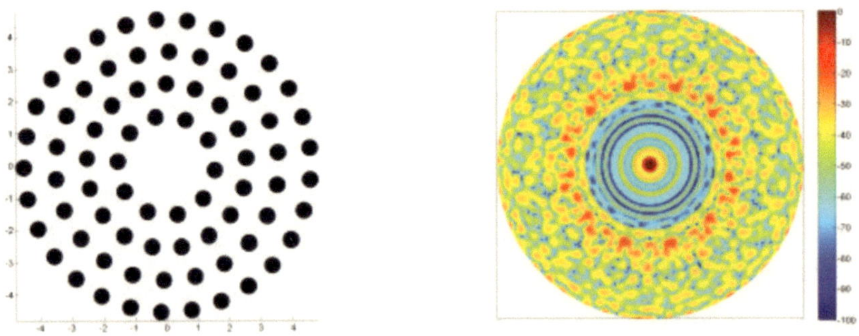

(b) AR = 1.

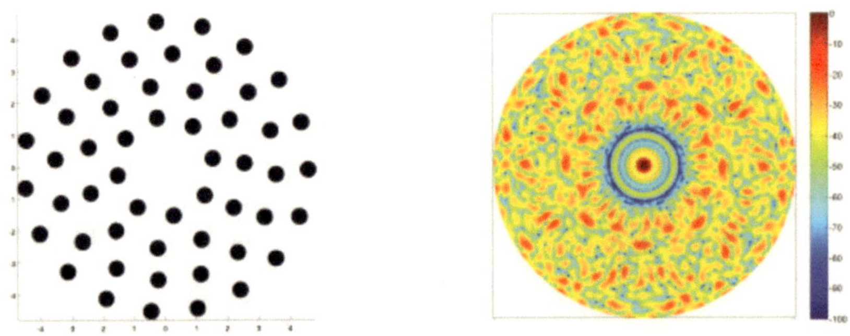

(c) AR = 1.5

Fig. 9. Aperture of $d_R = 2\lambda$ and $D = 20\lambda$ and Array Factor Lobe distribution with diferent Aspect Ratio.

4.2 Circular array design procedure

Circular apertures provide more freedom degrees to improve our design than spiral apertures. The study of Regular Apertures shows that grating lobe distribution can be controlled if radial and angular distances are properly chosen. Futhermore, elements that control grating lobe

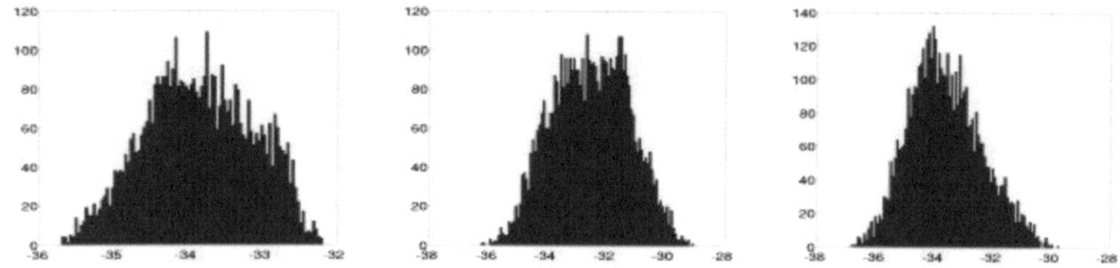

(a) AR = 0.5 (b) AR = 1 (c) AR = 1.5

Fig. 10. Distribution of grating Lobe values for 1000 different apertures wideband (60%). The three aspect ration are considered.

formation can be independently studied, which allows to divide the design process in several stages.

- Flattening emission beampattern, that is to say:
  - Dividing the aperture in equispaced radial regions and avoiding angular grating lobes generation. An optimization process is implemented to spot the rings distribution that produces lower grating lobes.
  - With the solution obtained, the aperture is composed with 128 elements. Different interelement distances are used in each ring in order to spread angular lobes over different elevation positions and reduce coincidences. After that, an optimization operation to find the most adequate phases alignment is performed.
- A complementary aperture is obtained. Using the previously obtained solution as a basis and as the emission aperture, the reception aperture for the pulse-echo process is composed by finding the new phases alignment that produces better beampattern

4.2.1 Reducing radial grating

At first stage the aperture with 60λ diameter and 128 elements is configured using an aspect ratio near to one to obtain a uniform distribution of the elements. A 9 ring configuration is obtained. Figure 10(b) shows how this configuration can produce, in function of its phases alignment, an intial 29dB to 36dB dynamic range .
Then, the number of elements per ring is increased to eliminate angular grating lobes using $d_A = \lambda/2$. An optimization process is initalized to find the new ring locations that minimize radial grating lobes. To avoid ring concentrations and other non adequate solutions some restrictions were applied to the optimization process. The outer ring has a fixed location to garantee lateral resolution. The other can expand or contract but only within their own regions. The minimun distance between rings is λ to allow the use of big elements.
However, we would like to emphasize that since the optimization process was not our objective, only a simple search algoritm was implemented. Figure 11 shows the results, our initial aperture and its lateral profile (minimum, mean and maximum secondary lobes at each elevation position) and the optimized aperture obtained. The grating lobes were initially located at 18°, and after the optimization process they spread over the 10° to 30° range. An improvement in the grating lobe level is obtained, it goes down from -54dB to -61dB. Table 3 shows the solution obtained.

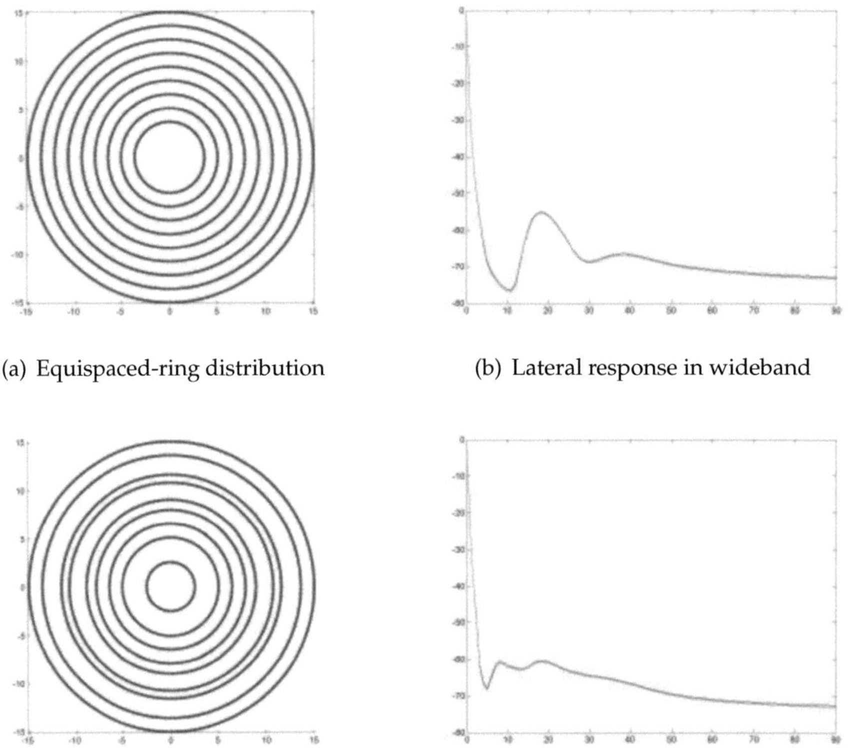

(a) Equispaced-ring distribution (b) Lateral response in wideband

(c) Improved-ring distribution (d) Improved lateral response in wideband

Fig. 11. Improved ring distribution to reduce radial grating lobes

4.2.2 Reducing angular grating lobes

To reduce grating angular lobes, the interelement distance varies from one ring to another. Distances increase a λ per ring to guarantee the distribution of angular grating lobes over a wide area. However, round operations to discretize the number of elements can cause a change in the estimated garting lobes positions. Obviously, the best solution is to avoid coincidences with the radial grating lobe region. Unfortunately this is not always posible since we are trying to get a wide dispersion. Table 3 shows the configuration and grating lobes positions.

RING	1	2	3	4	5	6	7	8	9
Radio (mm)	2.53	5.08	6.5	7.92	8.96	10.75	11.57	13.58	15
N^o elem.	11	13	14	15	14	15	15	16	15
d_A (mm)	1.45	2.45	2.91	3.31	4.02	4.5	4.84	5.33	6.28
GL_A. (deg)	20.16	11.73	9.86	8.6	7.13	6.37	5.92	5.37	4.56

Table 3. Element configuration of the optimized aperture.

The dynamic range obtained goes up 36dB. Then, an optimization algorithm is implemented to search a better phase alignement and thus improve the result. The new dynamic range goes up 40dB, that is to say a 4dB gain.

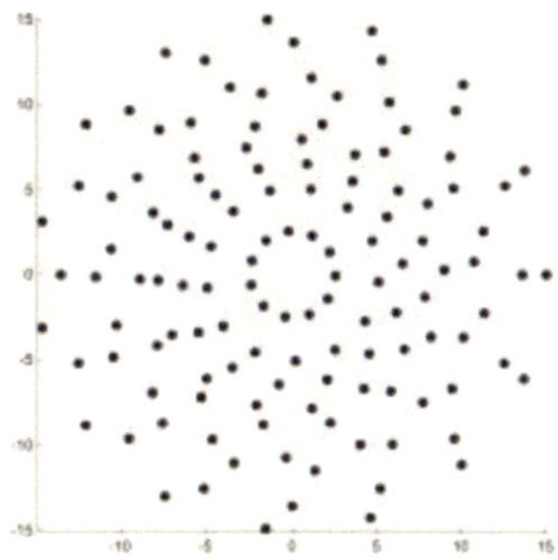

(a) Element distribution

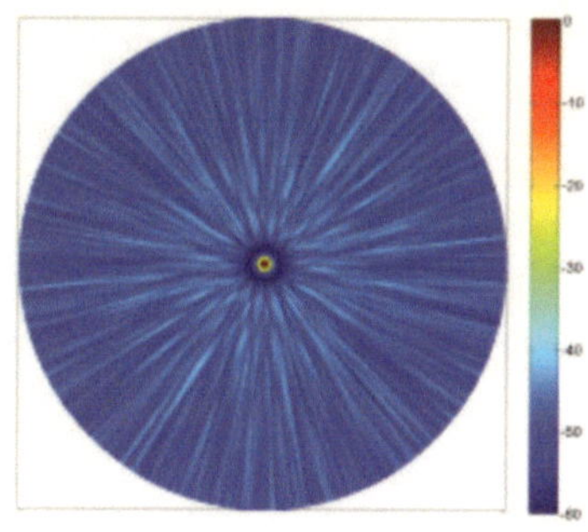

(b) Beampattern in the semisphere

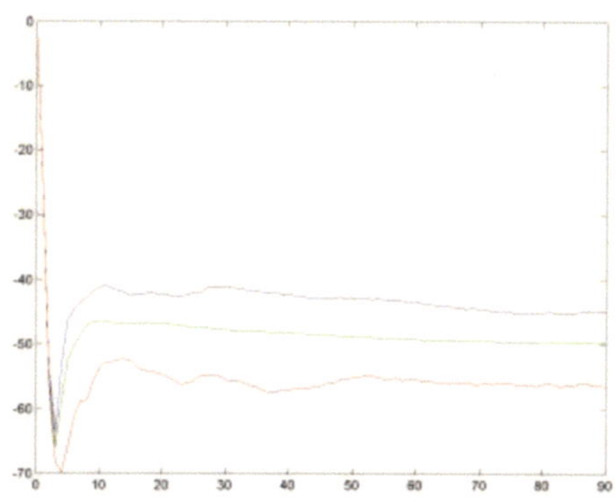

(c) Lateral profile. Maximum, mean and minimum side lobes in elevation are presented

Fig. 12. Best result for CA(128) is presented.

4.2.3 Complementary aperture

Finally, we need to find the complementary aperture that reduces the grating lobe in the pulse-echo response. With this aim, the CA(128) is used as reference and emission aperture and a new phase alignment is searched for the reception configuration. Figure 13 shows the solution obtained.

Table 4 shows CA(128) and CA(128,128) parameters. The dynamic range is improved by 4dB and the MSR is significantly better when complementary apertures are used. Both apertures present equal lateral resolution.

			Lat. Res.		MSR
Configuration	D	GL Level (60%)	-6dB	-40dB	-40dB
CA(128)	60λ	-40.5dB	1.0^o	2.7^o	10.8dB
CA(128,128)	60λ	-44.5dB	1.0^o	2.7^o	17.26dB

Table 4. Performance of the best CA(128) configuration and the CA(128,128).

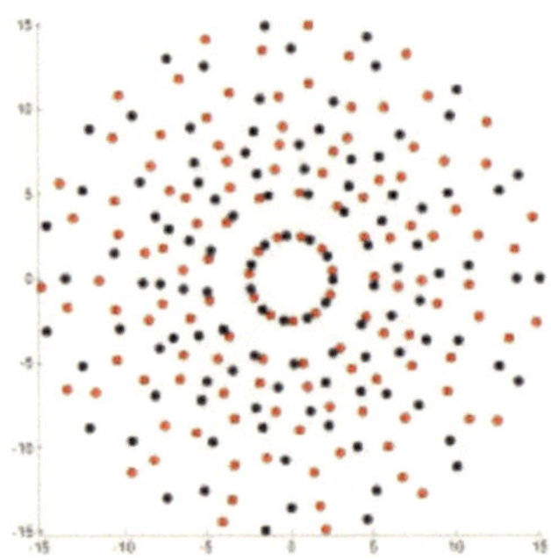

(a) Element distribution: in black emission aperture; in red reception aperture

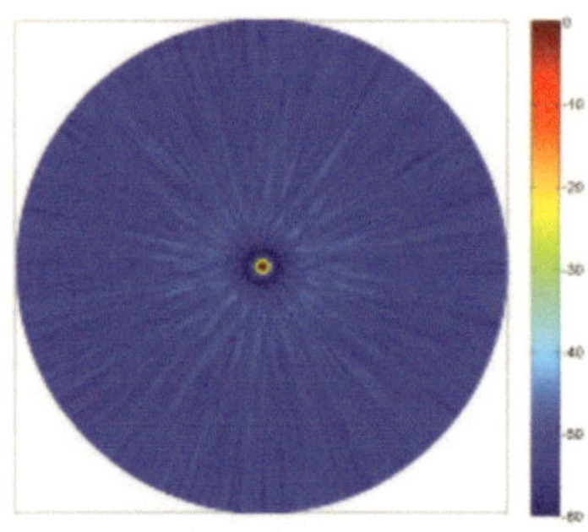

(b) Beampattern in the semisphere

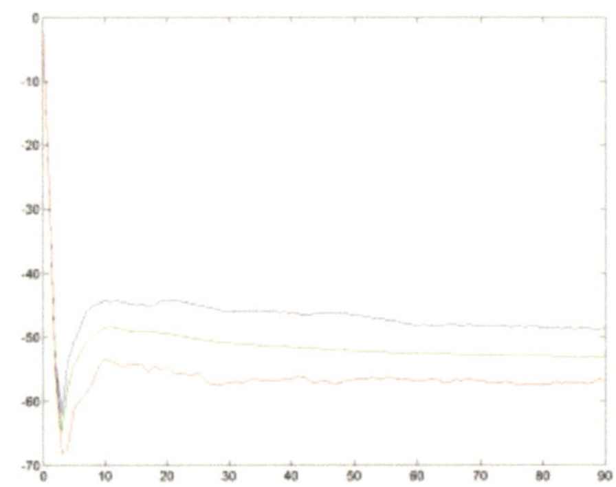

(c) Lateral profile. Maximum, mean and minimum side lobes in elevation are presented

Fig. 13. Best result for CA(128,128) is presented.

5. Conclusions

As this paper shows, both the Fermat Spiral and the Circular Apertures are interesting distributions for designing bidimensional sparse arrays. The mechanisms that determine the grating lobes formation were studied. For each configuration, two design strategies based on the multiplicative effect of the emission reception response were studied.
Both apertures produce similar results. Spiral apertures do slightly better in dynamic range whereas circular apertures, in turn, in lateral resolution. Both present adequate values to be used in some Non Destructive Testing applications, that is a dynamic range of near 45dB and 2.5^o of lateral resolution at (-40dB). However the strategies used to obtain the best solutions were different.

- In the Fermat Spiral design, since there are no constructive parameters we need to find the most adequate solutions by exhaustive computation in one of the identified regions. In this sense SP1, SP2 and SP3 regions offer good solutions with similar results. The main difference between them is the number of branches that organize element distribution.

Some solutions can be more easily implemented than others. Choosing the adequate solution could simplify the manufacturing process.

- In the Circular Apertures case, the solution is given by an optimization process. The elements that generate grating lobes were analysed. Taking into account this analysis the process was divided in several stages. At each stage, a particular constructive parameter was isolated and optimized. Although the optimization process was very simple, the procedure was able to improve the initial aperture by 10dB. Therefore we could assume that better results could be obtained if more sofisticated optimization process were employed.

To compare our results with other configurations we have used the existing examples in literature. Sumanaweera at Sumanaweera et al (1999) presents several examples for configurations with a 40λ diameter: a Archimedean Spiral SP(128,127) a random M(192,64) and a periodic M(128,127) with dynamic ranges of 40dB, 30dB and 15 dB respectively. Nivolov at Nikolov & Jensen (2000) studied 18λ apertures using different arragements based on matrix aperture and the convolution far field model of the pulse-eco in the complementary apertures design. He obtaned a dynamic range of 49dB with a M(256,256) configuration. Also, on the same basis, Austeng at Austeng & Holm (2002) studies different matrix configurations for 25λ. He extends the Vernier models in directions other than the main axes (radial, diagonal) and compares them with random configurations with different sparsing distribution functions (binned, polar). Although Austeng uses more elements than we do, we can compare our results with smaller apertures that achieve a dynamic range of: 39.9dB for Vernier M(421,208), 48.5dB for polar random distribution M(484,361) and 51.6 for binned random distribution M(447,447). More recently, Oliveri has presented a non-overlamping solution M(265,264) with a dynamic range of 40dB.
In general our results are better than those found in the literature. Although our dynamic range goes up to 45dB, we obtain a better lateral resolution (our aperture is bigger) with a number of elements that is significantly lower. Futhermore, when the number of elements is comparable, our apertures provide better dynamic range.

6. Acknowledgments

This study was partly supported by the Spanish Ministry of Science and Innovation under projects DPI2007- 65408-C02-01, DPI2007-65408-C02-02, and PSE-020000-2009-10 (PSS-020000-2009-25 subproject) which is co-supported by the ERDF (European Regional Development Fund).

7. References

S.W. Smith, H.G. Pavy and O.T. von Ramm (1991) High-speed ultrasound volumetric imaging system, Part I: Transducer design and beam steering. IEEE Tans. on UFFC. vol 38(2). pp. 101–108. ISSN: 0885-3010.

W.J Hendricks (1991) Totally random versus the bin approach for random arrays. IEEE Trans on Antennas and Propagation. vol 39(12). pp.1757–1761. ISSN: 0018-926X.

J.L. Schwartz and B.D. Steinberg, (1998) Ultrasparse, ultrawideband arrays. IEEE Tans. on UFFC. vol 45(2). pp. 376–393. ISSN: 0885-3010.

G.R. Lockwood and F.S. Foster, (1996) Optimizing the radiation pattern od sparse periodic two-dimensional arrays. IEEE Tans. on UFFC. vol 45(2). pp. 338–348. ISSN: 0885-3010.

A. Austeng and Sverre Holm. (2002) Sparse 2D arrays for 3D Phased Array Imaging Design Methods. IEEE Tans. on UFFC. vol 49(8). pp. 1073–1086. ISSN: 0885-3010.

S.I. Nikolov and J.A. Jensen (2000) Application of different spatial sampling patterns for sparse array transducer design. Ultrasonics. vol 37. pp. 667–671. ISSN: 0041-624X.

Y. Mendelsohn and E. Wiener-Avnear (2002) Simulations of circular 2D phase-array ultrasonic imaging transducers. Ultrasonics. vol. 39 (9). pp. 657–666. ISSN: 0041-624X.

Ullate LG, Godoy G and Martinez O. (2006) Beam steering with segmented annular arrays. IEEE Tans. on UFFC. vol 53 (10). pp. 1944–1954. ISSN: 0885-3010.

V. Bavaro, G. Caliano and M. Pappalardo. (2008) Element Shape Designo of 2D CMUT Arrays for Reducing Grating Lobes. IEEE Tans. on UFFC. vol 55(2). pp.308–318. ISSN: 0885-3010.

T.S. Sumanaweera, J. Schwartz and D. Napolitano (1999) A spiral 2D phased array for 3D imaging. 1999 IEEE Ultrasonics Symposium. Proceedings. pp.1271-1274.

O. Martínez-Graullera, C.J. Martín, Gregorio Godoy, Luis Gomez-Ullate (2010) 2D Array design based on Fermat Spiral for ultrasound imaging. Ultrasonics. vol. 50 (2). pp. 280-289. ISSN: 0041-624X.

B. Piwakowski and K. Sbai,(1999) A new approach to calculate the field radiated from arbitrarily structured transducer arrays, IEEE Trans. Ultrason., Ferroelect., Freq. Contr., vol. 46, n. 2, pp. 422-439. ISSN: 0885-3010.

Roger V. Jean, (1983) Mathematical Modeling in Phyllotaxis: The State of the Art. Mathematical Biosciences. vol 64. pp. 1–27. ISSN: 0025-5564.

J.N. Ridley. (1982) Packing Efficiency in Sunflower Heads. Mathematical Biosciences. vol 58. pp. 129–39. ISSN: 0025-5564

Giacomo Oliveri and Andrea Massa,(2010) ADS-based array design for 2-D and 3-D ultrasound imaging.. IEEE Tans. on UFFC. vol 57(7). pp. 1568-82. ISSN: 0885-3010.

3

Synthetic Aperture Method in Ultrasound Imaging

Ihor Trots, Andrzej Nowicki, Marcin Lewandowski and Yuriy Tasinkevych
Institute of Fundamental Technological Research
Poland

1. Introduction

Medical ultrasound imaging is a technique that has become much more prevalent than other medical imaging techniques since it is more accessible, less expensive, safe, simpler to use and produces images in the real time. However, images produced by an ultrasound imaging system, must be of sufficient quality to provide accurate clinical interpretation. The most commonly used image quality measures are spatial resolution and image contrast which can be determined in terms of beam characteristics of an imaging system: beam width and side-lobe level. In the design of an imaging system, the optimal set of system parameters is usually found as a trade-off between the lowest side-lobe peak and the narrowest beam of an imaging system.

In conventional ultrasound imaging system, when one transducer (in mechanical wobble) or linear array are used, the quality of images directly depends on the transducer acoustic field. Also in conventional ultrasound imaging the image is acquired sequentially one image line at a time that puts a strict limit on the frame rate that is important in real-time imaging system. Low frame rate means that moving structures (e.g. heart valves) are not easily imaged and diagnosis may be impaired. This limitation can be reduced by employing synthetic aperture (SA) imaging. The basic idea of the SA method is to combine information from emissions close to each other. The synthetic aperture method has previously not been used in medical imaging. This method is a contrast to the conventional beamforming, where only imaging along one line in receiving is used. This means that every image line is visualized as many times as the number of elements used. This will create an equal amount of low resolution images, which are summed up to create one high resolution image.

Problems with medical ultrasound include low imaging depth, and high resolution is achieved only in the region where the transducer is focused. Another problem is decreasing SNR with depth. The basic idea with synthetic aperture is to combine information from emissions close to each other. This is a contrast to the conventional beamforming, were only imaging along one line in receiving is used. This means that every image line is visualized as many times as the number of elements used. This will create an equal amount of low resolution images which are summed up to create one high resolution image.

One of the important processes in ultrasound imaging systems is beamforming. There are many different beamforming methods. In this work both the synthetic transmit aperture (STA) (Trots, et al. 2009) and the multi-element STA (Trots, et al. 2010) methods for medical ultrasound imaging system are discussed. In the case of the multi-element STA imaging method a small number of elements is used to transmit a pulse and all array elements receive the echo signals. The main objective of this method is to increase system frame rate and the penetration depth, maintaining the resolution of images, so that smaller objects can be distinguished. Larger penetration depth can be obtained by increasing transmitted energy that allows increasing the SNR and in its turn to improve the ultrasound image contrast.

Ultrasound imaging systems usually use from 64 to 128 transmit/receive channels. In order to lower the cost of the system, the number of channels should be reduced.

2. Synthetic aperture method

2.1 Synthetic transmit aperture method

As an alternate to the conventional phased array imaging technique the STA method (Hongxia, 1997; Trahey & Nock, 1992) can be used. It provides the full dynamic focusing, both in transmit and receive modes, yielding the highest imaging quality.

In the STA method at each time one array element transmits a pulse and all elements receive the echo signals, see Fig. 1. where data are acquired simultaneously from all directions over a number of emissions, and the full image can be reconstructed from these data. The advantage of this approach is that a full dynamic focusing can be applied to the transmission and the receiving, giving the highest quality of image.

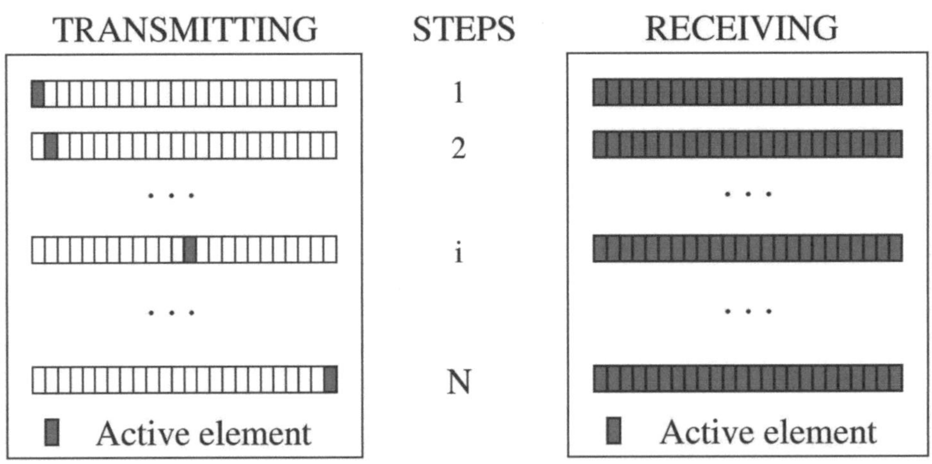

Fig. 1. Transmitting and receiving in STA method

In the STA method focusing is performed by finding the geometric distance from the transmitting element to the imaging point and back to the receiving element. The structure of the synthetic aperture and geometric relation between the transmit and receive element combination is shown in Fig. 2.

When a short pulse is transmitted by element m and the echo signal is received by element n, as shown in Fig. 2, a round-trip delay is

$$\tau_{m,n} = \tau_m + \tau_n , \tag{1}$$

where (m, n) is a transmit and receive element combination, $0 \le m, n \le N\text{-}1$.

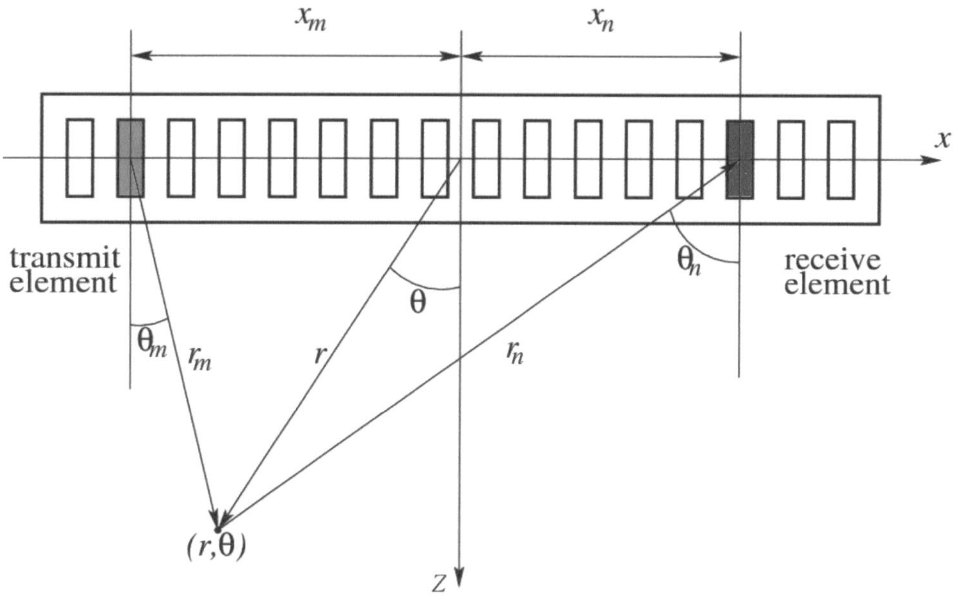

Fig. 2. Geometric relation between the transmit and receive element combination and the focal point

The delays for m'th element and n'th element are

$$\tau_m = \frac{1}{c}\left(r - \sqrt{x_m^2 + r^2 - 2x_m r \sin\theta}\right), \tau_n = \frac{1}{c}\left(r - \sqrt{x_n^2 + r^2 - 2x_n r \sin\theta}\right), \tag{2}$$

where x_m, x_n are the positions of the m'th and n'th elements, respectively and r is a distance between synthetic aperture centre and the point (r,θ). For an N-element array for each point in an image, the A-scan signal can be expressed as

$$A(r,\theta) = \sum_{m=0}^{N-1}\sum_{n=0}^{N-1} y_{m,n}\left(\frac{2r}{c} - \tau_{m,n}\right), \tag{3}$$

where $y_{m,n}(t)$ is the echo signal and $\tau_{m,n}$ is beamforming delay for the (m, n) receive and transmit element combination given in eq. (1). The first and second summations correspond to transmit and receive beamforming.

2.2 Multi-element synthetic transmit aperture

The multi-element STA imaging method represents the best solution in improving lateral resolution and penetration depth. It is known that the lateral resolution can be improved by increasing array length. Only a small number of elements are used to transmit a pulse but all array elements receive the echo signals. In practice, it is not very expensive to build a large transmit aperture, but it is very complex to form a large receive aperture. For a transmit pulse (from all transmit subaperture elements), the RF echoes for all receive elements are stored in memory. When all RF echo signals have been acquired, the total RF sum is formed by coherently adding them.

The multi-element STA method is proposed to increase the system frame rate and the speed of the image acquisition is determined by the number of transmissions M (Fig. 3). For an N-element aperture, M×N data recordings are needed for image reconstruction, where M<<N.

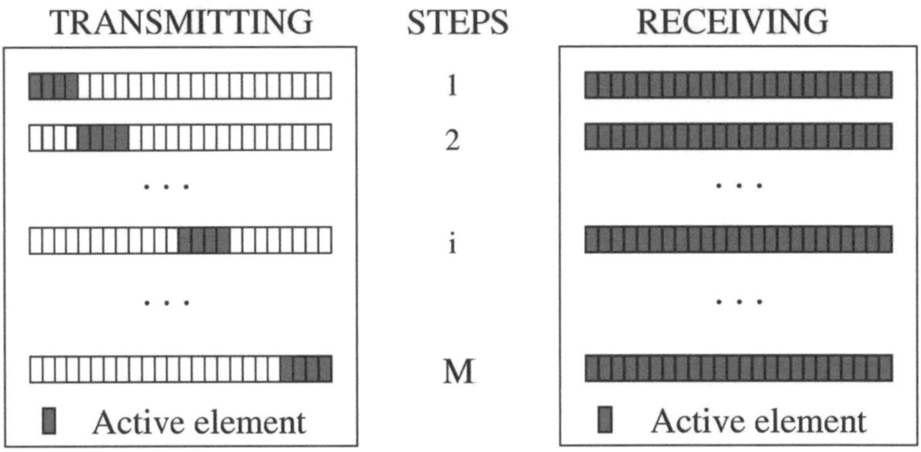

Fig. 3. Transmitting and receiving in multi-element STA method

The geometrical locations of the transmit elements in a multi-element array system impacts the radiation pattern of that system, which in its turn impacts lateral resolution of the image, whereas the number of active transmit elements directly influences the transmitted energy and the SNR. These parameters define the ultrasound image quality. Therefore, the optimization of a multi-element STA imaging system can be formulated as an optimization problem of the location and the number of the transmit elements. The main optimization criterion in the multi-element STA method is the minimal width of the main-lobe combined with the minimum side-lobe level. This optimization leads to increasing image penetration depth and high lateral resolution.

For an N-element array, the transmit aperture is split into Ns subapertures with K_t=N/Ns elements each (Hongxia, 1997). Each subaperture transmits a prefocused beam with focus point near the middle of the region of interest. Echo signals reflected from objects are received at a full or dynamically varying receive aperture with dynamic focusing, and stored in memory. Then data recordings must be focused synthetically with dynamic transmit focusing.

Fig. 4 shows the geometry of the transmission and the reception for the STA system, where $(r; \theta)$ is the point of focus.

The transmit delay has two parts. The first part is the delay to focus all the elements in the subaperture towards the focal point. The second part is the delay to focus all subapertures dynamically. The first part of the delay for the m'th element in the subaperture is

$$\tau_m = \frac{r_s - r_{tm}}{c} \tag{4}$$

$$r_{tm} = \sqrt{\left[\left(-\frac{K_t - 1}{2} + m\right)d\right]^2 + r_s^2 - 2\left(-\frac{K_t - 1}{2} + m\right)dr_s \sin\alpha}$$

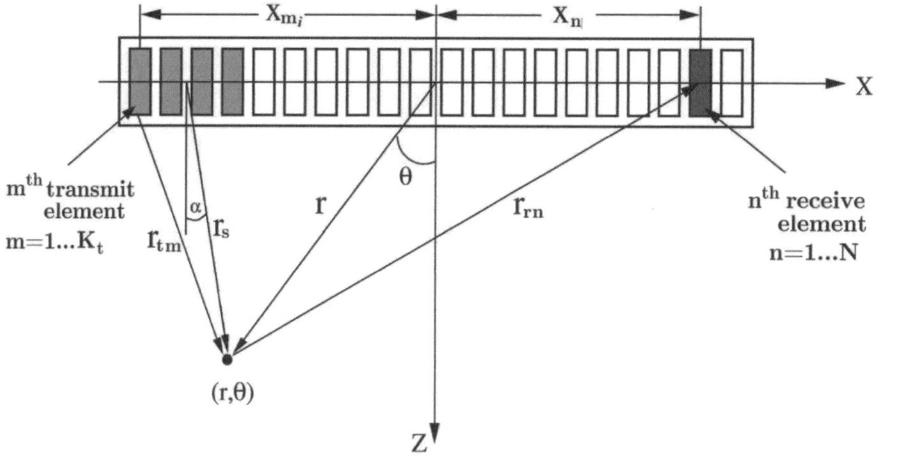

Fig. 4. Geometric relation between the transmit and receive element combination and the focal point

and

$$\alpha = \cos^{-1}\left(\frac{r\cos\theta}{r_s}\right).$$

The second part of the delay for the i'th subaperture is

$$\tau_i = \frac{r - r_s}{c} = \frac{1}{c}\left(r - \sqrt{(r\cos\theta)^2 + (xm_i - r\sin\theta)^2}\right) \tag{5}$$

$$= \frac{1}{c}\left(r - \sqrt{\left[K_t\left(-\frac{N_s - 1}{2} + i\right)d\right]^2 + r^2 - 2K_t\left(-\frac{N_s - 1}{2} + i\right)dr\sin\theta}\right)$$

The receive delay τ_n for the STA can be obtained in a similar way as for the phased array

$$\tau_n = \frac{(r - r_{rn})}{c}. \tag{6}$$

Thus, the total delay is $\tau_m + \tau_i + \tau_n$.

For each image point $(r; \theta)$, the A-scan signal is

$$A_{STA}(t) = \sum_{n=0}^{N-1}\sum_{i=0}^{N_s-1}\sum_{m=0}^{K_t-1} s_{K_t i+m,n}(t - \tau_n - \tau_i - \tau_m), \tag{7}$$

where $s_{m,n}(t)$ is the echo signal. The first summation corresponds to the receive beamforming, while the second and the third summations correspond to the transmit synthetic aperture beamforming.

3. Element directivity diagram influence

In the described above beamforming methods for each point in the resulting image every combination of transmit-receive pairs contributes according to the round-trip propagation time only. The angular dependence is not taken into account in the applied point-like source model. But when the width of the array element is comparable to the wavelength corresponding to the nominal frequency of the emitted signal, the point-like source model becomes inaccurate. The element directivity influences the partial contribution to the resulting signal $A(r, \theta)$ in eq. (3) depending on the mutual position of the imaging point and transmit- receive pair, determined by the angles θ_m, θ_n (see Fig. 2). Here, a modified STA imaging algorithm, which accounts for the element directivity function and its influence on $A(r, \theta)$, is developed (Tasinkevych, et al. 2010).

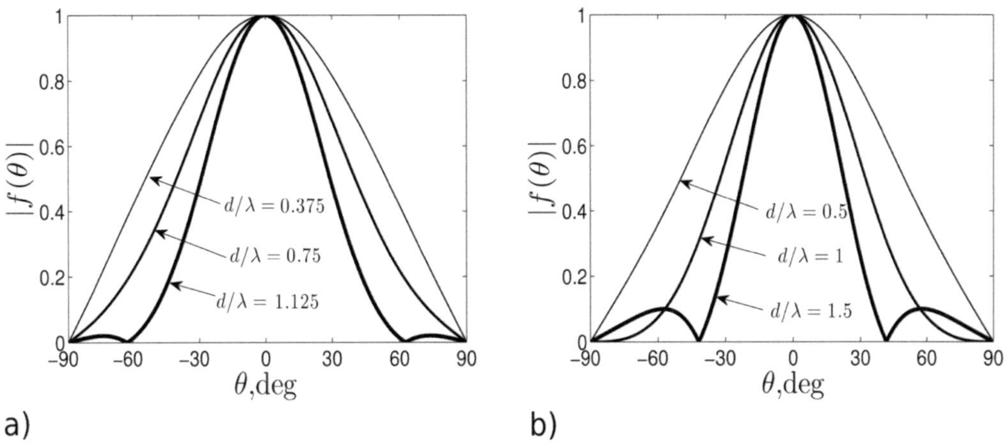

Fig. 5. Directivity function for different values of d/λ

The underlying idea can be illustrated on the following example, shown in Fig. 6. Here, it is assumed, that the same element transmits and receives signal. Two scatterers located at the points with polar coordinates (r_i, θ_i), i=1,2 such that r_{1m}=r_{2m} would contribute to the corresponding echo signal $y_{m,m}(t)$ simultaneously, since the round-trip propagation time $2r_{im}/c$, i=1,2 is the same (the corresponding numerical example is shown in Fig. 3 in the next section). Apparently, the contribution from the scatterer at the point (r_1, θ_1) would be dominant, since the observation angle θ_{1m} coincides with the direction of maximum radiation for the m-th element, whereas its transmit-receive efficiency at the angle θ_{2m} is much smaller for the case of the scatterer at the point (r_2, θ_2). Thereby, evaluating the value of $A(r_2, \theta_2)$ from eq. (3), the partial contribution of the echo $y_{m,m}(t)$, in addition to the correct signal from the obstacle located at (r_2, θ_2) (being small due to the large observation angle θ_{2m}), would also introduce the erroneous signal from the scatterer located at (r_1, θ_1). The latter signal is larger due to the small observation angle θ_{1m}. The larger observation angles appear in the imaging region close to the array aperture. Therefore, the most appreciable deviation from the point-like source model of the array element will occur there. A solution to the problem, which accounts for the observation angle in accordance with the array element directivity function, is proposed. Assume, that the dependence of the transmit-receive efficiency of a single array element versus the observation angle is known and is denoted by $f(\theta_m)$, where θ_m is measured from the line parallel to z-axis and passing through the m-th element center. Thus, in order to suppress the erroneous influence from the scatterer located at (r_1, θ_1) on the value of the resulting signal $A(r_2, \theta_2)$, the partial contribution of the echo $y_{m,m}(t)$ is weighted by the corresponding value of $f(\theta_{2m})$. This corresponds to the superposed signal correction in accordance with respective contributions of individual scatterers located at the points (r_1, θ_1) and (r_2, θ_2) (Fig. 6).

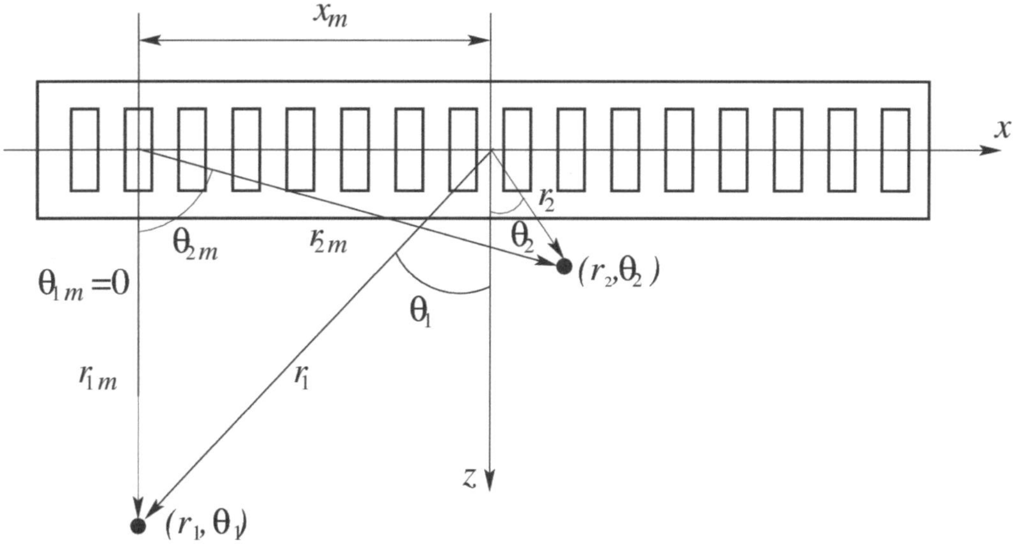

Fig. 6. Influence of the scatterer located at the point (r_1, θ_1) on the value of resulting signal $A(r_2, \theta_2)$ for imaging point (r_2, θ_2)

The above considerations lead to the following modification of the synthetic focusing imaging algorithm

$$A(r,\theta) = \sum_{m=1}^{N}\sum_{n=1}^{N} f(\theta_m) f(\theta_n) y_{m,n}\left(\frac{2r}{c} - \tau_{m,n}\right), \tag{8}$$

where $\theta_i(r, \theta)$, $i=m,n$ are the corresponding observation angles for the transmit-receive pair. The modification of the STA thus is expressed by weighted summation of properly delayed RF signals (as in the case of conventional STA). The corresponding weights $f(\theta_m)$, $f(\theta_n)$ in the transmit and receive modes are calculated by means of the single element directivity function. Note, that the angles depend on the spatial location of the imaging point (r, θ). The directivity function $f(\theta)$ can be calculated in the far-field approximation for a single element of the array transducer in analogous manner as in (Selfridge, et al. 1980) (see example in Fig. 5)

$$f(\theta) = \frac{\sin(\pi d / \lambda \sin\theta)}{\pi d / \lambda \sin\theta} \cos\theta \tag{9}$$

where d is the element width, and λ is the wavelength. Some examples of the directivity function evaluated for different values of the ratio d/λ are shown in Fig. 5. Note, in Fig. 5b the values of d/λ correspond to the case when the element width d=0.75*pitch, and the pitch is 0.5, 1, and 1.5 of the lambda, respectively. The above result applies to a narrow strip transducer with a time harmonic uniform pressure distribution along its width. It is obtained by means of the Rayleigh-Sommerfeld formula in the far-field region. The result is in a good agreement with experimental studies as shown by the authors in the cited work. For simplicity, eq. (9) is applied in the numerical results presented in the next section. It should be noted, that we use the angular response $f(\theta)$ in eq. (8) evaluated from eq. (9) for some fixed value of λ, which corresponds to the nominal frequency of the transmitted signal. The far-field approximation is admissible for the case of synthetic focusing algorithm discussed here. For the typical examples considered in the next section, the ratio d/λ =1.125 is assumed, and the coresponding element directivity function is depicted in Fig. 5b. The far-field limit $r_{min} \approx 2d^2/\lambda$ (Michishita, et al. 2000) is 2.5λ. This requirement is met in the considered numerical experiments.

4. Computer simulation

Simulation is a fundamental way of testing methods. This is done to confirm or reject a hypothesis in a controlled environment. Since it is possible to control all parameters in a simulation, one can set up a simple model and then gradually transform it into something more similar to reality. When this is done one can continue with measurements and confirm or reject the simulations for a real setup, in vivo or on a phantom. All simulations in this work are carried out with a powerful software, *Field II* (Jensen, 1999). The program is developed especially for investigating ultrasound fields, and gives the possibility to simulate and calculate ultrasound fields and defining one's own transducer. The accuracy is very high since *Field II* is based on numerical analysis. *Field II* runs under Matlab which makes it even more versatile and useful. This is the reason why *Field II* is used worldwide.

The numerical results presented in Fig. 7 and Fig. 8 were performed for a 48-element linear transducer array excited by one sine cycle burst pulse at a nominal frequency of 5 MHz. The element pitch is 1.5λ and the inter-element spacing is 0.25 of the pitch, where λ corresponds to the nominal frequency of the burst pulse. The STA algorithm is employed. The transmit and receive elements combinations give a total of 48×48 possible RF A-lines. All these A-lines echo signals are sampled independently at a frequency of 50 MHz and stored in RAM.

In Fig. 7 a numerical example explaining the discussion of the previous section is shown. Two point scatteres are placed at different depths: one in the immediate vicinity of the transducer element and another is located deeper, as depicted in Fig. 6.

The blurring of the scatterer placed near the aperture is significantly diminished in the case of introducing the directional diagram of element in synthetic focusing algorithm as compared to the algorithm without this correction, being in agreement with the above consideration of section 3.

In Fig. 8 the results of simulation of a wire phantom are shown. Thin wires are spaced equidistantly with raster of 6λ in the lateral and axial directions. Fig. 8a (left) corresponds to the algorithm eq. (8) with the angular directivity function calculated according to (9), whereas in Fig. 8a (right) the results corresponding to the algorithm eq. (3) are shown for comparison.

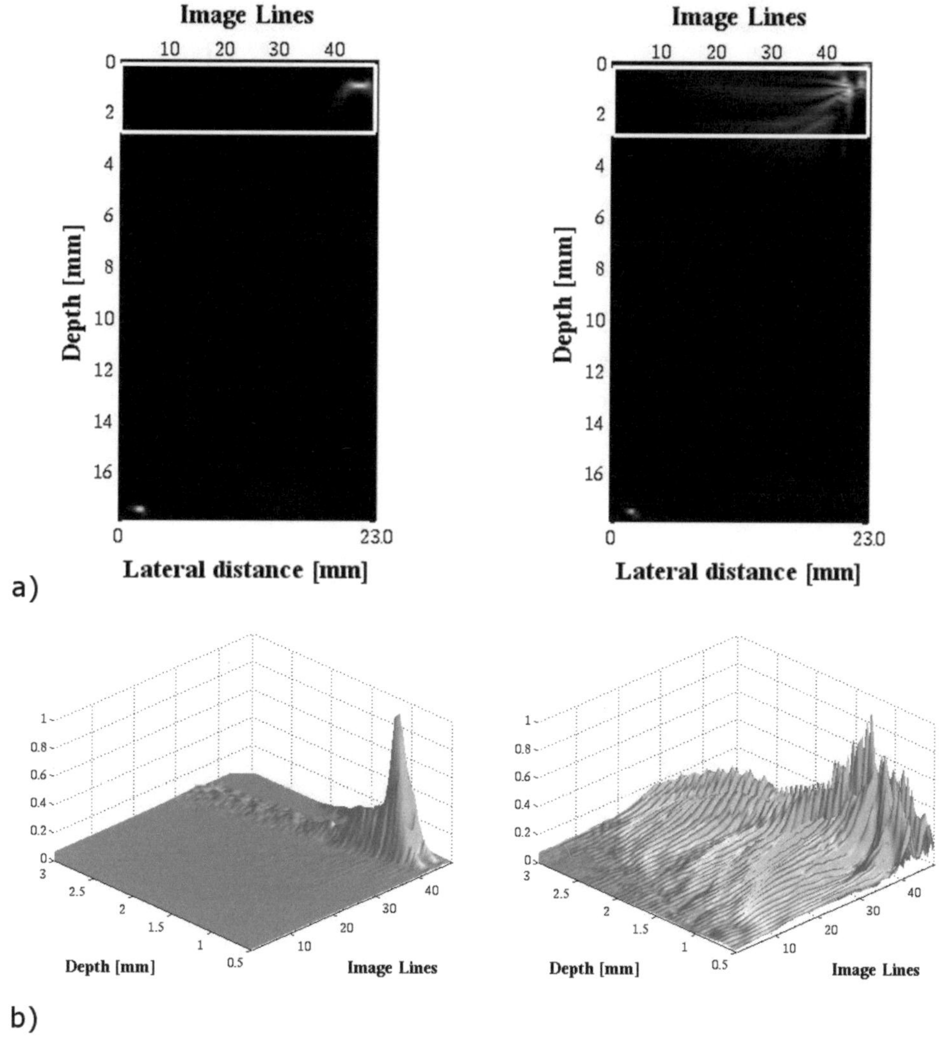

Fig. 7. Simulation of 2 point scatterers for 48-element linear array: a) left subplot - including directional diagram of element, right subplot - not including directional diagram of element; b) detailed view of the selected part of the images in (a), respectively. The magnitude of the scattered field in a linear scale is shown

The simulation results have shown distinguishable improvement of the imaging quality of the scatterers situated in the region near the transducer aperture. The artefacts in the form of hazy blurring, observable in the conventional STA algorithm are substantially suppressed in the case of the modified one. Besides, the imaging depth is also increased, which is the valuable advantage of the developed method.

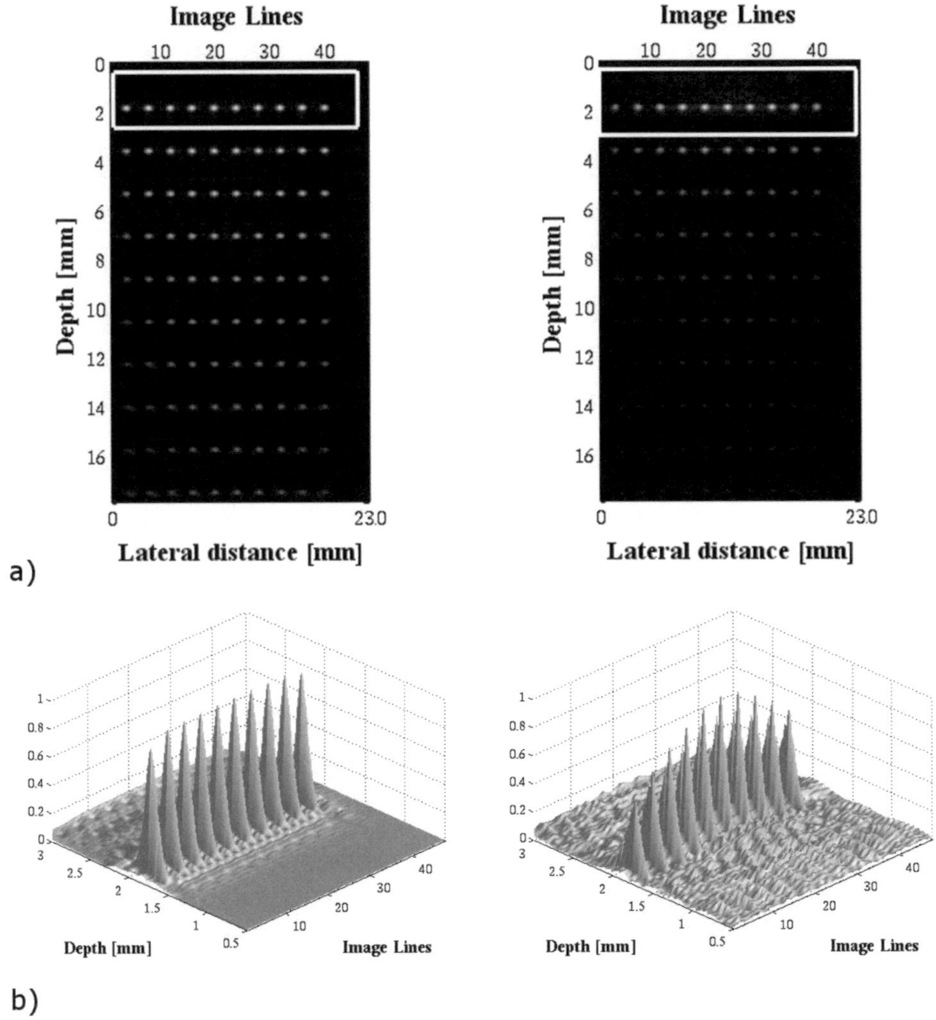

Fig. 8. Thin wire phantom simulation using a) left subplot - including directional diagram of element, right subplot - not including directional diagram of element; b) detailed view of the selected part of the phantom including and not including directional diagram of element, respectively. The magnitude of the scattered field in a linear scale is shown

In the next part of simulation the parameters used in the simulations are set to be similar to those of transducer used in the measurements. The medium in the simulations is homogeneous and its only variable parameter is the speed of sound. In the simulations no attenuation is considered. Even so, echoes far from the transducer become weaker and have lower amplitude because the energy is spread out. These simplifications do not affect the method in principle and in measurements these simplifications have been taken into account.

In Fig. 9 the 2D ultrasound images of phantom, obtained by computer simulation for the case of 32-element linear transducer array with 0.48 mm inter-element spacing and one-cycle burst pulse at nominal frequency 5 MHz, are shown. In the case of multi-element STA method every subaperture consists of the two elements and transmits an unfocused ultrasound wave. The phantom medium attenuation is 0.5 dB/[MHz×cm] and consists of the collections of point targets spaced 4 pitches apart laterally, and the collections are spaced axially 5 mm apart from each other.

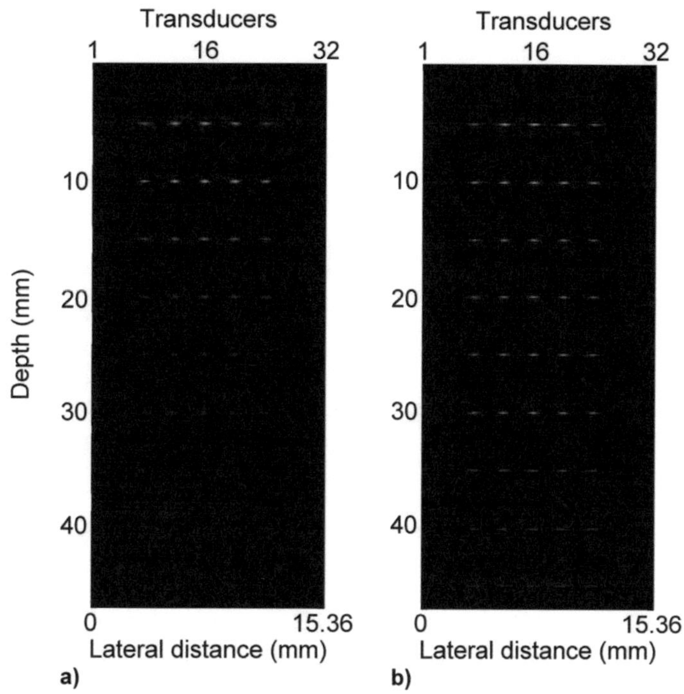

Fig. 9. The 2D ultrasound images of phantom with point targets for the STA method (a) and the multi-element STA (b)

It can be easily seen, that penetration depth increases in the case of the multi-element STA. For the objective comparison of the resolution the axial cross sections of the centre line and lateral cross sections in the depths 10 mm and 20 mm are shown in Fig. 10.

Fig. 10 shows that transmitted energy grows in the multi-element STA method and the penetration depth increases while lateral resolution is comparable in both cases.

The multi-element STA imaging method represents the best solution in improving penetration depth and maintaining lateral resolution.

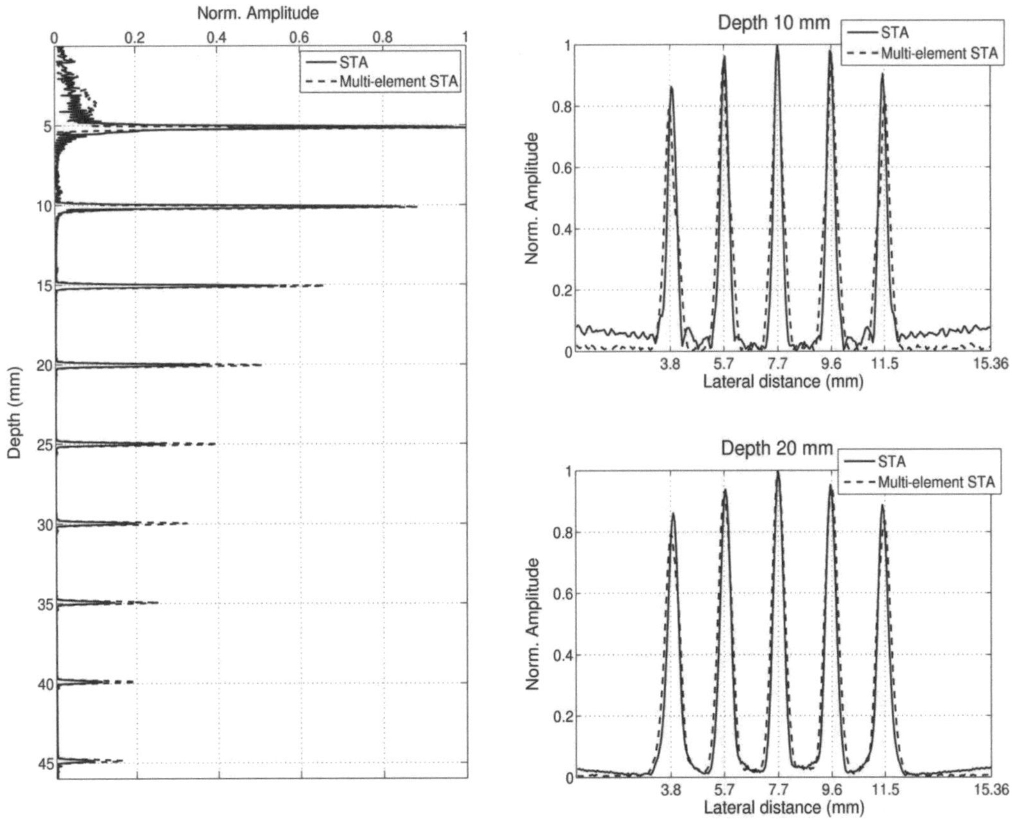

a) b)

Fig. 10. Comparison of the cross sections between STA method and multi-element STA method: a) axial cross section of the centre line; b) lateral cross section in depth 10 mm (top) and depth 20 mm (bottom)

5. Ultrasound imaging system

Synthetic aperture evaluation was performed using a simplified ultrasound imaging system which is shown in Fig. 11.

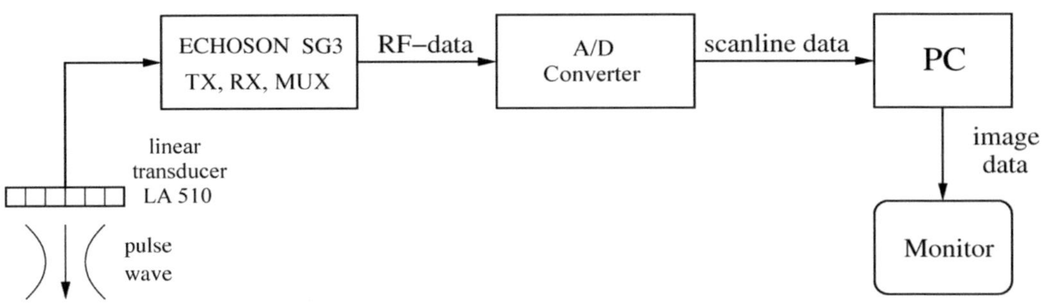

Fig. 11. Block diagram of the ultrasound imaging system

Linear transducer LA510 produced by Echoson (Echoson, Pulawy, Poland) transmits pulsed ultrasound waves, and receives reflected echo signals. Echoson SG3 transmitting/receiving system enables full control of selected 32 consecutive channels/transducers of a linear array transducer. Parameters of transmission and reception are programmable from a PC using a serial port (RS-232). Using the SG3 one can switch on arbitrary transmit and receive channels in the selected 32 channels aperture. The second block, A/D converter extracts the RF data, acquires it and sends to the PC. Next, the collected digital data were processed offline and displayed on the monitor. All post processing and display is done on the computer using Matlab™ software. The processing creates 2D ultrasound imaging focused in every point of image.

The system allows performing simulated multichannel acquisition for synthetic aperture imaging. Using a single channel digitizer and switching receiving transducers the system is capable of gathering the RF data for up to 32 lines. Repeating this procedure for each transmitted element of the N-element transducer the N×N data recordings are obtained with the STA method or the M×N data with the multi-element STA method, where M is subaperture number, needed for image reconstruction. These data are the input to the synthetic aperture algorithm.

Synthetic aperture image reconstruction requires considerable amount of data storage and processing power. The amount of raw RF data needed in the STA imaging for reconstruction of a single image is proportional to $D_{RF} * N^2$, and the number of delay-and-sum operations is $D_{RF} * N^3$, where D_{RF} is the number of samples in a single RF line. For 32 elements linear array with 15 cm penetration (D_{RF}=8000 at 40 MHz sampling frequency) storage requirements $\approx$ 8.2*10^6 samples, delay-and-sum operations $\approx$ 262*10^6 are obtained.

The multi-element STA method imaging allows to reduce the amount of raw RF data needed for reconstruction of a single image and is equal to $D_{RF} * M * N$ and the number of delay-and-sum operations is $D_{RF} * M * N^2$. For 32 elements linear array and 2 elements in subaperture (M=16) with 15 cm penetration storage requirements $\approx$ 4.1*10^6 samples, delay-and-sum operations $\approx$ 131*10^6 are obtained. It is two times less than in the case of classical STA method.

6. Experimental results and discussion

The 32-element linear transducer array with 0.48 mm inter-element spacing and a burst pulse with time duration of 100 ns (a half-cycle at nominal frequency 5 MHz) were used in experiments. The inter-element spacing is about 1.5λ. All elements are used for both the transmitting and receiving. An element in the transducer transmitting aperture was used to generate a spherical wave covering the full image region. The received echo signals were sampled independently at 50 MHz and then stored.

Firstly, the experiments were performed using the standard STA method in which one array element transmits a pulse and all elements receive the echo signals. In this experiments the wire phantom was used, that consists of 24 wires 0.1 mm in diameter, positioned axially every 2 mm at an angle of 75 degrees. This phantom allows to examine the axial and lateral resolution at various depths in the ultrasound image, as well as the focal and dead zone registration. Since the phantom was immersed in water, where there is almost no attenuation, high amplitude echo signals from the wires were obtained.

Three of 1024 (32x32) received RF echo signals, which were digitized and stored in the PC, are shown in Fig. 12.

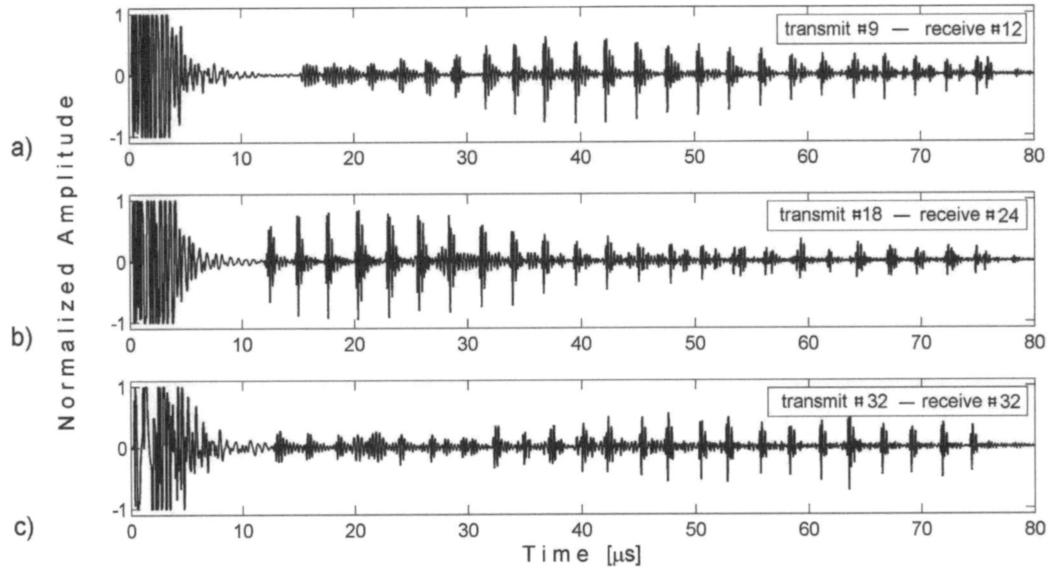

Fig. 12. The recorded by PC RF echo signals: a) element #9 is transmitting - element #12 is receiving, b) #18 transmitting - #24 receiving, c) #32 transmitting - #32 receiving

All these RF echo signals are different and echo time position and signal amplitude in every case depend on sound field and geometrical position of transmitted and received transducers. After all emissions the full set of the RF A-lines echo signals, needed to reconstruct one 2D B-mode ultrasound image, is obtained. For this aim the synthetic aperture algorithm calculates the time delays and weights resulting from the directivity function for every combination of transmit-receive pairs and current imaging points and from the RF-lines computes the final image.

As was mentioned above, a single element in the transducer aperture is used for transmitting a spherical wave covering the full image region. The received signals for all or part of the elements in the aperture are sampled for each transmission. This data can be used for producing low resolution images (Fig. 13a - 13c), which is only focused in the receive due to the unfocused transmission. Focusing is performed by compensating the geometric distance from the transmitting element to the imaging point and back to the receiving element and can be obtained from eq. (3). These low resolution images need to be added coherently to form the final high resolution image (Fig. 13d).

Fig. 13 presents the standard STA imaging method, where at each time one array element transmits and all elements receive. This method represents a good solution when small N-elements array transducers are used. In present ultrasound diagnostic the 128- or 192-elements array transducers are used and application of such STA method restricts the image acquisition considerably. For this purpose the multi-element STA method is proposed where two elements in subaperture transmit a flat ultrasound wave and are shifted by one subaperture that allows to increase the speed of the image acquisition.

To compare the multi-element STA method and standard STA method the tissue mimicking phantom, model 525 Danish Phantom Design, with attenuation of background material 0.5 dB/[MHz×cm], was used in experiments.

In Fig. 14 two of 512 (16x32) received RF echo signals, which were digitized and stored in the PC, are shown.

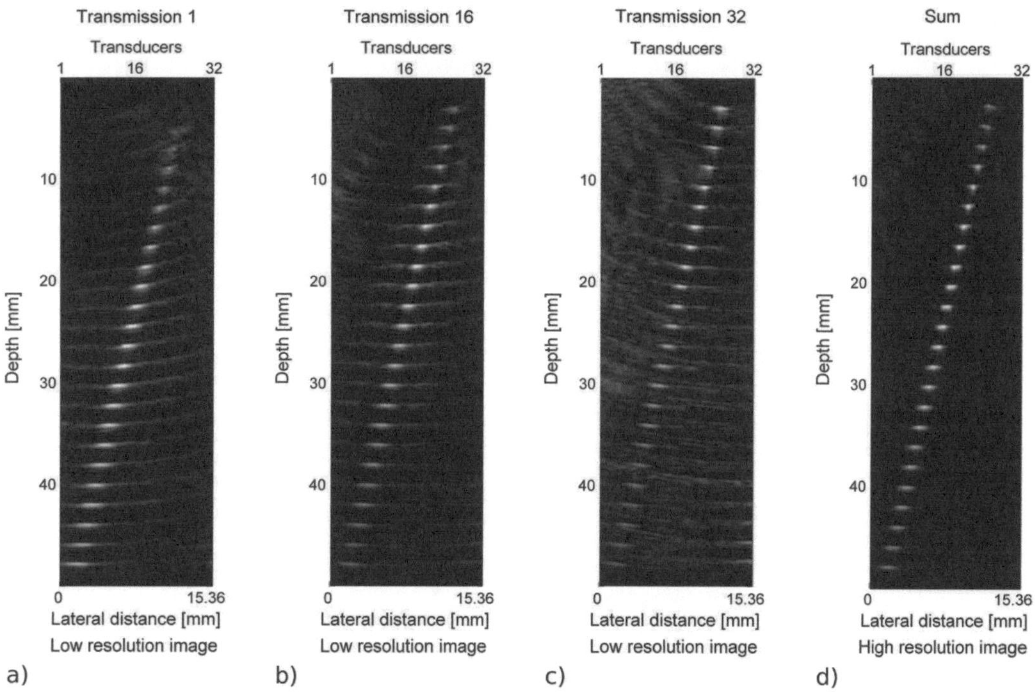

Fig. 13. Low resolution images combined to produce a high resolution image. One element transmit at the time, while all are used to receive. The images are then added into one high resolution image

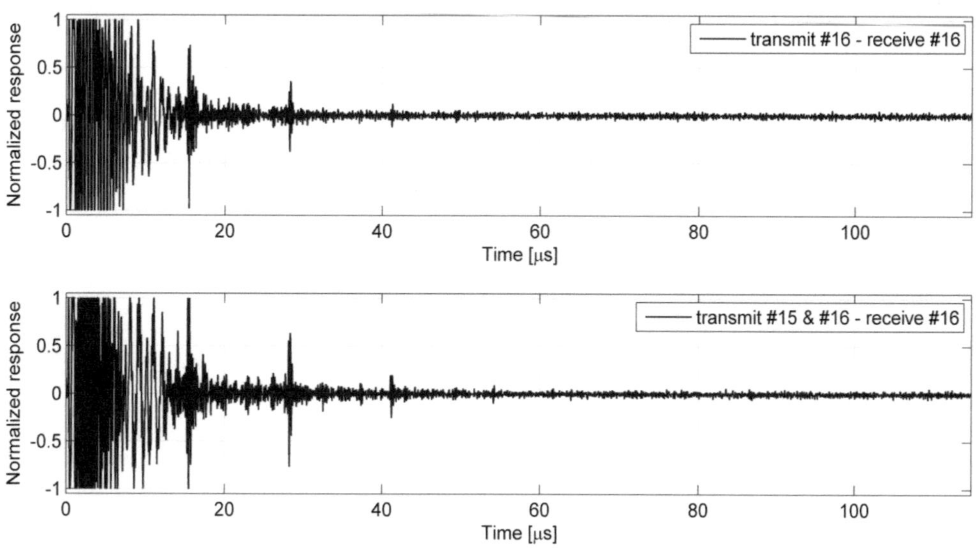

Fig. 14. The recorded echo signals: a) the STA method - element #16 is transmitting – element #16 is receiving, b) the multi-element STA method - elements #15 and #16 transmitting – #16 receiving

It can be easily seen, that the amplitude of the echo signals in the multi-element STA method is about two times higher.
The comparison of the 2D ultrasound images of the tissue phantom, obtained with the standard STA method and multi-element STA method, are shown in Fig. 15.

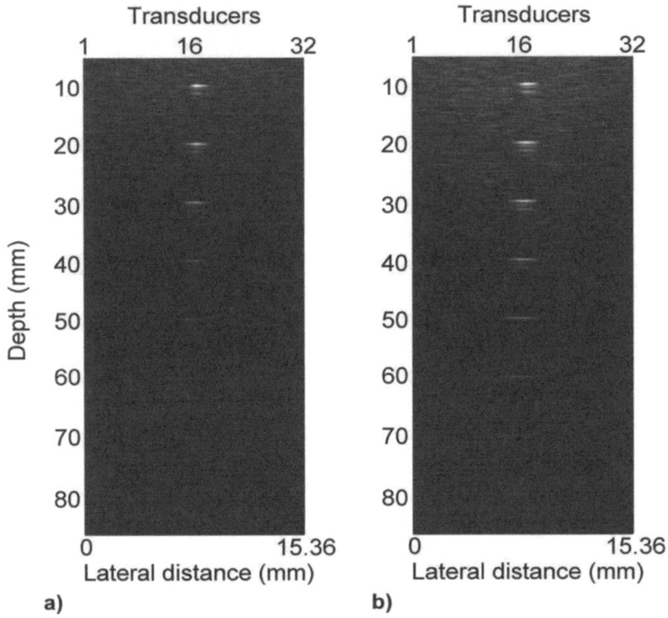

Fig. 15. 2D ultrasound images of tissue mimicking phantom: a) using STA method; b) using multi-element STA method

The obtained 2D ultrasound images clearly demonstrate the advantage of the multi-element STA method. With the elongation of the transmit aperture the acoustical power increases yielding a higher SNR, that leads to an increase in the penetration depth while maintaining both axial and lateral resolution. The last resolution depends on transducer acoustic field and is discussed in (Nowicki et al., 2007).
In order to compare quantitatively the SNR gain the central RF-lines of the 2D ultrasound images shown in Fig. 15 are in Fig. 16 and the SNR is calculated.
Fig. 16 shows that increasing transmitted aperture by one element improves the SNR by about 5 dB that in one's turn leads to improvement of the penetration depth and the contrast of the image.
The next part of the experiments was to compare the 2D B-mode ultrasound images obtained using the STA method and the standard linear array scanning method that is applied in commercial ultrasound scanner Antares (Siemens, Mountain View, CA, USA). In this experiments the wire phantom was used. In the STA method the linear transducer array (LA510) with 0.48 mm inter-element spacing and a burst cycle pulse at nominal frequency 5 MHz, while in the ultrasound scanner Antares the linear transducer array with 0.3 mm pitch (VF13-5) and a burst cycle pulse at nominal frequency 10 MHz, were used.
Focus principle in ultrasound scanner Antares is shown in Fig. 17.

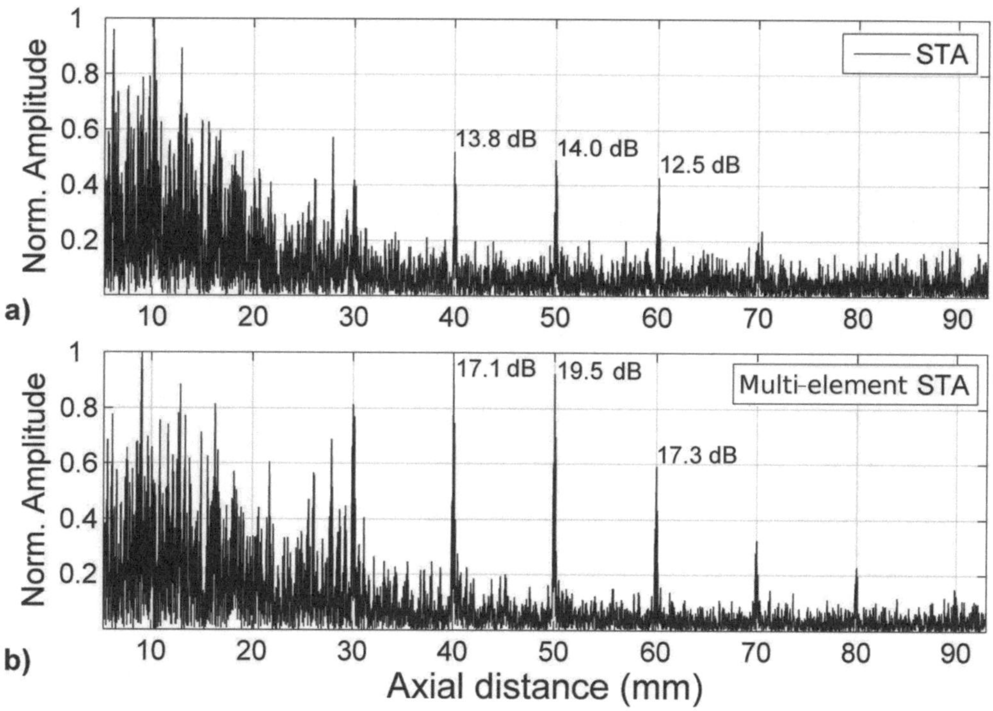

Fig. 16. The RF-lines of the tissue mimicking phantom: a) using STA method; b) using multi-element STA method

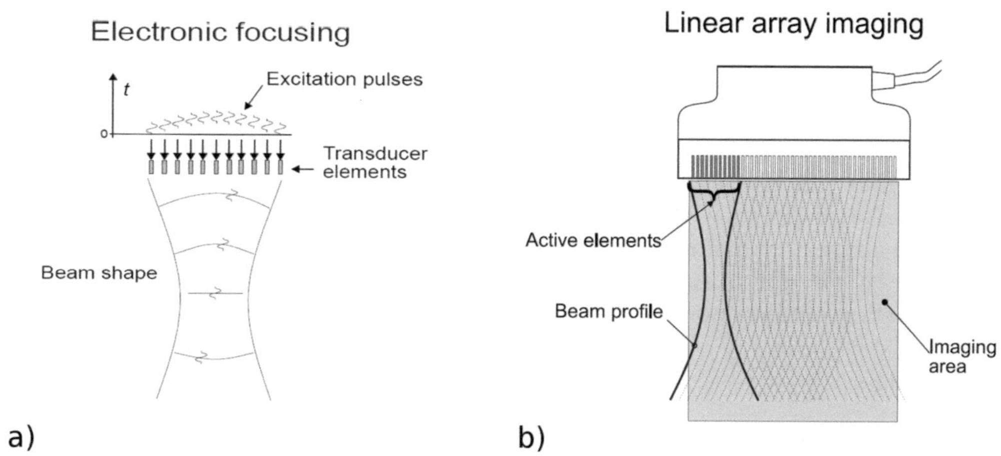

Fig. 17. a) electronic focusing principle; b) linear array transducer for obtaining a rectangular cross-section image

The comparison of the reconstructed wire phantom images, obtained using the STA method and standard linear array scanning with commercial ultrasound scanner Antares, is shown in Fig. 18. The maximum quantity of focal points, which were equal to 1 and 8, were chosen in the ultrasound scanner; they are marked by little triangles at the bar side.

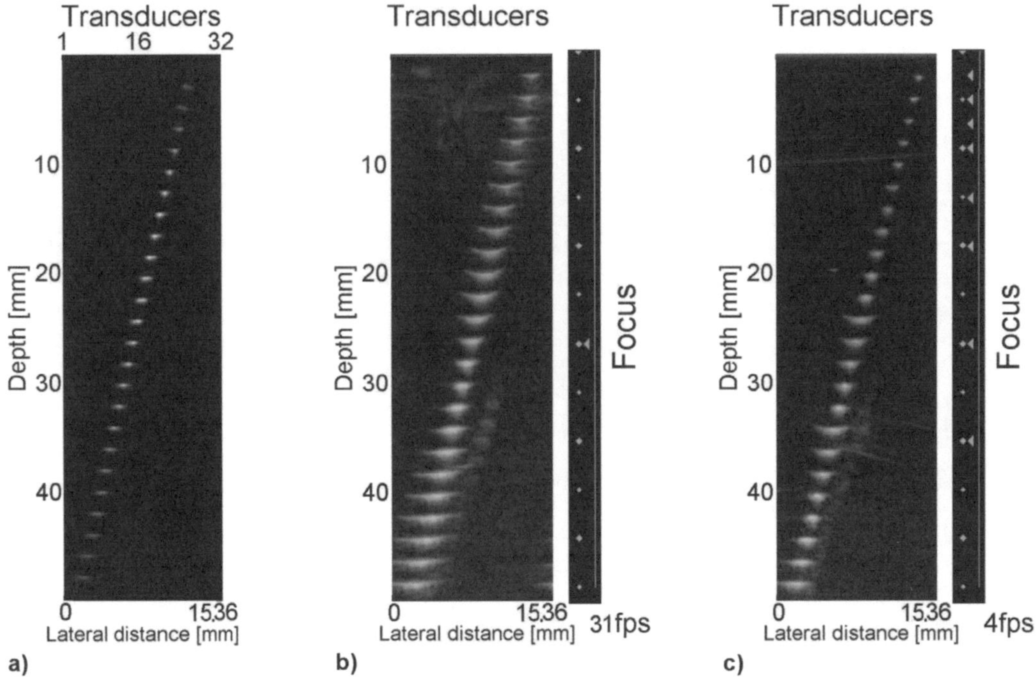

Fig. 18. The 2D ultrasound images of the wire phantom: a) using STA method; b) ANTARES ultrasound scanner with one focal point; c) ANTARES ultrasound scanner with 8 focal points

In Fig. 18 it can be easily seen, that axial and lateral resolutions at the top and at the bottom parts of the image are different and depend on the focal point quantity in these regions. It needs to be noted, that frame rate in the case 8 focal points dramatically decreases down to 4 fps (in the case of one focal point it is equal to 31 fps). Such frame rate is definitely insufficient to examine in a standard way the dynamically moving organs, such as heart, where high frame rate even up to 50 fps is required.

The obtained 2D images show that the STA method allows obtaining good resolution in the whole explored region maintaining the high frame rate. Also, the results show the effectiveness of the STA method and its resistance to the refraction, attenuation, and reflection of ultrasound waves.

7. Conclusion

The STA method, being a variety of the synthetic aperture approach, is discussed. Its development and investigation is presented. The main advantage of the STA method is the increase of the system frame rate and thus substantial improvement of the image quality. Numerous examples of how the medical SA ultrasound imaging can be acquired and processed are shown. The conventional STA method and multi-element STA imaging algorithm are compared. In the latter case, more than one elements are used in transmit mode but all array elements operate in receive mode. It is shown, that even for two element transmit aperture the SNR can be improved by about 5 dB maintaining the same imaging

resolution as compared to the conventional STA. This, in its turn, allows to improve the penetration depth and makes the ultrasound image more contrast.
Also, the modified STA algorithm is presented. This algorithm is based on the array element angular directivity function implementation into the conventional STA method and corresponding correction of the back-scattered RF signals of different transmit-receive pairs. It is shown that the far-field radiation pattern of a narrow strip transducer, calculated for the case of a time harmonic uniform pressure distribution over its width, can serve as a good approximation for the above directivity function. The results of numerical calculations using simulated data, as well as experimentally obtained ones for different phantoms, have shown distinguishable improvement of the imaging quality of the scatterers situated in the region near the transducer aperture, the hazy blurring artefacts, observable in the case of conventional STA algorithm, are substantially suppressed.
Finally, the comparison of the ultrasound images reconstructed, using the STA method and by commercial ultrasound scanner Antares, is shown. The images reconstructed by the STA system give the same image resolution as that from the conventional ultrasound system with an increased frame rate. The STA system offers higher image resolution than conventional system if the frame rate is the same in both cases. The synthetic transmit aperture method can be applied in a standard ultrasound scanner. Introduction of the STA method in medical ultrasound would increase the efficiency and quality of the ultrasound diagnostic.

8. Acknowledgements

Funding: The European Regional Development Fund under the Innovative Economy Operational Programme & Ministry of Science and Higher Education, Poland.

9. References

Jensen, J.A. Linear description of ultrasound imaging systems. (1999). *Notes for the International Summer School on Advanced Ultrasound Imaging,* Technical University of Denmark, June 10, 1999.

Hongxia, Y. (1997). *Synthetic aperture methods for medical ultrasonic imaging*. Thesis.

Michishita, K.; Sakagami,K,; Morimotgo, M.; Svensson, U.P. (2000). Sound radiation from an unbaffled elastic plate strip of infinite length. *Applied Acoustics,* Vol. 61, No. 1, pp. 45-63, S0003-682X(99)00067-5

Nowicki, A.; Klimonda, Z.; Lewandowski, M.; Litniewski, J.; Lewin, P.A.; Trots, I. (2007). Direct and post-compressed sound fields for different coded excitation, *Acoustical Imaging,* Vol. 28, No. 5, pp. 399–407, ISBN 978-1-4020-5720-5

Selfridge, A.R.; Kino, G.S.; Khuri-Yakub, B.T. (1980). A theory for the radiation pattern of a narrow-strip acoustic transducer. *Appl. Phys.Lett.,* Vol. 37, No. 1, pp. 35-36, ISSN 0003-6951

Tasinkevych, Y.; Nowicki, A.; Trots, I. (2010) Element directivity influence in the synthetic focusing algorithm for ultrasound imaging, *Proceedings of the 57th Open Seminar on Acoustics OSA 2010*, pp. 197-200, ISBN 978-83-931744-0-9, September 2010, Gliwice, Poland

Trahey, G.E.; Nock, L.F. (1992). Synthetic receive aperture imaging with phase correction for motion and for tissue ihomogeneities – part I: Basic principles. *IEEE Trans. Ultrason. Ferroelec. Freq. Contr.*, Vol. 39, No. 4, pp. 489–495, ISSN 0885-3010

Trots, I.; Nowicki, A.; Lewandowski, M. (2009). Synthetic transmit aperture in ultrasound imaging, *Archives of Acoustics*, Vol. 43, No. 4, pp. 685-695, ISSN 0137-5075

Trots, I.; Nowicki, A.; Lewandowski, M.; Tasinkevych, Y. (2010). Multielement synthetic transmit aperture in medical ultrasound imaging, *Proceedings of the 57th Open Seminar on Acoustics OSA 2010*, pp. 205-208, ISBN 978-83-931744-0-9, September 2010, Gliwice, Poland

Trots I., Nowicki A., Lewandowski M., Tasinkevych Y. (2010). Multi-element synthetic transmit aperture in medical ultrasound imaging, *Archives of Acoustics*, Vol. 35, No. 4, pp. 687 - 699, ISSN 0137-5075

4

Adaptive Beamforming by Phase Coherence Processing

J. Camacho and C. Fritsch
Consejo Superior de Investigaciones Científicas (CSIC), Madrid
Spain

1. Introduction

The quality of *phased array* and *synthetic aperture* ultrasonic images is limited by several factors determined by the sound propagation physics and diffraction laws. Image quality is mainly determined by:

1. *Resolution*, which depends on signal bandwidth (in the axial direction) and on the aperture extent (in the lateral direction).
2. *Dynamic range*, which is bounded by the ratio of the main to the sidelobes level and is related to the smallest features detection capability.
3. *Contrast*, which is the capability to differentiate among subtle changes in the acoustic impedance (i.e., different tissues in medical imaging).
4. *Signal-to-noise ratio*, where noise can be electrical (i.e., thermal, EMI, etc.) or *speckle*, also called *clutter* or *grain noise*, depending of the application field. Speckle results from interferences among unresolved *scatterers* in a *range cell*.
5. *Artifacts*, such as *reverberations*, *grating lobes* and others which blur the image and reduce the dynamic range.

Along the years, many research efforts have been devoted to find techniques that increase the image quality by addressing the above factors. Frequently, some characteristics are improved at the expenses of losses in some others. A typical example is *apodization*, used to reduce the sidelobe level, with an adverse effect in the lateral resolution [Szabo, 2004]. In medical imaging, where contrast is essential, this function is quite useful; however, in the NDT field, where resolution is more relevant, apodization provides marginal or no benefits at all.

As another example, lateral resolution is improved with larger apertures, which may be obtained with increased array inter-element pitch d. However, when $d>\lambda/2$ (*sparse apertures*) grating lobe artifacts appear. The condition $d>\lambda/2$ also arises with 2D arrays or in high frequency ultrasound imaging due to manufacturing constraints. Sparse apertures with randomly distributed elements reduce the grating lobes by spreading their energy among the sidelobes, whose level increases [Turnbull & Foster, 1991]; [Gavrilov et al., 1997].

In other cases, the concept of *effective aperture* allows to reduce the grating lobe levels by using different element distributions in emission and in reception, so that the compound radiation pattern equals that of a dense aperture [Lockwood et al., 1998]; [Nikolov & Jensen, 2000]; [Nikolov & Behar, 2005]. When a single focus is set in emission (as in phased array), some residual grating lobe artifacts remain in the image [Lockwood et al., 1996]. Furthermore, these approaches produce a lower signal-to-noise ratio.

As a final case example, speckle noise can be reduced by image compounding (*spatial diversity*), but this negatively affects resolution [Shankar & Newhouse, 1985]. *Frequency diversity* methods have been also proposed [Newhouse et al., 1982], but they critically depend on the selected parameters to work properly [Gustafson & Stepinski, 1993].
The conclusion is clear: there is no a *universal* method to improve the image quality by simultaneously addressing all the involved factors. This work is an exception to this rule, where *simultaneous improvements* in lateral resolution, side and grating lobe suppression, signal-to-noise ratio enhancement and artifacts cancellation, with the corresponding improvements on contrast and dynamic range, are obtained.
This is achieved by a new ultrasound imaging concept: *Adaptive Beamforming by Phase Coherence Processing*. The idea behind this approach is to consider the aperture data phases *explicitly* in the image formation process [Camacho et al., 2009].
Until now, this has not been applied in conventional ultrasonic imaging, whatever is the modality (phased array or synthetic aperture). Rather, the aperture data phases are only implicitly involved in the coherent sum, thus disregarding relevant information for the image formation. The aim of this work is to give the basis of the new technique and show its performances both, with simulated and experimental data.

2. The aperture data phases

The beamforming process is achieved by introducing delays that compensate the differences in the round-trip time-of-flight from the emitter to the focus and to every element. In the phased array modality, the emitter is considered at the array center, whereas in synthetic aperture imaging the actual emitter position is used to compute the delays. This way, dynamic focusing can be performed in reception only (phased array) or in emission and reception (synthetic aperture imaging).
From the simple geometry of Fig. 1, the round-trip time-of-flight from the array center O to the focus F and to element X is:

$$t_i^P = \frac{R_f + |\vec{r}_f|}{c} = \frac{1}{c}\left(R_f + \sqrt{R_f^2 + x_i^2 - 2R_f x_i \sin\theta}\right) \tag{1}$$

where c is the sound propagation velocity. The delay applied to signals received by element i for focusing at F is:

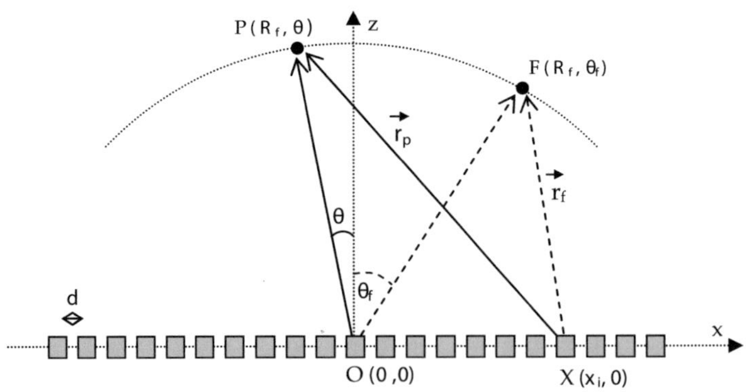

Fig. 1. Geometry for computing the focusing delays.

$$\tau_i = \frac{1}{c}\left(R_f - \sqrt{R_f^2 + x_i^2 - 2R_f x_i \sin\theta_f}\right) \quad 1 \le i \le N \tag{2}$$

Considering an emitted signal $e(t)=E\cdot\cos(\omega_s t)$, with $\omega_s=2\pi f_s$, the *aperture data* $s_i(t)$ that results after application of the focusing delay τ_i to the signal received by element i is:

$$s_i(t) = E\cos\left(\omega_s t - \omega_s\left(t_i^P + \tau_i\right)\right) \tag{3}$$

and the *unwrapped phase* of the aperture data i is:

$$\Phi_i(t) = \omega_s t + \frac{\omega_s}{c}\sqrt{R_f^2 + x_i^2 - 2R_f x_i \sin\theta_f} - \frac{\omega_s}{c}\sqrt{R_f^2 + x_i^2 - 2R_f x_i \sin\theta} \tag{4}$$

With the approximation $(1+a)^{1/2} \approx 1+a/2$, for a small and, with $R_f >> x_i$,

$$\Phi_i(t) \approx \omega_s t + \frac{\omega_s}{c} x_i\left(\sin\theta_f - \sin\theta\right) \tag{5}$$

The term $\omega_s t$ is equal for all the elements at a given time instant, so that the variability of the set $\{\Phi_i\}$ is only determined by the second term. On the other hand, for an N-element linear array with the coordinate origin at its center and inter-element spacing d,

$$x_i = [i-(N+1)/2]d \qquad 1 \le i \le N \tag{6}$$

Substituting in (5) and ignoring the time-dependent term:

$$\Phi_i \approx \frac{\omega_s d}{c}[i-(N+1)/2]\left(\sin\theta_f - \sin\theta\right) \tag{7}$$

Thus, for a point reflector at P (R_f, θ) with $\theta \neq \theta_f$, the unwrapped phases vary linearly along the aperture data. Only if P is located at the focus F ($\theta = \theta_f$), all the phases become equal. Therefore, by analyzing the dispersion of the aperture data phases, it can be realized when the received signals come from the focus or from some other region. To this purpose, any measurement of the statistical dispersion of the aperture data phases can be used (standard deviation, variance, etc.). For example, the standard deviation σ_Φ of the set of aperture data phases $\Phi = \{\Phi_i\}$ is computed from:

$$\sigma_\Phi = \sqrt{\frac{1}{N}\sum_{i=1}^{i=N}\left(\Phi_i - \frac{1}{N}\sum_{i=1}^{i=N}\Phi_i\right)^2} \tag{8}$$

After some mathematical manipulation, substitution of (7) in (8) yields,

$$\sigma_\Phi(\theta) = std(\Phi) = \frac{\pi}{\sqrt{3}}\frac{d}{\lambda}\sqrt{N^2-1}\left|\sin\theta_f - \sin\theta\right| \tag{9}$$

For $N>>1$ and with $D=N\cdot d$,

$$\sigma_\Phi(\theta) \approx \frac{\pi}{\sqrt{3}}\frac{D}{\lambda}\left|\sin\theta_f - \sin\theta\right| \tag{10}$$

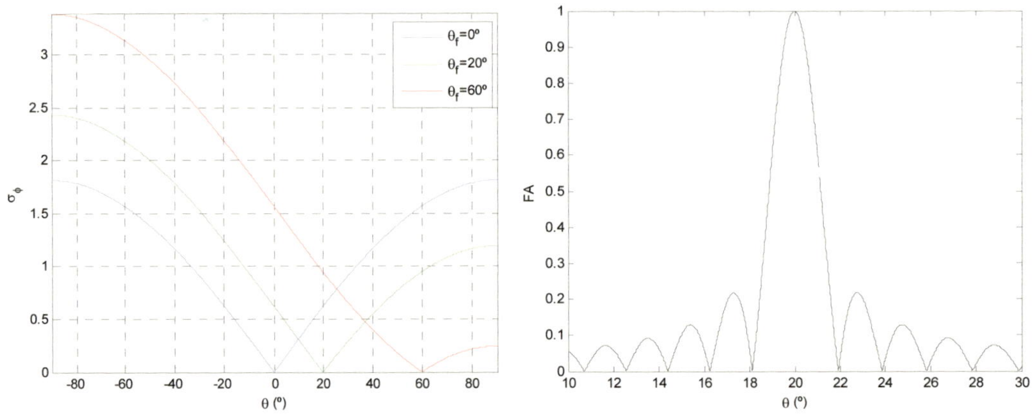

Fig. 2. Left: plot of σ_Φ in D/λ units for three steering angles. Right: $FA(\theta)$ around $\theta_f = 20°$.

Figure 2 (left) shows this function for three steering angles θ_f in D/λ units. It is seen that σ_Φ is zero only at the focusing direction, showing increasing values as θ separates from θ_f. This can be used to detect signals strictly coming from the focus ($\sigma_\Phi = 0$) or, with a more practical point of view, from *inside* the array main lobe.

The normalized radiation pattern of an array in continuous wave is[Steinberg, 1976]:

$$FA(\theta) = \left| \frac{\sin\left[\frac{\pi D}{\lambda}\left(\sin\theta_f - \sin\theta\right)\right]}{\sin\left[\frac{\pi d}{\lambda}\left(\sin\theta_f - \sin\theta\right)\right]} \right| \tag{11}$$

which is zero at

$$\sin\theta_{Zn} = \sin\theta_f \pm \frac{\lambda}{D} n \qquad n = 1, 2, ... \tag{12}$$

and unity at $\theta=\theta_f$. Figure 2 (right) shows an example for $D=32\lambda$, $d=\lambda/2$. The main lobe is bounded by the first zeroes of the radiation pattern (n=1) at:

$$\sin\theta_{z1} = \sin\theta_f \pm \lambda / D \tag{13}$$

Substitution of this value for $\sin\theta$ in (10) yields:

$$\sigma_\Phi(\theta_{z1}) = \frac{\pi}{\sqrt{3}} \tag{14}$$

Therefore, if the standard deviation of the aperture data unwrapped phases is $0 \le \sigma_\varphi \le \pi/\sqrt{3}$, it can be assumed that the received signals were originated inside the main lobe. This leads to a straightforward method for suppression of the side lobes, as it is explained next. The value $\sigma_0=\pi/\sqrt{3}$ equals the standard deviation of a uniform linear distribution in $(-\pi, \pi]$.

3. Phase coherence factors

The absolute phase coherence factor (*FCA*) is defined to take values in the [0, 1] interval as a function of the standard deviation of the aperture data unwrapped phases:

$$FCA = \max\left(0\,,1 - \frac{\sigma_\Phi}{\sigma_0}\right) \quad (15)$$

The term $f = 1\text{-}\sigma_\Phi/\sigma_0$ takes the unity at the main lobe axis, where σ_Φ=0, then monotonically decreases reaching zero at the main lobe limits θ_{z1}, where $\sigma_\Phi = \sigma_0$, and continues decreasing with negative values for angles θ outside the main lobe, where $\sigma_\Phi > \sigma_0$. As the function max(0, *f*) avoids negative values, the *FCA* is zero in the latter region (at the side lobes).
Figure 3a shows $FCA(\theta)$ over the normalized radiation pattern. It can be appreciated that the coherence factor has a narrower main lobe than the array factor and is free of side lobes. However, both reach unity at the focus steering angle θ_f.
In any conventional digital beamformer, the output is the coherent sum of the aperture data:

$$y(k) = \sum_{i=1}^{N} s_i(k) \quad (16)$$

where *k* is the sample index. Suppression of sidelobes can be achieved by weighting the beamformer output with the coherence factor obtained from the *k*-th aperture data set:

$$z(k) = y(k) \cdot FCA(k) \quad (17)$$

Besides suppressing sidelobes, this operation provides a narrower main lobe as shown in Figure 3b (compare, for example, the original and resulting main lobe width at -6 dB).

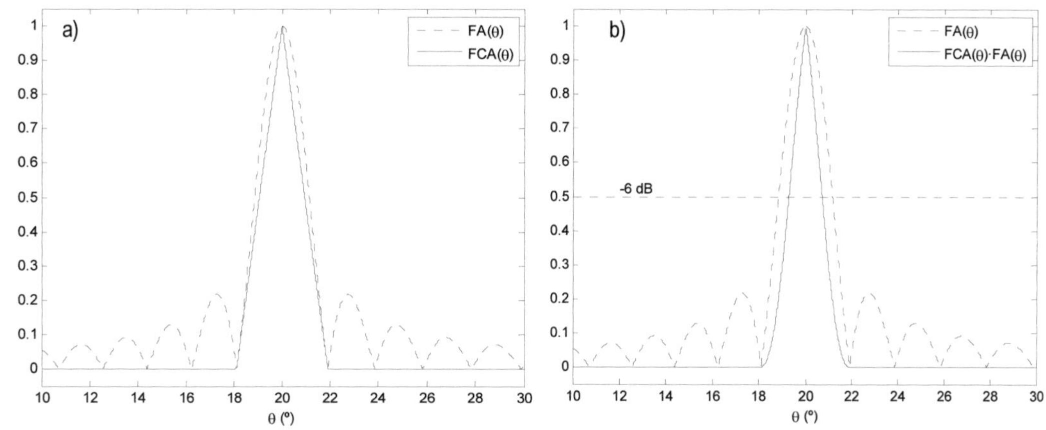

Fig. 3. a) $FCA(\theta)$ and FA(θ) for θ_f = 20°; b) Radiation pattern after the weighting operation

However, the unwrapped phase is not usually available. Instead, the *instantaneous phase* (wrapped phase) can be obtained from the signal analytical representation of the aperture data, $S_i(k) = Ae^{j\varphi_i(k)} = SI_i(k) + jSQ_i(k)$ as:

$$\varphi_i(k) = \tan^{-1}\left(\frac{SQ_i(k)}{SI_i(k)}\right) \quad (18)$$

being *SQ* and *SI* the quadrature and in-phase components, respectively. With $SI_i(k) = s_i(k)$, $SQ_i(k)$ can be obtained by means of a Hilbert transform, $SQ_i(k) = Hilbert[s_i(k)]$, [Oppenheim &

Schaffer, 1989], or by any other approximate process [Ranganathan et al., 2004]. If the former is used, the instantaneous phases can be obtained from the aperture data by:

$$\varphi_i(k) = \tan^{-1}\frac{Hilbert[s_i(k)]}{s_i(k)} \tag{19}$$

Then, the unwrapped phases Φ_i can be evaluated from φ_i. A common unwrapping algorithm scans the vector φ_i from i=2 to N, computing the increments $\Delta\varphi_i = \varphi_i - \varphi_{i-1}$; when $|\Delta\varphi_i| > \pi$, a value of sign($\Delta\varphi_i$)$\cdot 2\pi$ is subtracted to the successive phases, from i to N.
However, it is also possible to avoid the unwrapping process by using the value of the instantaneous phases to evaluate a different coherence factor. In this case, since the phases are circularly distributed in the $(-\pi, \pi]$ interval, a different function to obtain the standard deviation should be used [Fisher, 1993].
But, also, the circular distribution of the instantaneous phases can be considered that of vectors in the unit circle (module=1, angle=φ_i), represented as the complex $\cos\varphi_i + j\sin\varphi_i$. The standard deviation of a complex number σ_c is computed as the square root of the sum of the variances of the real and imaginary parts, that is:

$$\sigma_c = \sqrt{\text{var}(\cos\varphi_i) + \text{var}(\sin\varphi_i)} \tag{20}$$

In this case, $0 \le \sigma_c \le 1$, so that the complex phase coherence factor, *FCC* can be defined as:

$$FCC = 1 - \sigma_c \tag{21}$$

Furthermore, to avoid the complications involved in computing σ_c in the complex plane, it is possible to consider the phase having a linear distribution in the $(-\pi, \pi]$ interval. In such case,

$$\sigma_\phi = \sqrt{\frac{1}{N}\sum_{i=1}^{i=N}\left(\varphi_i - \frac{1}{N}\sum_{i=1}^{i=N}\varphi_i\right)^2} \tag{22}$$

However, it must be taken into account that, when the phases become grouped around $\varphi=\pm\pi$, a large σ_φ will be produced in spite of being very similar phases, a consequence of considering the phase a linear distribution. A general solution to this problem is given later.
When phases distribute uniformly in the $(-\pi, \pi]$ interval, the standard deviation is $\sigma_0=\pi/\sqrt{3}$. This happens when signals are just white noise and, approximately, at the sidelobes. This way, analogously to the *FCA*, the linear phase coherence factor *FCF* is defined as:

$$FCF = \max\left(0\,, 1 - \frac{\sigma_\varphi}{\sigma_0}\right) \tag{23}$$

4. Comparison of phase coherence factors

The phase coherence factors *FCA*, *FCC* and *FCF* share, in general, the same properties of sidelobe suppression and main lobe narrowing, but with some important differences. So, at the sidelobes, $\sigma_\varphi \approx \sigma_0 = \pi/\sqrt{3}$, which provides a $FCF(\theta)$ *near zero*, but with some small positive spikes at angles where $\sigma_\varphi < \sigma_0$. At angles where $\sigma_\varphi > \sigma_0$, it is $f = 1-\sigma_\Phi/\sigma_0 < 0$ and the function max(0, f) nulls the *FCF*. This behavior contrasts with that of $FCA(\theta)$, which is zero at the sidelobes, achieving their complete suppression (Fig. 4).

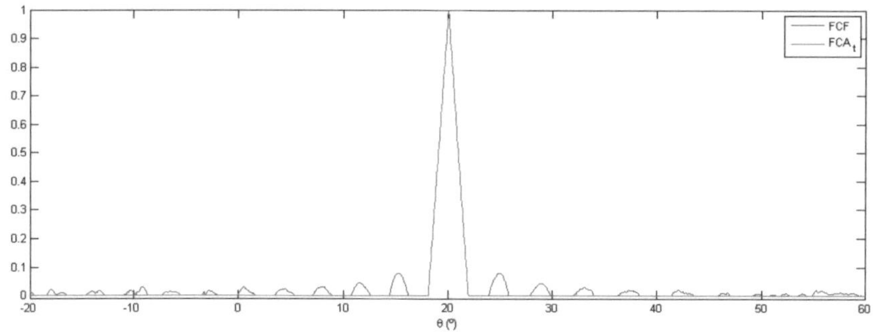

Fig. 4. Comparison among $FCF(\theta)$ and $FCA(\theta)$ for $\theta_f = 20^o$.

Another difference is a consequence of considering the instantaneous phases linearly distributed in $(-\pi, \pi]$. The effect is critical when the focus is located at an odd multiple of $\lambda/2$, where the standard deviation is zero just at θ_f since all phases are exactly π, but at angles $\theta \approx \theta_f$ (at both sides of the main lobe axis), phases group around $\varphi=\pm\pi$, producing a large σ_φ. Figure 5 compares $\sigma_\varphi(\theta)$ when the focus is located at an even or odd multiple of $\lambda/2$. This periodic effect appears in the image as a pattern, an artifact that must be avoided.

The complex coherence factor $FCC(\theta)$ does not present phase discontinuities and shows a smooth pattern. Figure 6 compares $FCC(\theta)$ with $FCF(\theta)$ for a focus at an even multiple of $\lambda/2$. The latter shows irregularities caused by the phase discontinuities that are not present in $FCC(\theta)$. Furthermore, the *FCC* provides higher side lobe suppression and a slightly narrower main lobe, whose width is independent of the focus axial position. The irregularities shown by $FCF(\theta)$ in the sidelobes region are of low level and, thus, have little impact on the image.

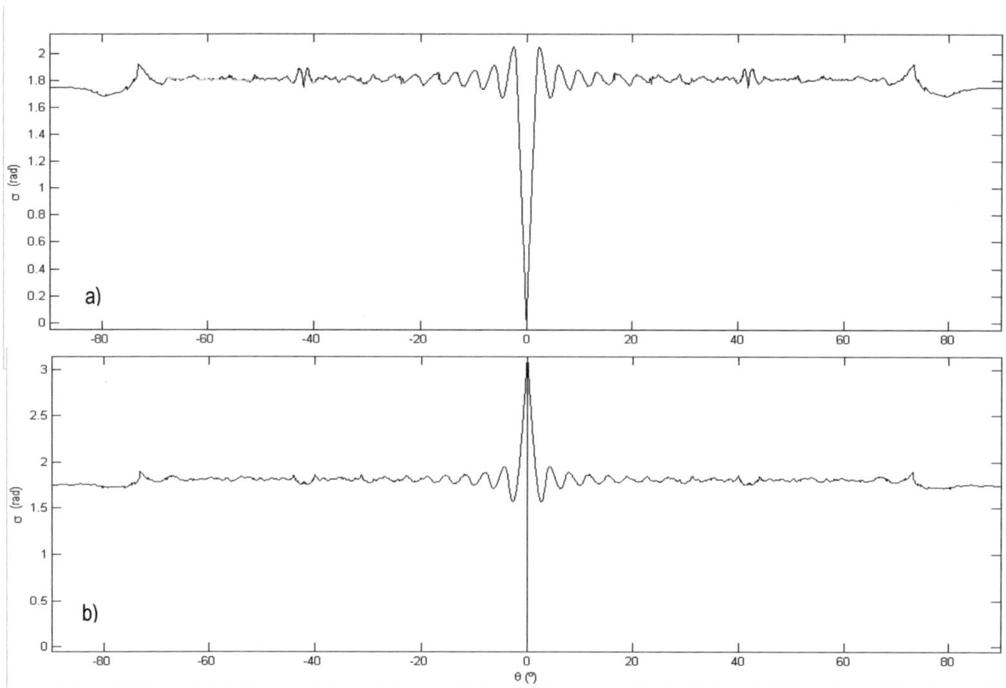

Fig. 5. Plot of $\sigma_\varphi(\theta)$: a) Focus at an even multiple of $\lambda/2$; b) Focus at an odd multiple of $\lambda/2$.

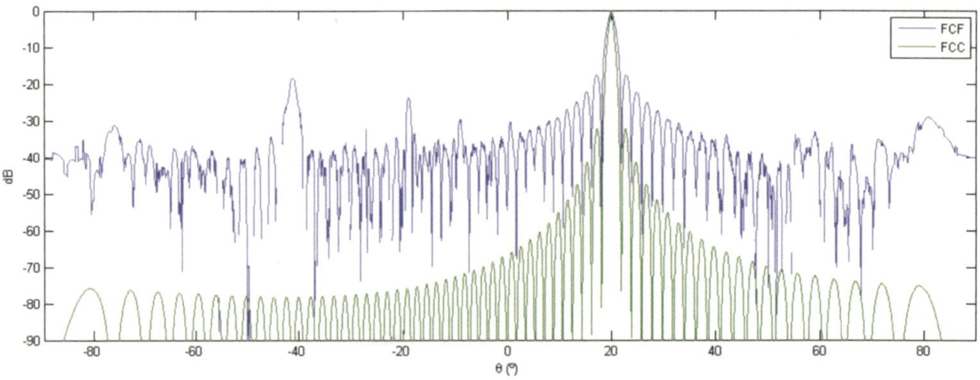

Fig. 6. Comparison between *FCC*(θ) and *FCF*(θ).

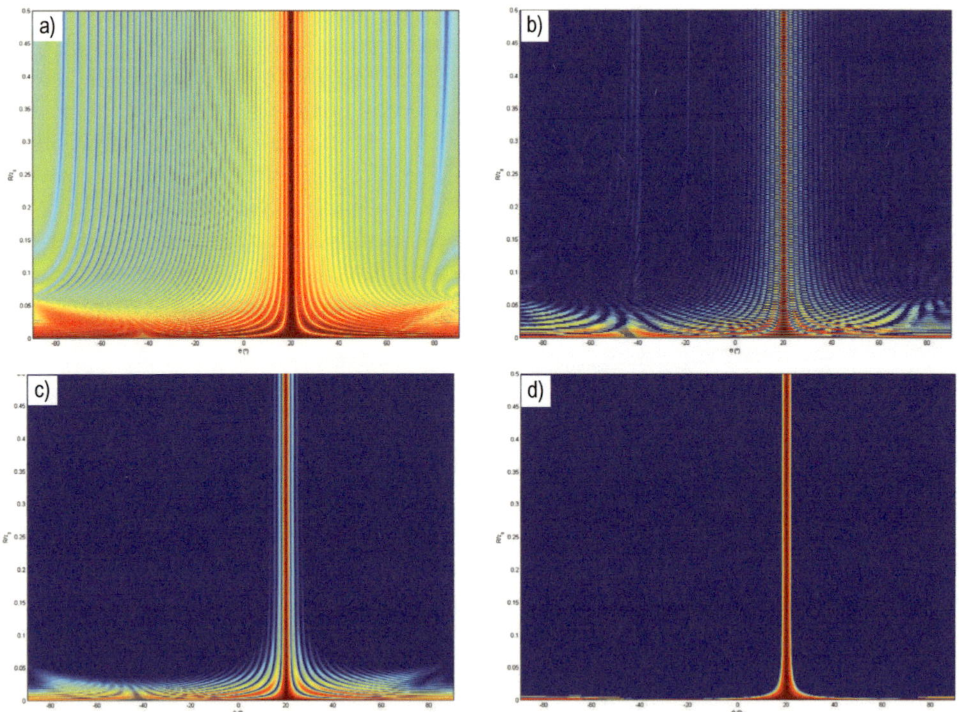

Fig. 7. Reception patterns: a) Conventional beamforming; b) Weighted by *FCF*; c) Weighted by *FCC*; d) Weighted by *FCA*. Dynamic range = 70 dB. Array: N=64, d= $\lambda/2$, θ_f = 20°.

Figure 7 shows the *reception pattern* with a 70 dB of dynamic range, considering continuous omnidirectional emission from the array center and dynamic focusing in reception, for an array with N=64 elements, d= $\lambda/2$ and processing with different coherence factors.
The side lobe indications shown by the original image in (a) become mostly suppressed with the phase coherence processing, whatever is the coherence factor used. However, weighting the beamformer output with the *FCF* (in b) produces the periodic pattern in the propagation direction discussed before. Also, some residual sidelobe indications remain.

In (c) the beamformer output is weighted with *FCC*, which shows a smooth beam without periodic artifacts and with higher sidelobe suppression. However, some sidelobe indications remain in the very near field (below 1/20 the far field limit) and near the main lobe (the first sidelobes), in agreement with the results shown in Fig. 6.
Finally, processing with the *FCA* (d) provides full sidelobe suppression, even in the very near field region, and a uniform main lobe pattern, which does not depend on depth.
These results have been obtained under the assumption of monochromatic wave and noise-free signals. The effect on wideband signals with noise is analyzed in the next Sections.

5. Phase quantization and the sign coherence factor FCS

In any digital implementation of the proposed method, the phase will be quantized. It is relevant to consider the errors involved as a function of the resolution used to represent the phases. Figure 8 shows the rms error in the computed *FCF* when the phase is quantized with a number *B* of bits, with regard to a 64-bits floating point representation.

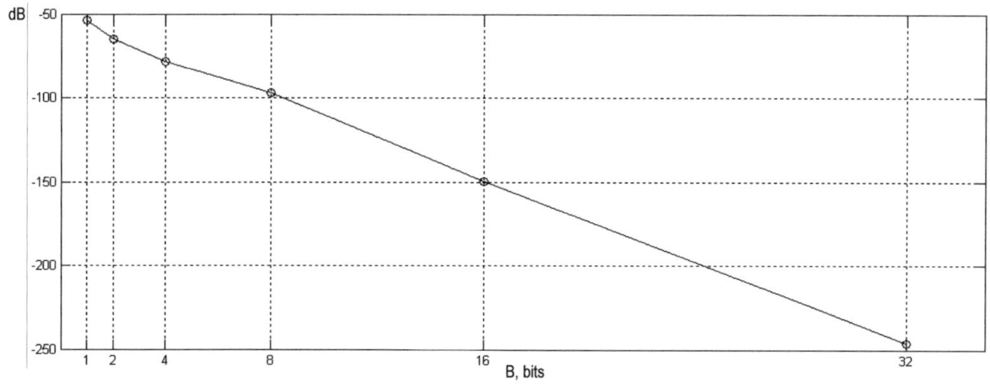

Fig. 8. *FCF* rms error as a function of the number of bits used to represent the phases.

It becomes apparent that the *FCF* is not very sensitive to the phase resolution. In fact, the rms error of computing the phases with only 4 bits instead of 64 bits is lower than 0.1%. In an extreme case, the phase can be coded with a single bit by breaking the (-π, π] interval in:

$$\Psi_i(k) = \begin{cases} \pi/2 & \text{for } \varphi_i(k) \in [0,\pi] \\ -\pi/2 & \text{for } \varphi_i(k) \in (-\pi,0) \end{cases} \tag{24}$$

For received signals of the form $s(t) = A(t)\sin(\varphi(t))$, with $A(t)>0$, these intervals correspond to the sign of $s(t)$, represented here by the discrete variable $b_i(k)$:

$$b_i(k) = \begin{cases} +1 & \text{for } s_i(k) \geq 0 \\ -1 & \text{for } s_i(k) < 0 \end{cases} \tag{25}$$

The variance of this variable is (omitting the sample index k):

$$\sigma_b^2 = \frac{N \sum_{i=1}^{N} b_i^2 - \left(\sum_{i=1}^{N} b_i \right)^2}{N^2} \tag{26}$$

and, since $\sum b_i^2 = N$,

$$\sigma_b^2 = 1 - \left(\frac{1}{N} \sum_{i=1}^{N} b_i \right)^2 \tag{27}$$

The Sign Coherence Factor, *FCS*, is defined as a function of the standard deviation of the aperture data signs:

$$FCS = 1 - \sigma_b = 1 - \sqrt{1 - \left(\frac{1}{N} \sum_{i=1}^{N} b_i \right)^2} \tag{28}$$

The sign coherence factor also takes values in the [0, 1] interval since $\sigma_b \leq 1$. One advantage of this function is its low computing cost, which allows a simple hardware implementation.
Figure 9 (left) shows $FCS(\theta)$ for an steering angle $\theta_f = 30°$. It reaches unity around the focus in the region where all the signals have the same polarity. Outside of this angular interval, $FCS(\theta)$ approaches zero.
The result of weighting the beamformer output with the sign coherence factor is shown in Figure 9 (right), together with the original radiation pattern. Both are equal around the steering angle, falling to low values (below -40 dB) at the sidelobe region. Note that the first sidelobe has been reduced by more than 26 dB and, simultaneously, the main lobe becomes narrower. The small irregularities in the resulting pattern are due to the discrete nature of the sign, but they have little impact on the image.

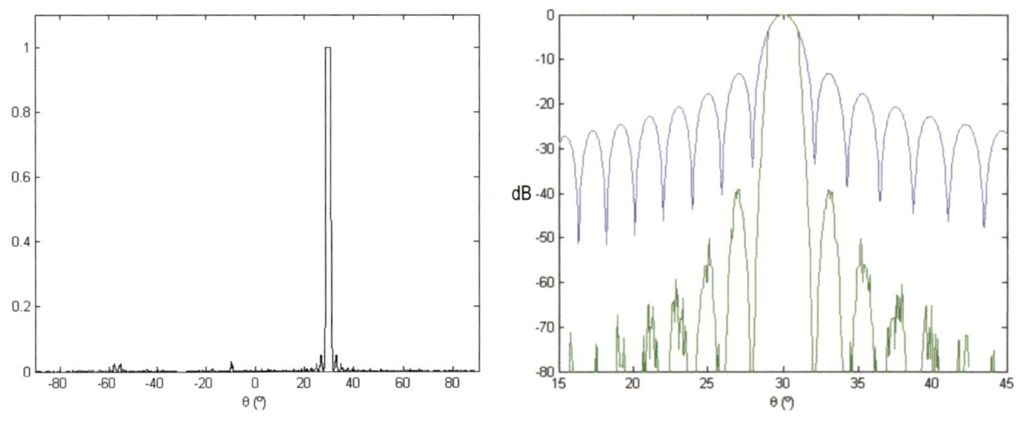

Fig. 9. Left: $FCS(\theta)$; Right: $FA(\theta)$ before (blue) and after (green) weighting by $FCS(\theta)$.

The $FCS(\theta)$ is a particular case of the $FCF(\theta)$, where the phases have been quantified with 1 bit. Therefore, it also shows the dependence with the focus position in the axial direction. In this case, the spatial period is $\lambda/2$, instead of λ.
Figure 10(a) shows the original reception pattern with a 70 dB of dynamic range, for an array with N=64, d= $\lambda/2$ and a steering angle at $\theta_f = 20°$ (the same case shown in Fig. 7a). The sidelobe indications become nearly suppressed when the beamformer output is weighted with the *FCS*, with residual values below -70 dB, as shown in (b). However, the image shows the periodic artifact caused by the dependence of $FCS(\theta)$ with the focus position, similar to that shown by $FCF(\theta)$ (see Fig. 7b), but of higher spatial frequency.

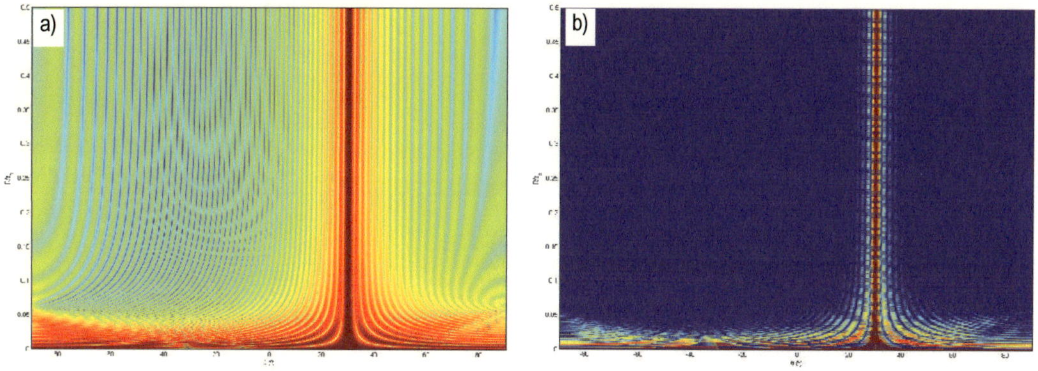

Fig. 10. Reception patterns: a) Conventional beamforming; b) Weighted by *FCS*. Image dynamic range = 70 dB. Array: N=64, $d=\lambda/2$, $\theta_f = 20°$.

6. Wideband and noisy signals

Until now, monochromatic and noise-free signals have been considered. This allowed obtaining closed expressions that may be useful to understand the main properties of adaptive beamforming by phase coherence processing. However, real images are obtained from wideband signals, which also include some amount of noise. For the sake of simplicity, Gaussian pulses are considered, of the form:

$$s(t) = e^{-t^2 / 2g^2} \cos(\omega_S t + \varphi) \tag{29}$$

where the parameter g determines the bandwidth at -6 dB as a function of the relative bandwidth BW and the fundamental frequency as:

$$g = \frac{\sqrt{8\ln(2)}}{\omega_S \cdot BW} \approx \frac{2.355}{\omega_S \cdot BW} \tag{30}$$

Furthermore, signals are contaminated with noise, considered white with a Gaussian distribution. From the point of view of phase coherence processing, the duration of the ultrasonic pulse T_P relative to the signal period T_S is determined by its bandwidth and the signal-to-noise ratio. It has been shown [Camacho, 2010] that this relationship is:

$$\frac{T_P}{T_S} \approx \frac{1}{BW}\sqrt{\ln\left(\frac{SNR}{2.1}\right)} \tag{31}$$

Figure 11 shows an example for an array with N=64 elements, $d=\lambda/2$, f_S = 5 MHz, BW=0.6 and SNR = 30 dB. The signal received by an element is shown in (a), with its instantaneous phase in (b). The *FCC* obtained from the set of 64 signals is shown in (c). The red lines delimit the pulse duration as indicated by (31). It is seen that *FCC* is higher than 0.5 within this interval, reaches unity at the center of the pulse and is nearly zero in other positions.

It must be highlighted that, for phase coherence processing, noise plays an important role: it provides information when some of the aperture data contain only noise whereas other show echo signals. This happens, for example, in the grating lobes for wideband signals.

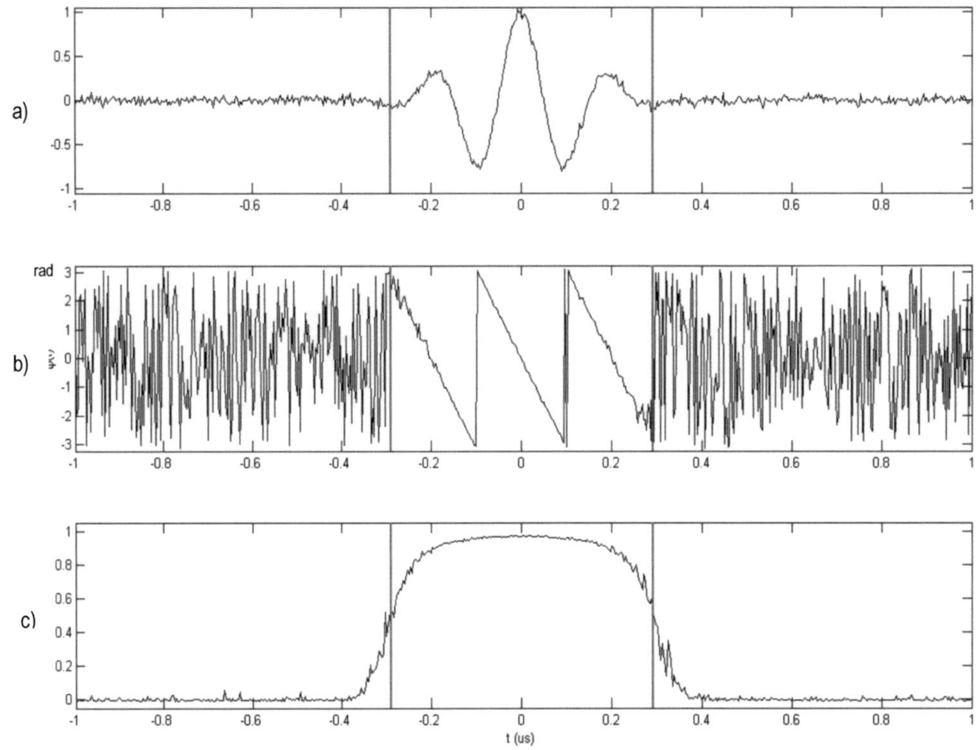

Fig. 11. a) Signal received by an element; b) Instantaneous phase; c) *FCC* of 64 signals.

Thus, since the phase dispersion of only-noise channels is high (even for low amplitude noise), the coherence factor will be small and the indication will be suppressed. This subject is further discussed in Section 8.

Figure 12 shows the 70 dB dynamic range images of a point reflector located at the far field limit ($R = D^2/4\lambda$) and $\theta=0^o$, produced by conventional beamforming (a) and after processing with *FCF* (b), *FCS* (c) and *FCC* (d). They are synthesized for an array with N=64 elements, $d=\lambda/2$, f_S = 5 MHz, BW=0.5 and with a signal-to-noise ratio SNR = 60 dB in every channel.

The sidelobe indications in the original image are suppressed by more than 50 dB with phase or sign coherence processing. Besides, the -6 dB lateral resolution has improved by nearly 50%. Processing with the complex coherence factor *FCC* (d) produces a smooth image of the point reflector. However, the images obtained after processing with the *FCF* (b) and *FCS* (c) show a periodic pattern in the main lobe as well as in the residual side lobes.

Noise is not visible in these images, since it falls below the image dynamic range after beamforming of the 64 channels.

7. Filtering out the periodic artifacts

The lateral patterns of phase $FCF(\theta)$ and sign $FCS(\theta)$ coherence factors depend on the focus position as it has been shown. To analyze more in detail this effect, Figure 13 shows the beamformed A-scan signal (blue) together with the *FCF* (green) and *FCS* (red) for the example above at θ= 0.9^o, which corresponds to half the angle of the first main lobe zero (θ_{z1}).

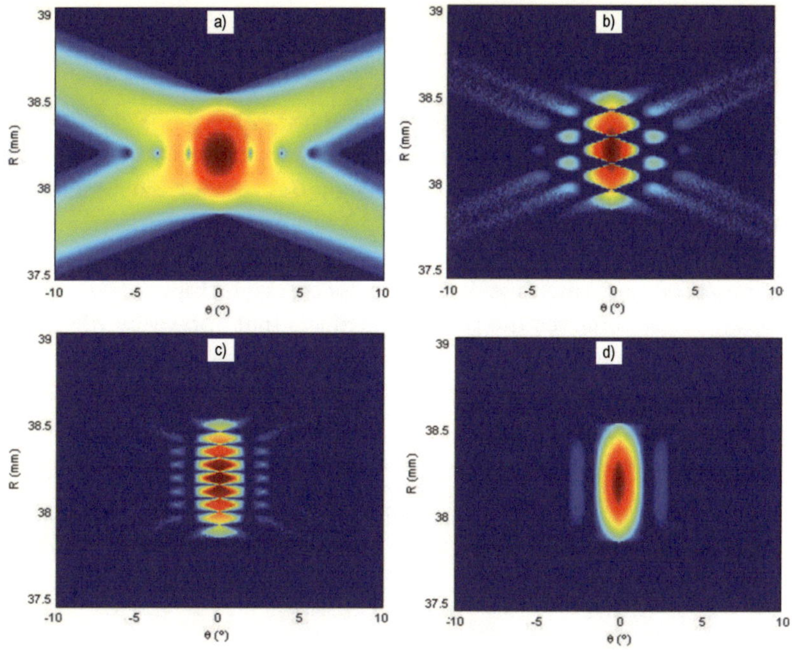

Fig. 12. Images of a point reflector obtained with conventional beamforming (a) and after processing with *FCF* (b), *FCS* (c) and *FCC* (d). Dynamic range 70 dB; N=64 elements, $d=\lambda/2$, f_S = 5 MHz, *BW*=0.5 and *SNR* = 60 dB per channel.

The amplitude of both factors changes with depth, which influences the image as shown in Fig. 12 b) and c). It can be observed that the *FCF* period of oscillation equals to that of the signal, whereas *FCS* oscillates at twice the signal frequency. This suggests that these oscillations could be reduced by a simple low-pass filter. However, low-pass filtering would provide the *average* of the coherence factors, while the *maximum* is required to keep the amplitude of the indications within the main lobe independent of depth.

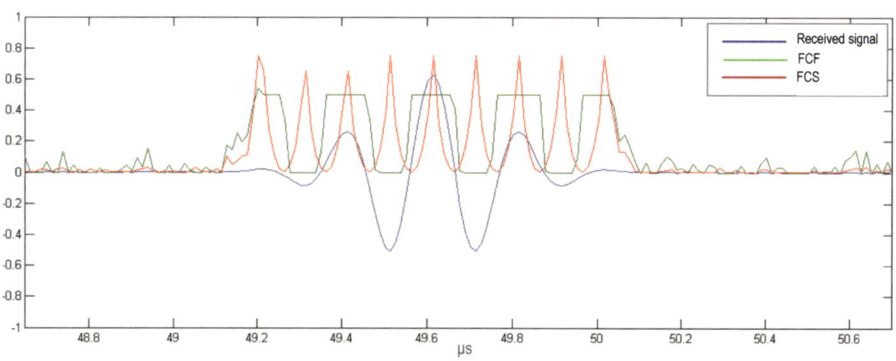

Fig. 13. Received signal (blue) and coherence factors *FCF* (green) and *FCS* (red).

A filter of ordered statistics that extracts the moving maximum [Pitas & Venetsanopoulos, 1990] seems an adequate choice. The filter output is the maximum of M consecutive samples of the coherence factor, where M is adapted to the signal frequency by means:

$$y[n] = F_v(x[n]) = \max(x[n-M+1], \ldots, x[n]), \quad M = round\left(h\frac{f_m}{f_s}\right) \tag{33}$$

being f_m the sampling frequency, h=1 for the *FCF* and h=1/2 for the *FCS*.

This non-linear filter has abrupt transitions that may be softened by means of a low-pass filter with a cutoff frequency equal to that of the signal. A moving average filter can be used with this purpose, building a combined moving maximum-average filter.

Figure 14 compares the images obtained for the same example than above without and with a moving maximum-average filter applied to the coherence factors output. The combination of both filters completely removes the periodic artifacts that appear by direct application of *FCF* and *FCS*, the lateral resolution and the sidelobe suppression remains similar to that achieved without these filters. This way, *FCF* and *FCS* behave similarly to *FCA* and *FCC*.

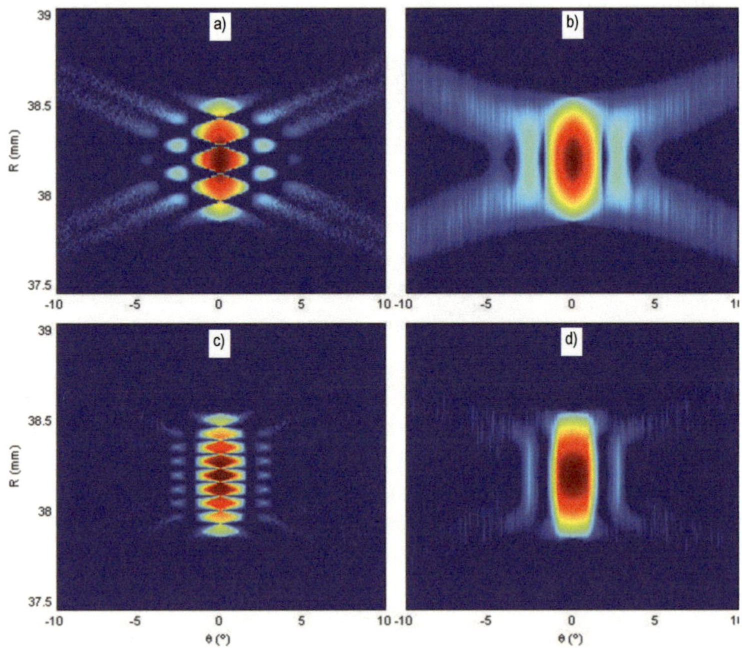

Fig. 14. 70 dB images of a point reflector: a) *FCF* processing; b) *FCF* processing with filters; c) *FCS* processing; d) *FCS* processing with filters. Filters (moving maximum + average).

8. Grating lobes suppression

When the inter-element distance is $d>\lambda/2$, grating lobe artifacts appear as a consequence of the spatially undersampled aperture (an aliasing effect). In the far field with monochromatic wave, a grating lobe is indistinguishable from the main lobe, since all the array elements contribute to its formation with the same phase at a given angular direction. With wideband signals and in the aperture near field, only a subset of the array elements produces the grating lobe at a given location. This way, with wideband signals, grating lobes spread over a large region and their amplitude is significantly lower.

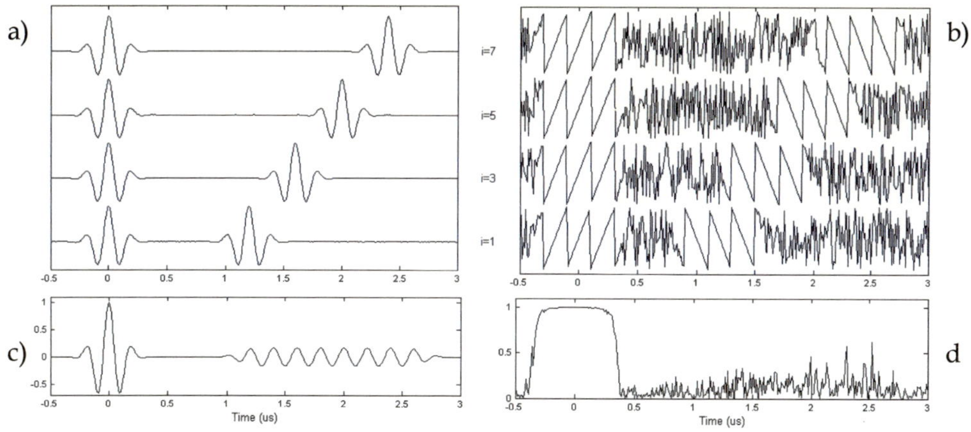

Fig. 15. Principles of grating lobes suppression: a) Aperture data amplitudes and b) phases; c) beamformer output; d) Phase coherence factor *FCF*

In fact, at a grating lobe, most of the aperture data are noise and only a few elements contribute constructively to the coherent sum. This opens an opportunity to cancel the grating lobe artifacts by phase coherence processing. To demonstrate its operation, Figure 15a) shows the aperture data corresponding to 4 channels of an 8-element array. At the left part of the A-scans, a true scatterer is located at the focus, whereas the rightmost indications correspond to a grating lobe. It is seen that all the aperture data contribute constructively to form the output A-scan in the true scatterer, but only a fraction of the aperture data adds constructively at the grating lobe (Fig. 15c).

In conventional beamforming, grating lobes show as relatively low level indications that spread out spatially (over directions and time). However, consider the aperture data phases for the same example (Fig. 15b). They are perfectly aligned at the true scatterer position, showing a large disparity at the grating lobe indications, mainly caused by noise. The coherence factor will be large (near unity) at the true scatterer and low (near zero) at the grating lobe, as it is shown for the *FCF* in the lower trace (Fig. 15d).

The grating lobe suppression level is a function of the signal bandwidth and number of aperture data used to compute the coherence factor. Figure 16 shows these results for an array with inter-element pitch of 1.5λ. It is seen that, for *N*=128 and *FCC* or *FCS* processing, the grating lobes become suppressed by about 40 dB if the signal BW > 60%.

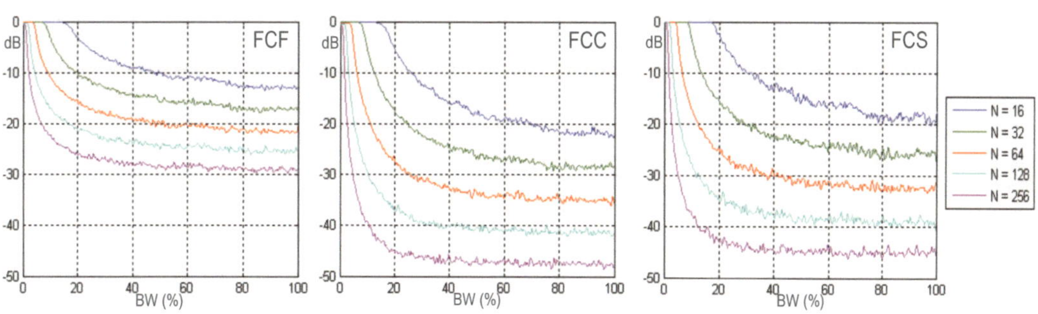

Fig. 16. Grating lobes attenuation level as a function of the signal bandwidth and number *N* of aperture data channels used to compute the different coherence factors.

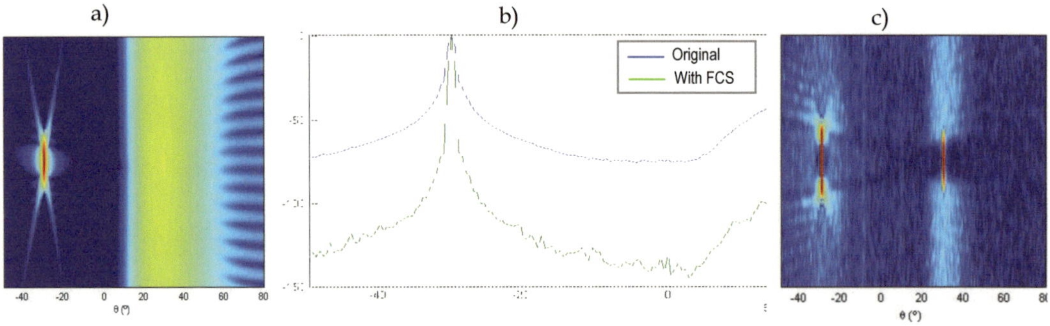

Fig. 17. a) Conventional STA image of two reflectors of 0 dB and -43 dB amplitude, obtained with a 64-element array, $d=\lambda$; b) LSF of the original and processed images; c) *FCS* image.

Figure 17a) shows the 70 dB dynamic range conventional image of two point reflectors of different amplitudes: 0 dB and -43 dB, located at angles of -30° and +30°, respectively. The images were obtained by simulation of a 5 MHz, 64-element array, $d=\lambda$, BW=50% and rms noise level of -60 dB. The modality is Synthetic Transmit Aperture (STA) [Gammelmark & Jensen, 2003], with a complete data set was used for beamforming.

It is seen that the grating lobe created by the high intensity point reflector completely hides the presence of the low-level one. This is made more evident by plotting the LSF (maximum amplitude at all depths), shown in Fig. 17b). In the original image, the grating lobe reaches a level similar to the amplitude of the smaller reflector, so that, its indication becomes literally buried in this artifact. But, after processing with the *FCS*, both point reflectors appear about 40 dB above the residual sidelobe level at, approximately, -80 dB.

Figure 17c) shows the image of the sign coherence factor, *FCS*, also with a 70 dB dynamic range. It is seen that it reaches unity (0 dB) at *both* reflector positions. Although this image gives no amplitude information, it determines the presence of true reflectors, even in the case of their signal amplitudes being below the grating lobe level.

By the way, the resulting lateral resolution produced by phase coherence processing of this 64-element sparse aperture is higher than that obtained with a 128-element dense aperture.

9. Limits on the grating and sidelobes suppression level

Out of the main lobe, the aperture data phases behave as a random variable, uniformly distributed in $(-\pi, \pi]$. The coherence factors have been defined to be zero when the phases distribute uniformly, so that they approach zero in the sidelobe region. However every coherence factor tends to this limit differently as a function of the number n of the phase values involved in its evaluation (in *phased array* $n=N$, the number of aperture data samples). This dissimilar behavior explains the differences in the sidelobe and grating lobe suppression levels achieved by every coherence factor.

For the phase coherence factor *FCF*, defined in (23) as:

$$FCF = \max\left(0\,,1-\frac{\sigma_\varphi}{\sigma_0}\right) \quad \sigma_\phi(n)=\sqrt{\frac{\sum_{i=1}^{n}(\varphi_i-\bar{\varphi})^2}{n}} = f(n^{-1/2}) \tag{34}$$

$$\lim_{n\to\infty}\sigma_\varphi(n)=\sigma_0 \tag{35}$$

$$FCF\big|_{sidelobes} \to 0 \quad as \quad f(n^{-1/2}) \tag{36}$$

For the complex coherence factor *FCC*, defined in (20) and (21) as,

$$FCC = 1 - \sqrt{\text{var}(\cos\varphi) + \text{var}(\sin\varphi)} \tag{37}$$

$$\text{var}(\cos\varphi) = \frac{1}{n}\sum_{i=1}^{n}\cos^2\varphi_i - \frac{1}{n^2}\left(\sum_{i=1}^{n}\cos\varphi_i\right)^2 \tag{38}$$

$$\text{var}(\sin\varphi) = \frac{1}{n}\sum_{i=1}^{n}\sin^2\varphi_i - \frac{1}{n^2}\left(\sum_{i=1}^{n}\sin\varphi_i\right)^2 \tag{39}$$

$$\text{var}(\cos\varphi) + \text{var}(\sin\varphi) = \frac{1}{n}\sum_{i=1}^{n}(\sin^2\varphi_i + \cos^2\varphi_i) - \frac{1}{n^2}\sum_{i=1}^{n}(\sin\varphi_i + \cos\varphi_i) \tag{40}$$

With $\sin^2 x+\cos^2 x=1$ and $|\sin x+\cos x| \le \sqrt{2}$ the second term is bounded by κ/n, κ=constant and,

$$\text{var}(\cos\varphi) + \text{var}(\sin\varphi) = 1 - \frac{\kappa}{n} \tag{41}$$

$$FCC = 1 - \sqrt{1 - \frac{\kappa}{n}} \approx \frac{\kappa}{2n} = f(n^{-1}) \tag{42}$$

The sign coherence factor, *FCS*, was defined in (28) as:

$$FCS = 1 - \sqrt{1 - \left(\frac{1}{n}\sum_{i=1}^{n} b_i\right)^2}$$

Among the aperture data polarity bits b_i, there will be p positive values and n-p negative values. Then,

$$B = \frac{1}{n}\sum_{i=1}^{n} b_i = \frac{p-(n-p)}{n} = \frac{2p}{n} - 1 \tag{43}$$

$$FCS = 1 - \sqrt{1 - B^2} = 1 - \frac{2p}{n}\sqrt{\frac{n}{p} - 1} \tag{44}$$

For uniform phase distributions, $p \to n/2$ and the square root term tends to unity. Therefore,

$$FCS \to 1 - \frac{2p}{n} = f(n^{-1}) \tag{45}$$

In summary, *FCC* and *FCS* approach zero following a function $f(n^{-1})$, which is stronger than the trend towards zero shown by *FCF* as $f(n^{-1/2})$.

10. Experimental verification

The validity of the adaptive beamforming technique to improve lateral resolution, dynamic range, signal-to-noise ratio and artifact suppression is experimentally demonstrated.

In a first arrangement, an aluminum block with 10 pairs of 1.5 mm Ø side drilled holes (SDH) was used (Fig. 18). This part is mainly intended to test the resolution improvement together with sidelobe and reverberation artifacts reduction.

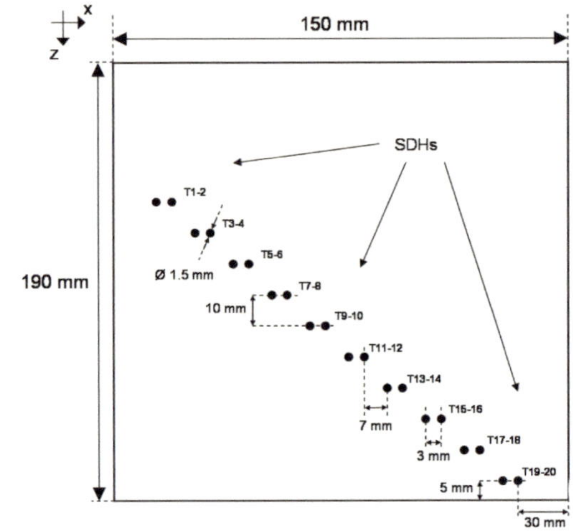

Fig. 18. Aluminum block with several pairs of side drilled holes.

A 5 MHz, 128-element array with d=0.6 mm (≈$\lambda/2$) (Imasonic, Besançon, France) was used in contact with the part upper surface. A SITAU 128:128 full parallel phased array system (Dasel, Madrid, Spain), was used to generate and acquire ultrasound data. The STA modality was applied for imaging, with dynamic focusing in emission and in reception.

Figure 19 shows the 80 dB dynamic range image obtained by conventional beamforming. Besides the indications of the SDHs, the image shows the sidelobes and reverberations produced among them and the part walls. Also, a small amount of noise is seen above the SDH indications (electrical noise). The bottom echo of the part is also clearly visible.

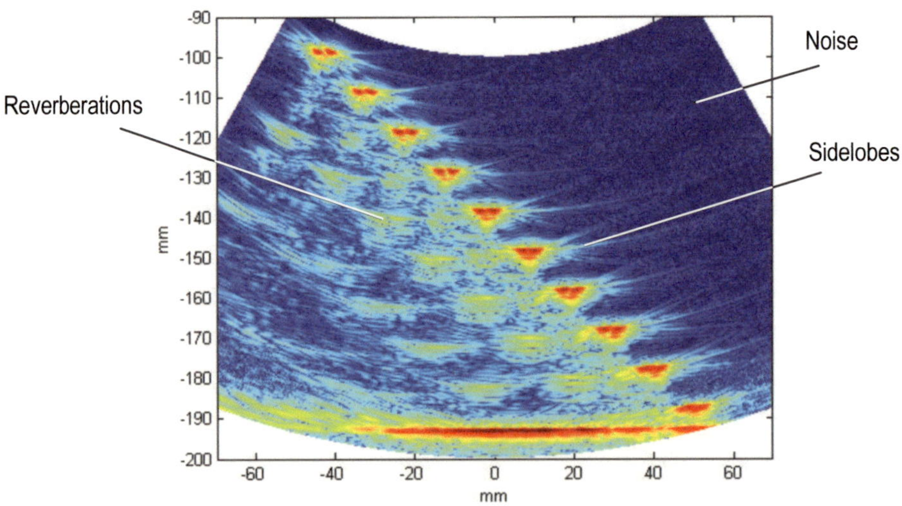

Fig. 19. STA image of the aluminum block with SDH obtained with 80 dB dynamic range

Coherence factors were computed from the aperture data following the procedures described in this paper, being applied to the whole set of N^2 signals provided by the STA imaging modality.

Figure 20 shows the 80 dB dynamic range images that result after weighting the beamformer output with a) *FCF*, b) *FCC*, c) *FCA* and d) *FCS*. The following observations can be made:

1. All the coherence factors provide a large suppression of the noise and reverberation artifacts, being moderate with *FCF* and complete with *FCA*.
2. Sidelobe indications get also fully suppressed with *FCA*, leaving some residual traces with *FCC* and *FCS* and slightly higher with *FCF*.
3. In the negative side, the *FCA* completely removes the bottom echo and its nearest SDH indications. This is due to the mutual interferences between the corresponding echoes that lower the strict coherence factor *FCA*, applied to 128^2 aperture data phases. This effect also causes some amplitude loss in the bottom echo with *FCC, FCS* and *FCF*.

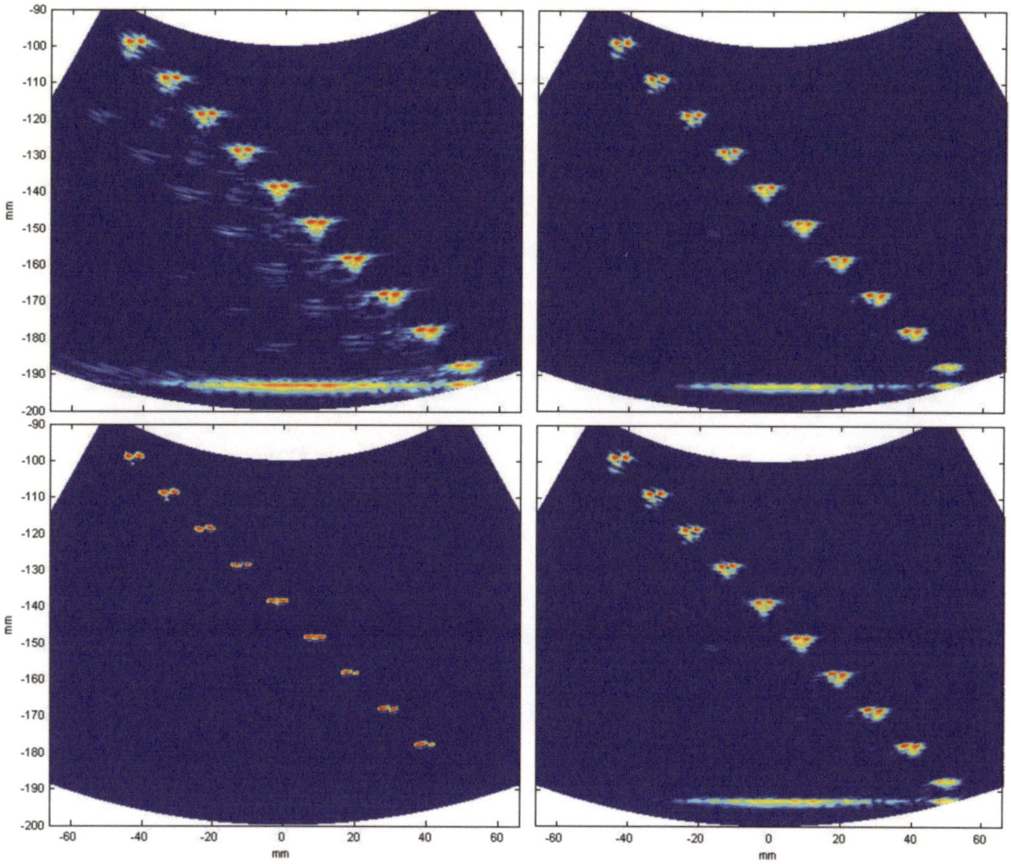

Fig. 20. Images obtained after processing with the coherence factors: a) *FCF*, b) *FCC*, c) *FCA* and d) *FCS*. Dynamic range: 80 dB.

The last observation advises of not using global processing with the STA imaging modality, due to the risk of losing some indications (especially with *FCA*). It seems better to apply the phase coherence processing to every one of the *N* partial images and keep the maximum coherence found to perform the weighting operation, at the expenses of a lower sidelobe and artifact reduction.

With regard to the lateral resolution improvement achieved by the adaptive beamforming technique, Figure 21 shows the images (in a linear color scale) before and after the weighting operation with different coherence factors for the three central pairs of SDH, where the angular interval between two holes is about 1.1°. Since the theoretical main lobe width is, for this aperture, about 1.8°, the original image cannot fully resolve their indications.

However, after the weighting operation with the different coherence factors, the SDH indications become separated, due to the narrowing effect on the main lobe width (discussed in Section 3).

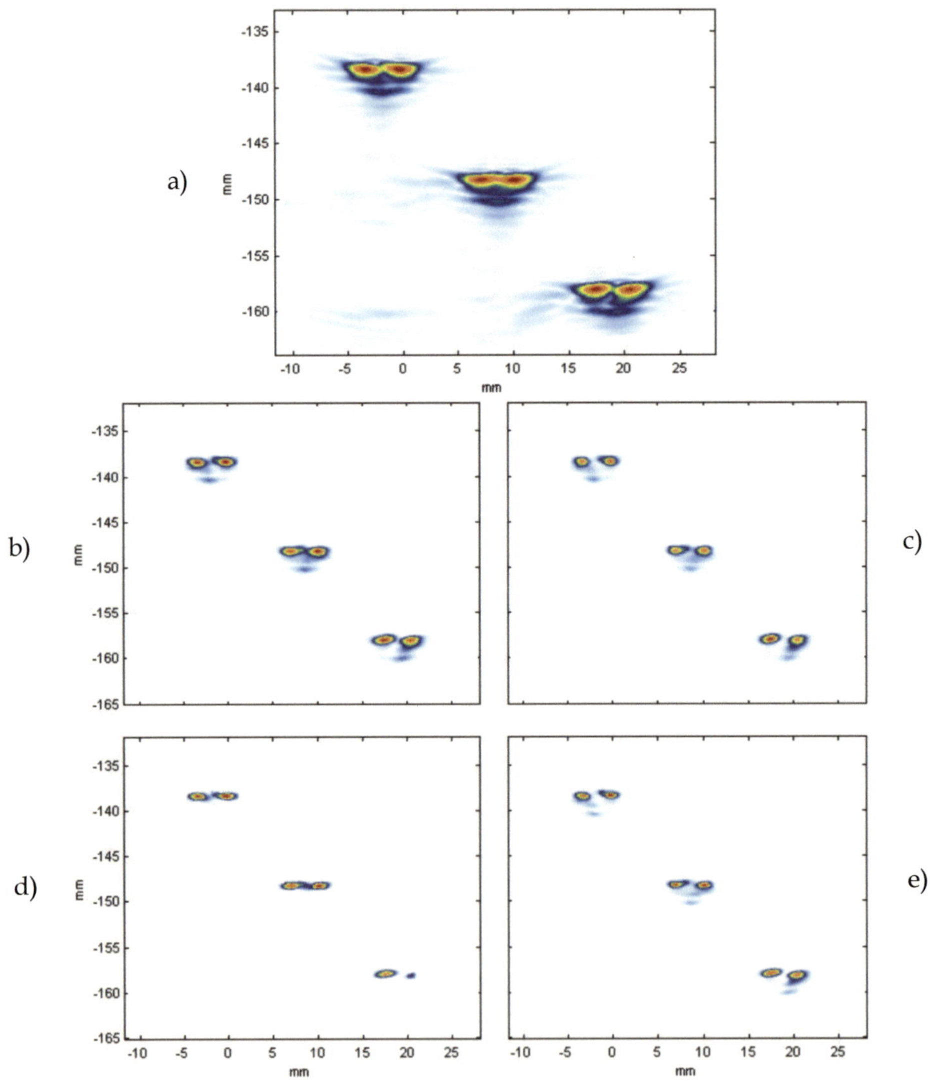

Fig. 21. Images of the three central pairs of SDH in linear scale: a) Original and processed with: b) *FCF*; c) *FCC*; d) *FCA*; e) *FCS*.

Table 1 shows the number of SDH pairs which become resolved at a given threshold.

	Number of SDH pairs resolved			
	-3 dB	***-6 dB***	***-12 dB***	***-20 dB***
Original	9	7	1	0
FCF	10	10	8	2
FCC	10	10	9	5
FCA	9	9	8	7
FCS	10	10	9	4

Table 1. Number of SDH resolved at a given threshold.

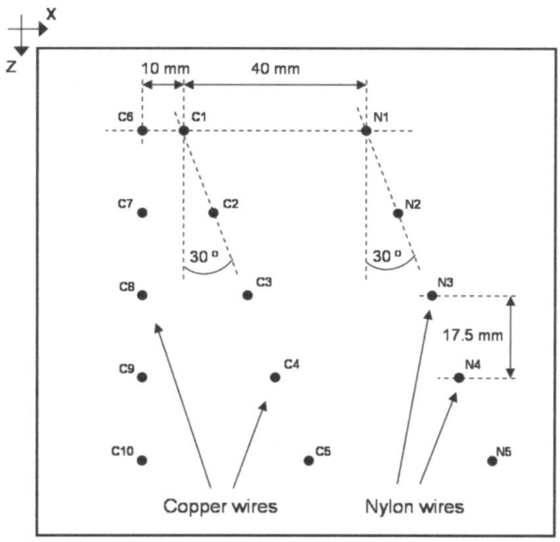

Fig. 22. Wire phantom.

Processing with any coherence factor (except *FCA*), resolves all the SDH pairs at -6 dB, whereas in the original image 3 pairs remain unresolved. At -20 dB, processing with the *FCA* resolves 7 pairs of SDH, while all pairs get unresolved in the original image.

The aim of a second experiment is to demonstrate the capabilities of the new technique to suppress grating lobes. To this purpose, a phantom with several nylon and copper wires was built (Fig. 22). The test is performed in water immersion with a 5 MHz, 96-element array with an inter-element pitch d = 0.5 mm ≈ 1.7λ. The SITAU 128:128 full parallel phased array system was used to generate and acquire the ultrasound data.

Figure 23a shows the image generated with the STA technique with a 90 dB dynamic range. The grating lobe artifacts created by the copper wires show at the right as large diffuse regions that hide the presence of some nylon wires. Conversely, the grating lobes created by the nylon wires appear at the left of the image. In this case their level is not enough to hide the presence of the copper wires. Sidelobe indications are also present, as well as some electrical noise.

The coherence factors were computed from the aperture data, using the whole set of N^2 signals and following the procedures presented in this paper. As an example, figure 23b) shows the 90 dB image of the *FCS*, before performing the weighting operation. It can be appreciated the high intensity (nearly 0 dB) at the wire positions and the high level of suppression of the grating lobes, even in a larger degree than the side lobes.

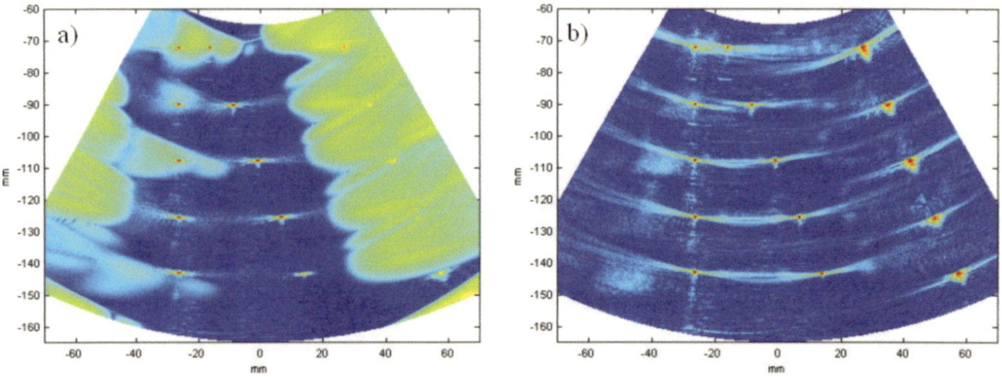

Fig. 23. a) STA image of the wire phantom; b) FCS image. Dynamic range = 90 dB

Figure 24 summarizes the images obtained after application of the different coherence factors. As expected, the grating and side lobe suppression level is higher with *FCA*, which also loses several target indications. As before, *FCA* processing is not advisable with STA. In the reverse side, the *FCF* provides lower grating and sidelobe suppression levels, in agreement with the behavior discussed in Section 9. Both, *FCC* and *FCS*, suppress grating

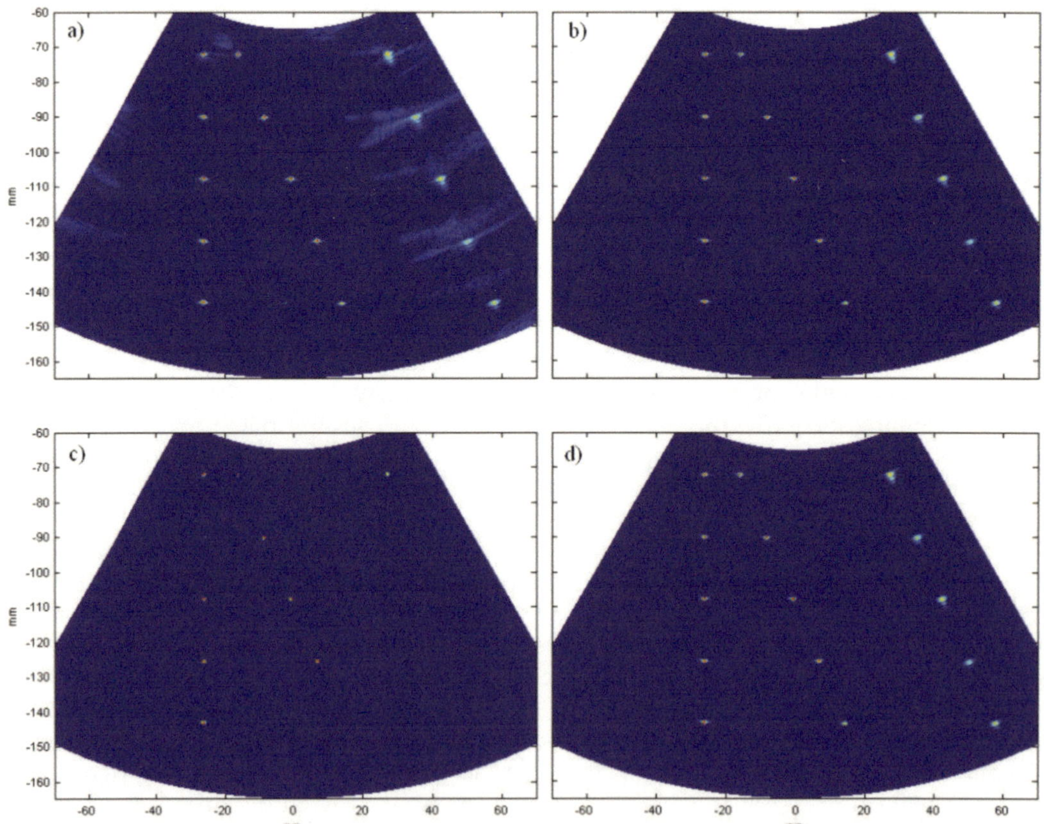

Fig. 24. Images after processing with the coherence factors: a) *FCF*, b) *FCC*, c) *FCA*; d) *FCS*.

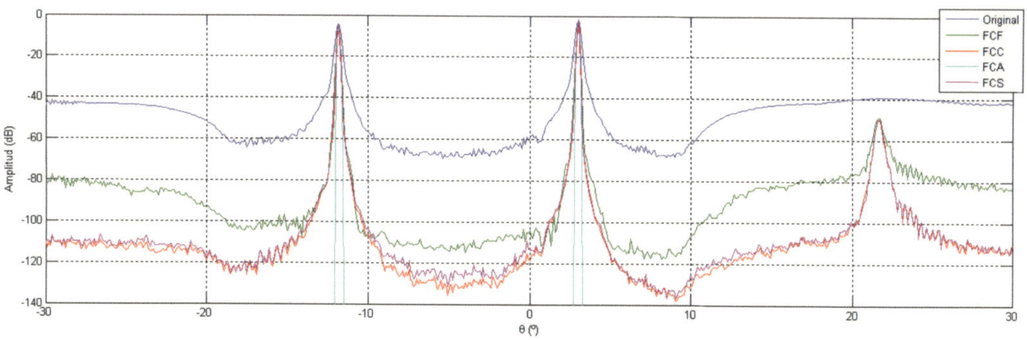

Fig. 25. LSF of the images before and after processing with different coherence factors.

and side lobe indications to well below -90 dB. It is worth to note these similarities in spite of the very different real-time implementation complexity involved.

Dramatic contrast improvements are obtained, as shown explicitly by the LSF applied to the fourth wire row (Fig. 25). The similarities in the results provided by *FCC* and *FCS* processing are made more evident, achieving a signal-to-grating lobe ratio enhancement approaching 60 dB. On average the signal-to-grating lobe ratio is raised to 63, 84 and 83 dB with *FCF*, *FCC* and *FCS* processing, respectively, from an original value of 28.5 dB.

11. Conclusion

This work describes a new ultrasonic imaging modality by means of adaptive beamforming with phase coherence processing. From the aperture data phases dispersion, it extracts a coherence factor with values in the [0, 1] interval that provides a quantitative measurement of the focusing quality: It yields a high value (≈ 1) if the received signals come from the focus and a low value (≈ 0) if they proceed from other regions. The coherence factors modify the behavior of the beamformer by weighting its output. This way, the indications produced by side and grating lobes, as well as other artifacts such as reverberations and noise, become suppressed. Besides, lateral resolution improvements are also obtained.

Four coherence factors have been defined, namely: the absolute phase coherence factor *FCA*, which operates on unwrapped phases, the complex phase coherence factor *FCC*, which considers the phases having a circular distribution, the phase coherence factor *FCF*, which regard the phases having a linear distribution in $(-\pi, \pi]$, and the sign coherence factor *FCS*, which quantify the aperture data phases with a single bit. Their main properties, including the grating and side lobe suppression degree provided by the different coherence factors have been analyzed for monochromatic, noise-free waves, as well as for wideband, noisy signals. Experimental results agree with theory.

12. Acknowledgements

Work supported by projects Artemis (2010-0607) funded by the Community of Madrid and DPI2010-17648 funded by the Spanish Ministry for Science and Innovation.

13. References

Camacho, 2009: J. Camacho, M. Parrilla, C. Fritsch, Phase Coherence Imaging, *IEEE Trans. UFFC*, 56, 5, pp. 958-974, 2009.

Camacho, 2010: J. Camacho, Imagen ultrasónica por coherencia de fase, Ph. D. Thesis, *Univ. Complutense*, Madrid, 2010.

Fisher, 1993: N.I. Fisher, Statistical analysis of circular data, Cambridge Univ. Press, 1993.

Gammelmark, 2003: K. L. Gammelmark, J. A. Jensen, Multielement Synthetic Transmit Aperture Imaging using Temporal Encoding, *IEEE Trans. Medical Imaging*, 22, 4, pp. 552-563, 2003.

Gavrilov, 1997: L. R. Gavrilov, J. W. Hand, P. Abel and C. A. Cain: A Method of Reducing Grating Lobes Associated with an Ultrasound Linear Phased Array Intended for Transrectal Thermotherapy, *IEEE Trans. Ultrason., Ferroelect., Freq. Contr.*, 44, 5, pp. 1010-1017, 1997.

Gustafsson, 1993: M. G. Gustafsson, T. Stepinski, Split-Spectrum Algorithms Rely on Instantaneous Phase Information- A Geometrical Approach, *IEEE Trans. UFFC*, 40, 6, pp. 659-665, 1993.

Lockwood, 1996: G. R. Lockwood, P. C. Li, M. O'Donnell, F. S. Foster, Optimizing the Radiation Pattern of Sparse Periodic Linear Arrays, *IEEE Trans. UFFC*, 43, 1, pp. 7-14, 1996.

Lockwood, 1998: G. R. Lockwood, J. R. Talman, S. S. Brunke, Real-time Ultrasound 3D-Imaging Using Sparse Synthetic Aperture Beamforming, *IEEE Trans. UFFC*, 45, 4, pp. 980-988, 1998.

Newhouse, 1982: V. L. Newhouse, N. M. Bilgutay, J. Saniie, E. S. Furgason, Flaw-to-grain echo enhancement by split-spectrum processing, *Ultrasonics*, 20, pp. 59-68, 1982.

Nikolov, 2000: S. I. Nikolov, J. A. Jensen, Application of different spatial sampling patterns for sparse array transducer design, *Ultrasonics*, 37, pp. 667-671, 2000.

Nikolov, 2005: M. Nikolov, V. Behar, Analysis and optimization of synthetic aperture ultrasound imaging using the effective aperture approach, *Int. J. Information Theory & Applications*, 12, pp. 257-265, 2005.

Oppenheim, 1989: A. Oppenheim, R. Schaffer, Discrete-time signal processing, *Prentice Hall*, 1989.

Pitas, 1995: I.Pitas, A. N. Venetsanopoulos: Non linear digital filters, *Kluwer Academic Publishers*, Massachusetts, 1995.

Ranganathan, 2004: K. Ranganathan, M. K. Santy, T. N. Blalock, J. A. Hossack, W. F. Walker, Direct Sampled I/Q Beamforming for Compact and Very Low-Cost Ultrasound Imaging, *IEEE Trans. UFFC*, 51, 9, pp. 1082-1094, 2004.

Shankar, 1985: P. M. Shankar, V. L. Newhouse, Speckle Reduction with Improved Resolution in Ultrasound Imaging, *IEEE Trans. Son. Ultrason.*, 32, 4, pp. 537-543, 1985.

Steinberg, 1976: B. D. Steinberg, Principles of Aperture and Array System Design, *John Wiley & Sons*, 1976.

Szabo, 2004: T. L. Szabo, Diagnostic ultrasound imaging, *Elsevier Academic Press*, 2004.

Turnbull, 1991: D. H. Turnbull and F. S. Foster, Beam steering with pulsed two-dimensional transducer array, *IEEE Trans. UFFC.*, vol. 38, no. 4, pp. 320–333, 1991.

5

Real-Time Speckle and Impulsive Noise Suppression in 3-D Ultrasound Imaging

Francisco J. Gallegos-Funes, Jose M. de-la-Rosa-Vazquez,
Alberto J. Rosales-Silva and Suren Stolik Isakina
National Polytechnic Institute of Mexico
Mexico

1. Introduction

Ultrasound imaging is considered one of the most powerful techniques for medical diagnosis and is often preferred over other medical imaging modalities because of noninvasive, portable, versatile and low-cost properties (Webb, 2002; Abd-Elmoniem, 2002; Porter, 2001; Shekhar, 2002). A fundamental problem in the field of ultrasound imaging is the speckle noise influence, which is a major limitation on image quality in ultrasound imaging. Imaging speckle is a phenomenon that occurs when a coherent source and a noncoherent detector are used to interrogate a medium, which is rough on the scale of the wavelength. Speckle noise occurs especially in images of the liver and kidney whose underlying structures are too small to be resolved using long ultrasound wavelength. The presence of speckle noise affects the human interpretation of the images as well the accuracy of computer-assisted diagnostic techniques (Nikolaidis, 2000; Kim & Park, 2001)
The goal of this chapter is the capability and real-time processing features of the robust MM-L (Median M-type L) filters to remove speckle and impulsive noise in 3-D ultrasound images (Gallegos-Funes et al., 2008, Varela-Benitez et al., 2007). The Texas Instruments DSP TMS320C6711 is used to implement the algorithms (Texas Instruments, 1998; Kehtarnavaz, 2001). Based on the processing time values of each a 3-D filter, different configurations of sweeping cubes (voxels) are used to obtain a balance between the processing time and quality of the restoration of 3-D images (Nikolaidis, 2000). The criteria used to measure the performance of filters are: the peak signal-to-noise ratio (PSNR) to characterize the noise suppression, and the mean absolute error (MAE) to evaluate the preservation of edges and fine details (Bovik, 2000; Astola & Kuosmanen, 1997; Kotropoulos & Pitas, 2001; Pitas & Venetsanopoulos, 1990). Extensive simulation results have demonstrated that the proposed filters can consistently outperform other filters used as comparative by balancing the tradeoff between noise suppression, detail preservation, and processing time.

2. Problem formulation

All coherent imaging that include laser, SAR, and ultrasound imagery are affected by speckle noise (Abd-Elmoniem, 2002; Bovik, 2000; Kotropoulos & Pitas, 2001). Speckle may appear distinct in different imaging systems but it is always manifested in granular pattern due to image formation under coherent waves. A general model for ultrasound speckle noise can be written as (Abd-Elmoniem, 2002),

$$x(i,j) = S(i,j)\eta_m(i,j) + \eta_a(i,j) \quad (1)$$

where $x(i,j)$ is a noisy observation (i.e., the recorded ultrasound image) of the two-dimensional (2-D) function $S(i,j)$ (i.e., the noise-free image that has to be recovered), $\eta_m(i,j)$ and $\eta_a(i,j)$ are the corrupting multiplicative and additive speckle noise components, respectively, and i and j are variables of spatial locations that belong to 2-D space of all real numbers $(i,j) \in \Re^2$. Generally, the effect of the additive component (such as sensor noise) of the speckle in ultrasound images is less significant than the effect of the multiplicative component (coherent interference). Thus, ignoring the term $\eta_a(i,j)$, can be rewritten (1) as (Abd-Elmoniem, 2002),

$$x(i,j) = S(i,j)\eta_m(i,j). \quad (2)$$

To transform the multiplicative noise model into the additive noise model, we apply the logarithmic function on both sides of (2)

$$\log x(i,j) = \log S(i,j) + \log \eta_m(i,j), \quad (3)$$

or

$$x^l(i,j) = S^l(i,j)\eta_m^l(i,j), \quad (4)$$

where $\eta_m^l(x,y)$ is approximated as additive white noise. We assume here that the speckle pattern has a white Gaussian noise model. Therefore, the acquisition or transmission of digitized images through sensor or digital communication link is often interfered by impulsive noise (Astola & Kuosmanen, 1997; Pitas & Venetsanopoulos, 1990). Thus, the impulsive noise is added to the model (2) as follows (Astola & Kuosmanen, 1997)

$$x(i,j) = \eta_i(S(i,j)\eta_m(i,j)) \quad (5)$$

where $\eta_i(f(i,j))$ is the functional $\eta_i(f(i,j)) = \begin{cases} \textit{random valued spike with probability } P \\ f(i,j) \quad \textit{otherwise} \end{cases}$.

3. 3-D Median M-type L-filters

Consider the monochromatic 3-D image $x(i,j,k)$ where i and j are the 2-D spatial axes and k is the time axis or may be the third dimension for 3-D images (Nikolaidis & Pitas, 2000; Kim & Park, 2001). When the current pixel location is (i,j,k), a 11-point window $W(i,j,k)$, is defined as follows (Kim & Park, 2001):

$$\begin{aligned} W(i,j,k) = \{&x(i-1,j-1,k), x(i,j-1,k), x(i+1,j-1,k), x(i-1,j,k), x(i,j,k), x(i+1,j,k), \\ &x(i-1,j+1,k), x(i,j+1,k), x(i+1,j+1,k), x(i,j,k+1), x(i,j,k-1)\} \end{aligned} \quad (6)$$

From eq. (6), the window $W(i,j,k)$ includes a 3x3 window centered at the current pixel of the current frame and the current pixel's corresponding pixels in the previous and the next frames, as shown in Figure 1.

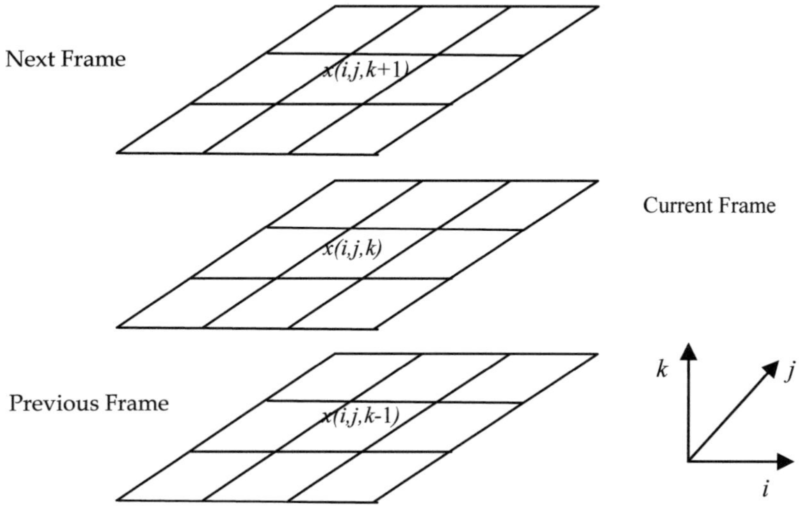

Fig. 1. The elements of the 11-point window $W(i,j,k)$.

A 3-D image can be considered as a 3-D matrix $x[i][j][k]$ or $x(i,j,k)$ of dimensions $N_1 \times N_2 \times N_3$ where i, j, k denote row, column, and slice (image) coordinates, respectively (Nikolaidis & Pitas, 2000). The 3-D representation is depicted in Figure 2. Each a voxel (volume elements) has physical size $di \times dj \times dk$ physical units (e.g. mm^3 or μm^3).
Recently (Gallegos & Ponomaryov, 2004; Gallegos et al., 2005), we proposed the combined RM (Rank M-type) -estimators for applications in image noise suppression. These estimators use the *M*-estimator combined with the *R*-estimator, such as the median or ABST (Ansari-Bradley-Siegel-Tukey) estimator. It was demonstrated that the robust properties of the RM-estimators exceed the robust properties of the base *R*- and *M*- estimators for the impulsive and speckle noise suppression (Gallegos & Ponomaryov, 2004). The RM-estimator used in the proposed 3-D filtering scheme is presented in such a form (Gallegos & Ponomaryov, 2004; Gallegos et al., 2005):

$$\theta_{\mathbf{medM}} = \mathrm{MED}\left\{X_p \tilde{\psi}\left(X_p - \mathrm{MED}\{\vec{\mathbf{X}}\}\right),\ p=1,\ldots,N\right\} \tag{7}$$

where θ_{medM} is the Median M-type (MM) estimator, X_p are data samples, $p = 1,\ldots,N$, $\tilde{\psi}$ is the normalized function ψ : $\psi(X) = X\tilde{\psi}(X)$, and $\vec{\mathrm{X}}$ is the primary data sample.
The MM-L type filter has been designed using the MM-estimator to increase the robustness of the *L*-filter. The detail description of such a filtering scheme is presented in recent works (Gallegos-Funes et al., 2008; Varela-Benitez et al., 2007), and in here we propose its modifications for 3-D imaging applications. So, the 3-D MM-L (Median M-type L) filter is defined as follows:

$$\hat{f}_{RM\text{-}L}(i,j,k) = \frac{\mathrm{med}\left\{a_p\left[X_p \cdot \psi\left(X_p - \mathrm{med}\{\vec{\mathrm{X}}\}\right)\right]\right\}}{a_{\mathrm{med}}}, \tag{8}$$

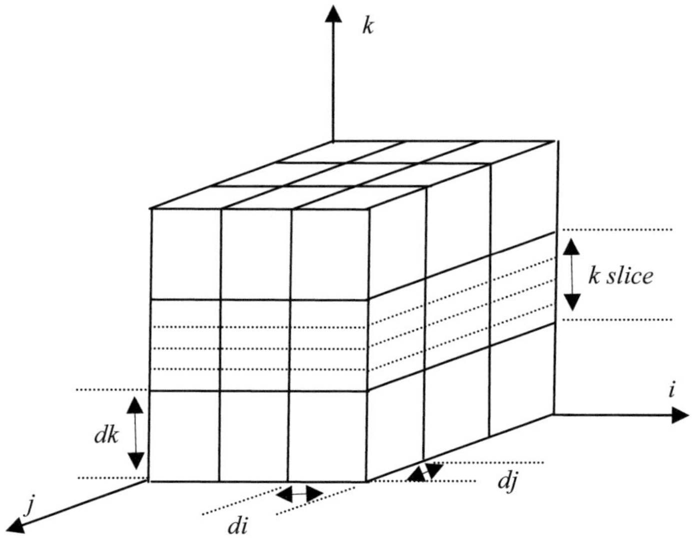

Fig. 2. 3-D representation as a 3-D array.

where $X_p \cdot \psi\left(X_p - \text{med}\{\vec{X}\}\right)$ represent the selected pixels in accordance with the influence function into a rectangular 3-D grid of voxels, $a_p = \int_{p-1/n}^{p/n} h(\lambda)d\lambda \Big/ \int_0^1 h(\lambda)d\lambda$ are the weighted coefficients where $h(\lambda)$ is a probability density function, a_{med} is the median of coefficients a_p, the filtering 3-D grid size is $N_1 \times N_2 \times N_3$, $N_p = (2L+1)^2$ and $l_p, m_p, n_p = -L,\ldots,L$, and X_p is the input data sample from the $x(i,j,k)$ of the 3-D image contaminated by noise in the rectangular 3-D grid where i and j are the 2-D spatial axes and k is the time axis (or third dimension). We use in the proposed 3-D filter the Tukey biweight influence function defined as (Hampel et al., 1986; Huber, 1981),

$$\psi_{\text{bi}(r)}(X) = \begin{cases} X^2\left(r^2 - X^2\right), |X| \le r \\ 0, |X| > r \end{cases} \tag{9}$$

where r is connected with the range of $\psi(X)$.

To improve the properties of impulsive noise suppression of the proposed MM L-filter we introduced an impulsive detector, this detector chooses if that voxel is filtered. The impulsive detector used here is defined as (Aizenberg et al., 2003):

$$\left[\left(rank\left(X_{ijk}\right) \le T_1\right) \vee \left(rank\left(X_{ijk}\right) \ge N_p - T_1\right)\right] \wedge \left|X_{ijk} - \text{MED}\left(\vec{X}\right)\right| \ge T_2, \tag{10}$$

where X_{ijk} is the central voxel in the 3-D grid, T_1>0 and T_2≥0 are thresholds.

We noted that the weighted coefficients of proposed 3-D filter are calculated using the exponential, Laplacian, and Uniform distribution functions (Pitas & Venetsanopoulos, 1990; Hampel et al., 1986) by each sliding filter window because the influence function selects

which pixels are used and then compute the weighted coefficients of *L*-filter according with the number of pixels used into the filtering window.
The parameters of the 3-D MM L-filters were found after numerous simulations by means of use a 3x3x3 grid (i.e., $N_1 \times N_2 \times N_3 = 27$, $l,m,n = -1,\ldots,1$, and $N_p = (2L+1)^2 = 9$). The idea was to find the parameters values when the criteria PSNR and MAE should be optimum. The optimal parameters of proposed filters are: $T_1=3$ and $T_2=15$ for the impulsive detector, and $r=15$ for Tukey influence function.
Processing times may change when we use other values for the parameters, increasing or decreasing processing times. The PSNR and MAE values change within the range of ±(5-10)%, it is due to the proposed fixed parameters that can realize the real-time implementation of the 3-D MM L-filters.

4. Experimental results

The objective criteria employed to compare the performance of noise suppression of different filters was the *peak signal to noise ratio* (PSNR) and for the evaluation of fine detail preservation the *mean absolute error* (MAE) (Bovik, 2000; Pitas & Venetsanopoulos, 1990):

$$\mathrm{PSNR} = 10 \cdot \log\left[\frac{(255)^2}{\mathrm{MSE}}\right], \ \mathrm{dB} \tag{11}$$

$$\mathrm{MAE} = \frac{1}{N_1 N_2 N_3} \sum_{i=0}^{N_1-1} \sum_{j=0}^{N_2-1} \sum_{k=0}^{N_3-1} \left| S(i,j,k) - \hat{f}(i,j,k) \right| \tag{12}$$

where $\mathrm{MSE} = \frac{1}{N_1 N_2 N_3} \sum_{i=0}^{N_1-1} \sum_{j=0}^{N_2-1} \sum_{k=0}^{N_3-1} \left[S(i,j,k) - \hat{f}(i,j,k) \right]^2$ is the *mean square error*, $S(i,j,k)$ is the original free noise 3-D image, $\hat{f}(i,j,k)$ is the restored 3-D image, and N_1, N_2, N_3 are the sizes of the 3-D image.
The runtime analysis of the 3-D MM L-filters and other concerned filters used as comparative were implemented by using the Texas Instruments DSP TMS320C6711 (Texas Instruments, 1998). This DSP has a performance of up to 900 MFLOPS at a clock rate of 150 MHz. The filtering algorithms were implemented in C language using the BORLANDC 3.1 for all routines, data structure processing and low level I/O operations. Then, we compiled and executed these programs in the DSP TMS320C6711 applying the Code Composer Studio 2.0. The processing time in seconds includes the time for acquisition, processing, and storing data.
The described 3-D MM L-filters with Tukey biweight influence function and different distribution functions have been evaluated, and their performance has been compared with different nonlinear 2-D filters which were adapted to 3-D. The filters used as comparative were the *modified a-Trimmed Mean* (Astola & Kuosmanen, 1997; Bednar & Watt, 1984), *Ranked-Order* (RO) (Astola & Kuosmanen, 1997; Pitas & Venetsanopoulos, 1990), *Multistage Median* (MSM1 to MSM6) (Arce, 1991), *Comparison and Selection* (CS) (Astola & Kuosmanen, 1997; Pitas & Venetsanopoulos, 1990), *MaxMed* (Nieminen & Neuvo, 1988), *Selection Average* (SelAve) (Astola & Kuosmanen, 1997; Pitas & Venetsanopoulos, 1990), *Selection Median* (SelMed) (Astola & Kuosmanen, 1997; Pitas & Venetsanopoulos, 1990), *Lower-Upper-Middle* (LUM, LUM Sharp, and LUM Smooth) (Hardie & Boncelet, 1993), and *Rank M-type K-nearest*

Neigbour (RM-KNN) (Ponomaryov et al., 2006) filters. These filters were computed according to their references and were adapted to 3-D imaging. Several experiments were realized to investigate the performances of the different techniques in 3-D imaging (Varela-Benitez et al., 2007).

4.1 Experiment 1

Figure 3 shows the 3-D space used to reconstruct the human organ as an object into 3-D space with its real measures. The coordinate *z* represents each a 2-D image of the sweeping in the 3-D space, and the coordinates *x* and *y* represent the height and width of the 2-D image, respectively. Having the 3-D image, one can carry out courts in the different plane *yz*, *xy*, and *xz*.

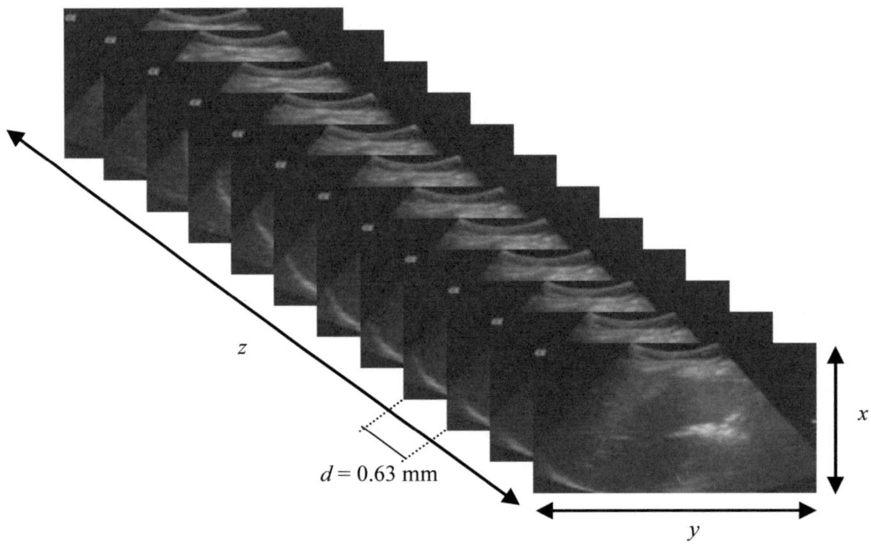

Fig. 3. 3-D ultrasound image representation.

The experiment 1 was realized by degraded an ultrasound sequence of 640x480 pixels with 90 frames (3-D image of 640x480x90 voxels) with 5 and 20% of impulsive noise and with the natural speckle noise of the 3-D image.

Table 1 presents the performance results of proposed filters and the comparative results of different non linear filters applied to a frame of the original sequence. From Table 1 we observe that when the noise corruption is 5%, the proposed filters almost have the same performances that other filters in terms of noise suppression and detail preservation, but when the noise corruption is high the best results are given by the MM-KNN filters. It can be seen from Table 1 that the processing time for proposed filters is less in comparison with the MM-KNN filters but the times of proposed ones are large in comparison with other filters. It is easy to see that the processing time values for MM L-filters are decreased but the performance criteria PSNR and MAE are sufficiently acceptable (see Table 1) in comparison with other RM filters such as the RM-KNN (Median, Wilcoxon, and ABST –KNN) filters and other filters proposed as comparative.

3-D Filters	Impulsive noise percentage					
	5%			20%		
	PSNR	MAE	Time	PSNR	MAE	Time
LUM Smooth	29.94	2.75	4.122	25.26	4.87	5.754
LUM Sharp	17.36	17.28	4.224	15.90	20.17	5.867
LUM	18.53	15.51	4.317	17.59	17.68	5.984
MaxMed	27.10	6.24	1.1981	23.24	9.20	1.1981
Modified Trimmed Mean	24.90	7.04	2.1716	24.71	7.35	2.1716
MSM1	28.92	4.25	0.5846	26.68	5.30	0.5846
MSM2	28.13	5.06	0.5773	26.18	6.00	0.5773
MSM3	27.46	5.94	1.2681	26.88	6.46	1.2681
MSM4	27.94	5.33	1.2367	27.13	5.81	1.2367
MSM5	29.44	3.77	1.2198	25.98	5.17	1.2198
MSM6	28.29	5.06	1.1667	27.67	5.45	1.1667
SelAve	26.83	6.97	1.9620	22.34	14.33	1.9620
SelMed	27.43	5.63	2.3240	26.31	6.37	2.3240
RO	26.50	6.67	1.6836	26.27	6.94	1.6836
MM-KNN Cut	28.83	4.27	20.49	27.91	5.14	20.63
MM-KNN Hampel	28.79	4.31	20.51	27.89	5.16	21.26
WM-KNN Hampel	22.75	10.91	38.54	21.98	11.59	45.06
ABSTM-KNN Hampel	27.45	5.21	34.14	26.77	6.00	38.00
MM-L TUKEY Uniform	28.30	4.77	3.7731	25.93	5.69	3.7732
MM-L TUKEY Laplacian	28.03	5.00	3.7733	25.80	5.83	3.7733
MM-L TUKEY	27.52	5.63	3.7732	24.84	7.01	3.7737

Table 1. Performance results of different filters in a frame of ultrasound sequence degraded with impulsive noise.

Figure 4 displays the visual results in terms of restored images obtained by the use of different filters according to Table 1 by means of use the xz plane. In Figure 4, we can see that the proposed MM L-filters provide good results in noise suppression and detail preservation.

4.2 Experiment 2

The experiment 2 was performed in the same sequence but it was degraded with 0.05 and 0.1 of variance of speckle noise added to the natural speckle noise of the sequence. The performance results are depicted in Table 2 by use of a frame in the xy plane of the sequence. From Table 2 we observe that the 3-D MM L-filters provide the best results in comparison to other comparative filters proposed. Figure 5 exhibits the visual results of restored images obtained by use of different filters according to Table 2, we observe that the proposed filters provide the best results in speckle noise suppression and detail preservation in comparison with other filters used.

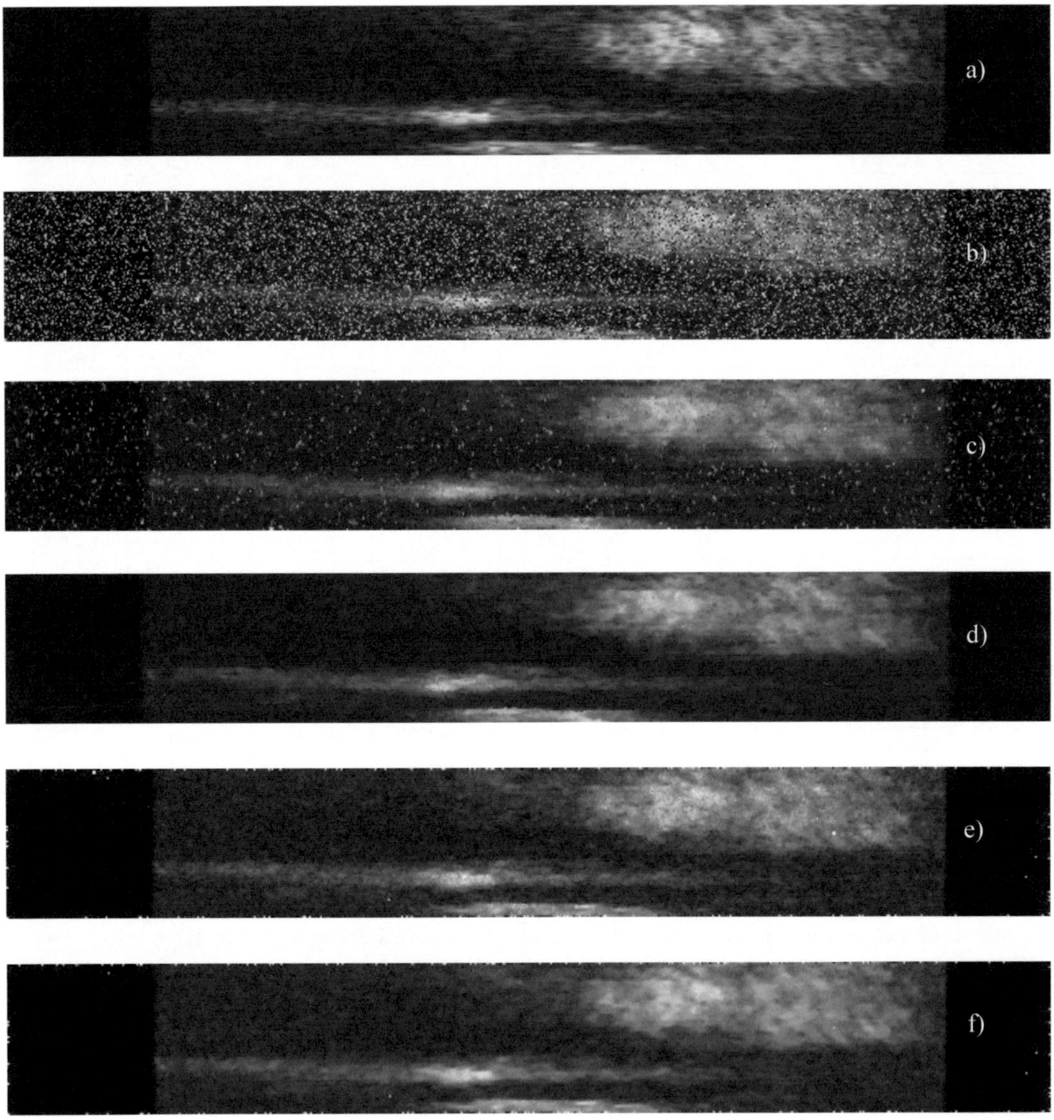

Fig. 4. Visual results in a frame of ultrasound sequence. a) original frame, b) frame degraded by 20% of impulsive noise, c) restored frame by MSM5 filter, d) restored frame by MM-KNN (Hampel) filter, e) restored frame by MM L-filter (Exponential), f) restored frame by MM L-filter (Laplacian).

3-D Filters	Speckle noise variance			
	0.05		0.1	
	PSNR	MAE	PSNR	MAE
CS	15.44	32.88	13.84	39.78
LUM Smooth	17.92	25.14	15.44	33.82
LUM Sharp	15.63	30.93	14.44	36.43
LUM	15.52	31.43	14.38	36.75
MaxMed	18.56	24.21	15.92	32.91
Modified α-Trimmed Mean	20.42	15.12	19.10	18.66
MSM1	20.57	17.62	18.06	23.68
MSM2	20.48	17.79	18.04	23.73
MSM3	22.42	14.21	20.26	18.46
MSM4	21.70	15.40	19.35	20.35
MSM5	19.55	20.21	16.96	27.44
MSM6	22.08	14.69	19.74	19.37
SelAve	21.18	17.65	19.19	22.81
SelMed	20.84	15.75	19.01	20.09
RO	21.59	14.520	19.80	18.18
MM-KNN Hampel	21.57	15.169	19.04	20.80
MM-L TUKEY Uniform	29.88	5.016	28.618	5.743
MM-L TUKEY Laplacian	28.80	5.646	28.19	6.020
MM-L TUKEY Exponential	28.03	6.261	26.30	7.666

Table 2. Performance results of different filters in a frame of ultrasound sequence degraded with speckle noise.

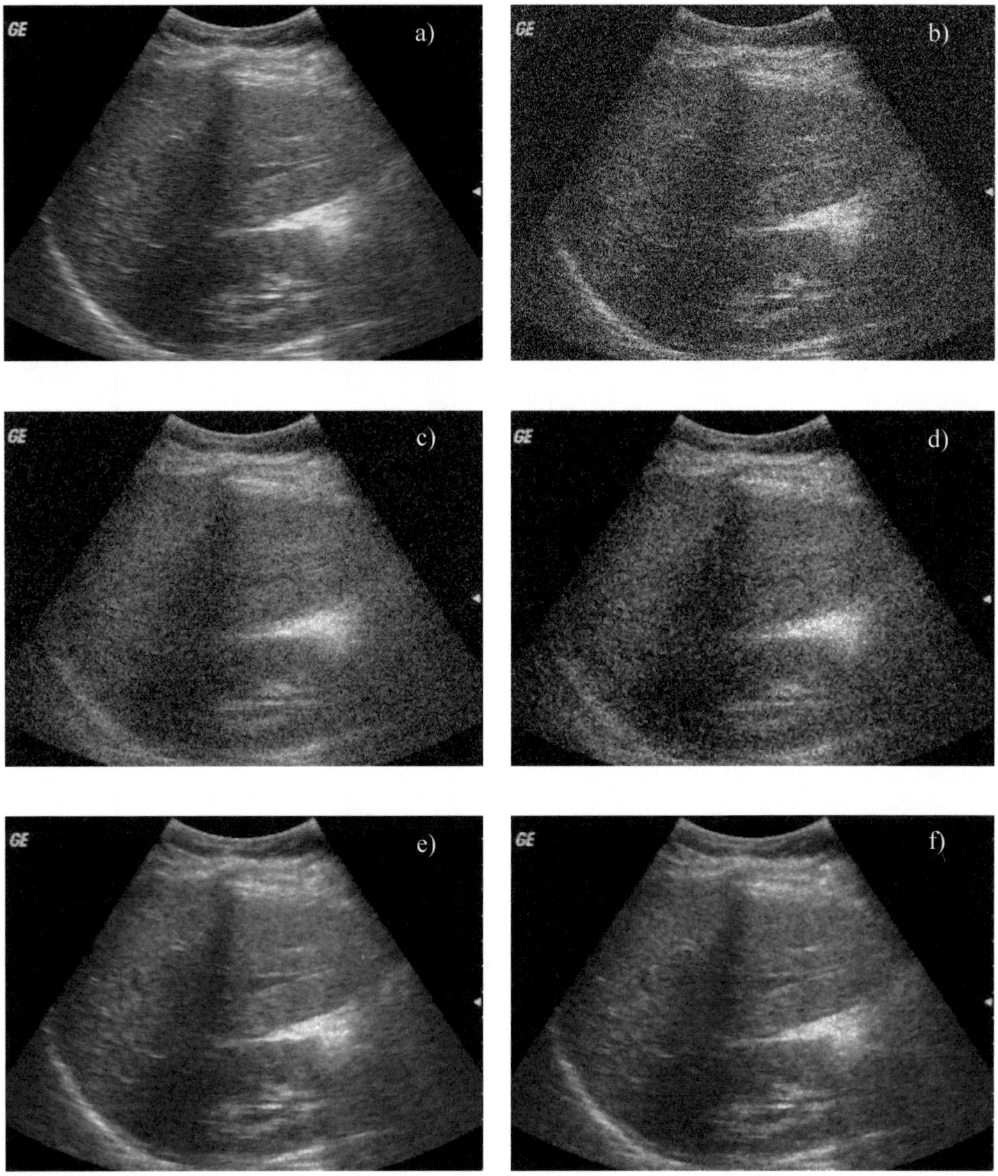

Fig. 5. Visual results in a frame of ultrasound sequence. a) Original frame, b) frame degraded by 0.05 of variance of speckle noise, c) restored frame by MSM6 filter, d) restored frame by MM-KNN filter, e) restored frame by MM L-filter (Uniform), f) restored frame by MM-L filter (Laplacian).

4.3 Experiment 3

Experiment 3 is related to different voxels cube configurations to provide better noise reduction. Figure 6 shows nine configurations of voxels used in the proposed 3-D filtering algorithms. It is obvious that by using less voxels in the different cube configurations the processing time can be decreased. In this experiment the ultrasound sequence was degraded

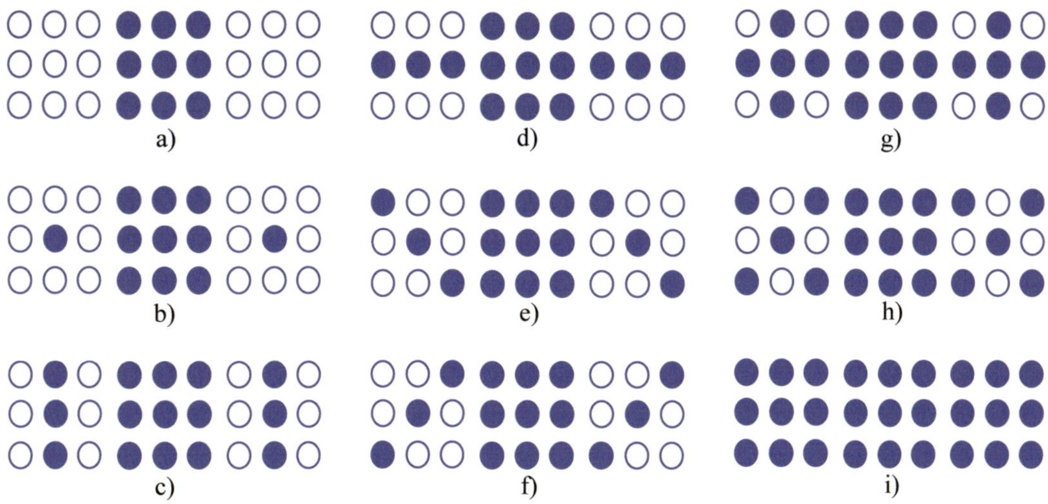

Fig. 6. Different configurations of processing cube.

with 20% of impulsive noise. Then, we implemented different cube configurations in the α-Trimmed Mean, MM-KNN, and MM L filters.

Table 3 presents the performance results of different filters in the case of use different cube configurations in the *xy* plane of the sequence. From this Table, the MM-KNN and α-Trimmed Mean filters provide better results in terms of PSNR in comparison with the MM L-filter but in the MAE performance the proposed filter provides the better results. About the processing time of the algorithms, the proposed MM L-filter has less processing time in comparison with the MM-KNN filter.

4.4 Discussion of results in ultrasound imaging

From the results presented in this chapter (see Tables 1-3) we conclude that the proposed MM L-filters can suppress the speckle noise with detail preservation better than other filters proposed in the literature. In the case of impulsive noise suppression the proposed filters have good performance in comparison with other filters proposed in the literature. Finally, the processing time of MM L-filters is acceptable to process 3-D images in real time applications because the proposed filters can process QCIF video format with standard film velocity for computer vision systems.

4.5 Experiment 4

We also process real video sequences to demonstrate that the proposed method potentially can provide a solution to quality video transmission. In the case of this test we use one frame of the video sequences "Carphone" and "Miss America" that were corrupted by mixed noise of 20% of impulsive noise and 0.1 of variance of speckle noise. The PSNR and MAE performances are depicted in Table 4. The visual results of the processing frames in the case of a frame of video sequence "Carphone" are displayed in Figure 7 according with Table 4.

Voxel Configuration	20% of impulsive noise					
	MM-KNN filter			Modified α-trimmed mean filter		
	PSNR	MAE	Time (secs.)	PSNR	MAE	Time (secs.)
a	28.41	4.54	1.6425	26.32	6.98	0.6398
b	29.41	4.42	1.9082	28.24	5.69	0.7127
c	28.77	5.28	4.8228	28.75	5.49	0.8267
d	28.86	5.16	5.1989	28.88	5.35	0.8269
e	28.71	5.29	4.8159	28.68	5.49	0.8267
f	28.68	5.30	4.8297	28.66	5.50	0.8268
g	28.43	5.23	10.0552	28.30	5.68	1.3775
h	28.19	5.38	10.0775	28.04	5.85	1.3769
i	27.92	5.14	20.6575	25.75	7.76	2.1716
	MM L-filter Uniform					
	PSNR	MAE	Time (secs.)			
a	26.83	5.81	1.1485			
b	27.67	5.00	1.1627			
c	27.57	5.06	2.3251			
d	28.30	4.31	2.3247			
e	27.53	5.10	2.3289			
f	27.54	5.11	2.3254			
g	28.07	4.55	3.4934			
h	27.44	5.21	3.4993			
i	27.77	4.85	4.7732			

Table 3. Performance results by use different cube configurations in a frame of ultrasound sequence degraded with impulsive noise.

Filters	20% of impulsive noise and 0.1 of variance of speckle noise			
	Carphone		Miss America	
	PSNR	MAE	PSNR	MAE
MM L Exponential, ND	18.8798	20.4191	21.5452	15.0880
MM L Laplacian, ND	20.4120	16.1230	24.1252	9.1169
MM L Uniform, ND	20.8869	15.1964	24.5764	8.4784
MM L Exponential, D	19.5138	18.6947	22.4313	12.6873
MM L Laplacian, D	20.7843	15.5185	23.9603	9.9071
MM L Uniform, D	21.1308	14.8694	24.5236	8.5236

Table 4. Performance results in a frame of video sequences "Carphone" and "Miss America" degraded with 20% of impulsive noise and 0.1 of variance of speckle noise by the use of different filters, where ND is without noise detector and D is with noise detector.

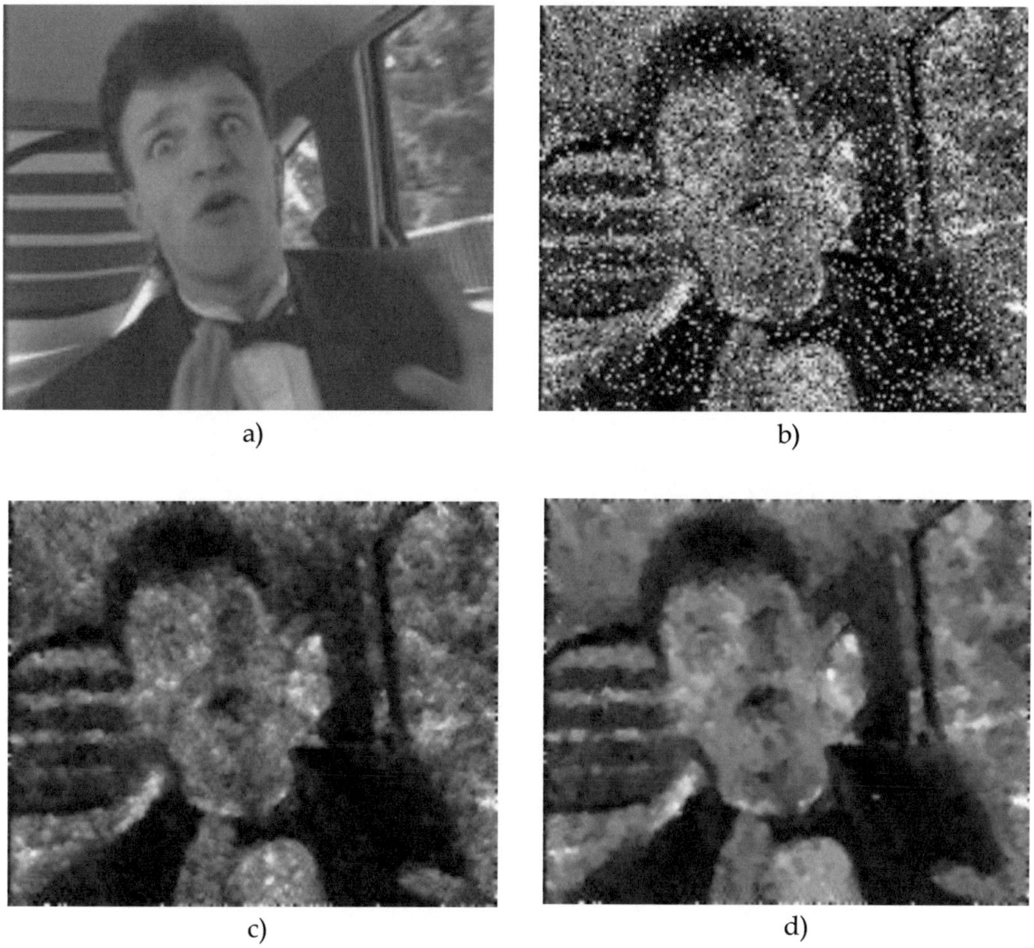

Fig. 7. Visual results in a frame of video sequence "Carphone", a) Original frame of "Carphone", b) Frame degraded with mixed noise of 20% of impulsive noise and 0.1 of variance of speckle noise, c) Restored frame with the proponed filter without noise detector, d) Restored frame with the proposed filter with noise detector.

4.6 Experiment 5

To demonstrate the performance of the proposed filtering scheme we apply it for filtering of the SAR images, which naturally have speckle noise. The results of such a filtering are presented in the Figure 8 in the case of the SAR image "Pentagon". It is possible to see analyzing the filtering images that speckle noise can be efficiently suppressed, while the sharpness and fine feature are preserved using the proposed MM L-filter.

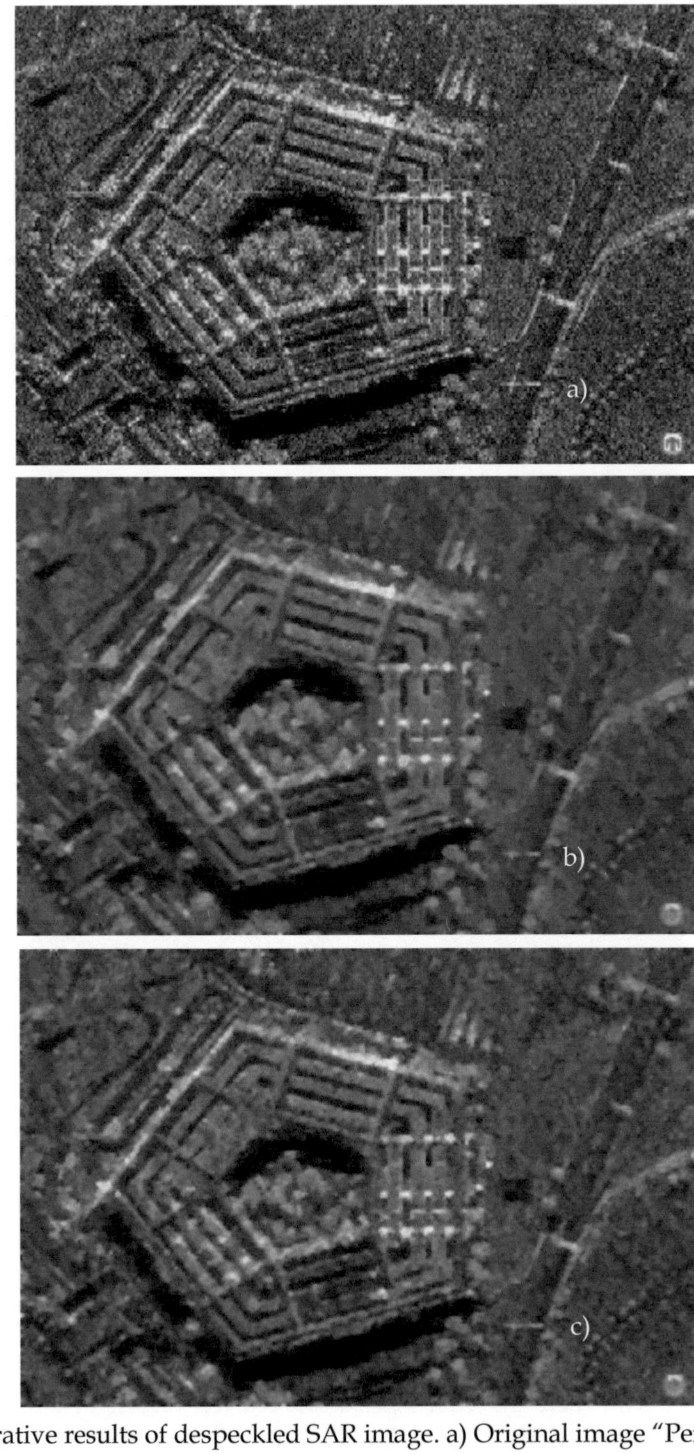

Fig. 8. Comparative results of despeckled SAR image. a) Original image "Pentagon", resolution 1m, source Sandia National Lab., b) Despeckled image with the MM L-filter without noise detector, c) Despeckled image with the MM L-filter with noise detector.

5. Conclusions

In this chapter is presented a real-time implementation of the 3-D MM L-filter for impulsive and multiplicative noise suppression with good detail preservation by means of use of DSP TMS320C6711. Different simulation results have demonstrated that the proposed filters consistently outperform other filters by balancing the tradeoff between speckle and impulsive noise suppression, detail preservation, and processing time. The proposed filter potentially provides a real-time solution to quality video transmission. The use of the linear combinations of order statistics (*L*-filter) with the MM-estimator provide to proposed 3-D MM L-filter better performance in terms of speckle noise in comparison with the 3-D RM-KNN filtering algorithm. In the case of impulsive noise the proposed filter provides good results in comparison with different filters found in scientific literature.

6. References

Abd-Elmoniem, K. Z., Youssef, A. M., & Kadah, Y. M. (2002). Real-Time speckle reduction and coherence enhancement in ultrasound imaging via nonlinear anisotropic diffusion. *IEEE Trans. Biomed. Eng.* Vol.49, No.9, 997-1014, ISSN:0018-9294

Aizenberg, I., Astola, J., Bregin, T., Butakoff, C., Egiazarian, K., & Paily, D. (2003). Detectors of the Impulsive Noise and new Effective Filters for the Impulsive Noise Reduction, *Proc. SPIE Image Process., Algorithms and Syst. II*, Vol. 5014, ISBN: 9780819448149, pp. 419-428, San Jose, Ca, USA

Arce, G. R. (1991). Multistage order statistic filters for image sequence processing. *IEEE Trans. Signal Process.* Vol.39, No.5, 1146-1163, ISSN:1053-587X

Astola, J. & Kuosmanen, P. (1997). *Fundamentals of Nonlinear Digital Filtering,* CRC Press. ISBN:0-8493-2570-6, Boca Raton-New York, USA

Bednar, J. B., & Watt, T. L. (1984). Alpha-trimmed means and their relationship to median filters. *IEEE Trans. Acoust., Speech, and Signal Process,* Vol.ASSP-32, 145-153, ISSN: 0096-3518

Bovik, A. (2000). *Handbook of Image and Video Processing,* Academic Press., ISBN:0121197921, San Diego CA

Gallegos, F., & Ponomaryov, V. (2004). Real-time image filtering scheme based on robust estimators in presence of impulsive noise. *Real Time Imaging,* Vol.8, No.2, 78-90, ISSN:1077-2014

Gallegos-Funes, F., Ponomaryov, V., & De-La-Rosa J. (2005). ABST M-type K-nearest neighbor (ABSTM-KNN) for image denoising. *IEICE Trans. Funds. Electronics Comms. Computer Science,* Vol.E88A, No.3, 798-799, ISSN:0916-8508

Gallegos-Funes, F., Varela-Benitez, J., & Ponomaryov, V. (2008). Rank M-Type L (RM L)-Filter for Image Denoising, *IEICE Trans. Funds. Electronics, Comms. Computer Sciences,* Vol.E91A, No.12, 3817-3819, ISSN:0916-8508

Hampel, F. R., Ronchetti, E. M., Rouseew, P. J. & Stahel, W. A. (1986). *Robust Statistics. The approach based on influence function.* Wiley ISBN:0-471-73577-9, New York, USA

Hardie, R. C., & Boncelet, C. G. (1993). LUM filters: a class of rank order based filters for smoothing and sharpening. *IEEE Trans. Signal Process.* Vol.41, 1061-1076, ISSN:1053-587X

Huber, P.J. (1981). *Robust Statistics,* Wiley, ISBN:0-471-65072-2, New York, USA

Kehtarnavaz, N., & Keramat, M. (2001). *DSP System Design using the TMS320C6000*, Prentice Hall, ISBN:0-13-091031-7, Upper Saddle River, NJ, USA.

Kim, J. S., & Park, H. W. (2001). Adaptive 3-D median filtering for restoration of an image sequence corrupted by impulsive noise. *Signal Processing: Image Communication*, Vol.16, 657-668, ISSN: 0923-5965

Kotropoulos, C. & Pitas, I. (2001). *Nonlinear Model-Based Image/Video Processing and Analysis*, John Wiley & Sons, ISBN:0-471-37735-X, New York

Nieminen, A., & Neuvo, Y. (1988). Comments of theoretical analysis of the max/median filter. *IEEE Trans. Acoust., Speech, and Signal Process.* Vol.ASSP-36, 826-827, ISSN: 0096-3518

Nikolaidis, N., & Pitas, I. (2001). *3-D Image Processing Algorithms*, John Wiley & Sons, ISBN:0-471-37736-8, New York, USA

Pitas, I., & Venetsanopoulos, A. N. (1990). *Nonlinear Digital Filters: Principles and Applications*, Kluwer Academic Publisher, ISBN: 0792390490, Boston, USA

Ponomaryov, V., Gallegos-Funes, F., Sansores-Pech, R., & Sadovnychiy, S. (2006). Real-time Noise suppression in 3D ultrasound Imaging based on Order Statistics. *IEE Electronics Letters*, Vol.42, No.2, 80-82, ISSN:0013-5194

Porter, B. C., Rubens, D. J., Strang, J. G., Smith, J., Totterman, S., & Parker, K. J. (2001). Three-dimensional registration and fusion of ultrasound and MRI using major vessels as fiducial markers. *IEEE Trans. Med. Imag.* Vol.20, No.4, 354-359, ISSN: 0278-0062

Shekhar, R., & Zagrodsky, V. (2002). Mutual information-based rigid and nonrigid registration of ultrasound volumes. *IEEE Trans. Med. Imag.* Vol.21, No.1, 9-22, ISSN: 0278-0062

Texas Instruments (1998). *TMS320C62x/67x Programmer's Guide, SPRU198D*, Texas Instruments Incorporated. Dallas, USA

Varela-Benítez, J. L., Gallegos-Funes, F. J., & Ponomaryov, V. I. (2007). Real-time speckle and impulsive noise suppression in 3-D imaging based on robust linear combinations of order statistics, *Proc. SPIE Real-Time Image Processing 2007*, Vol.6496, ISBN:9780819466099, pp. 64960H, San Jose, USA

Webb, A. G. (2002). *Introduction to Biomedical Imaging*, Wiley-IEEE Press, ISBN: 0471237663, *Hoboken, New Jersey*, USA

6

Tissue Harmonic Imaging with Coded Excitation

Masayuki Tanabe[1,2], Takuya Yamamura[2], Kan Okubo[2] and Norio Tagawa[2]
[1]*JSPS Research Fellow*
[2]*Graduate School of System Design, Tokyo Metropolitan University*
Japan

1. Introduction

It becomes more important to obtain medical ultrasound images with higher signal-to-noise ratio (SNR) and higher spatial resolution. In the last decade, tissue harmonic imaging (THI) and coded excitation to medical ultrasound imaging have been investigated. Coded excitation can overcome the trade-off between spatial resolution and penetration, which occurs when using the conventional pulse (Chiao, 2005), (Hu et al., 2001), (Tanabe et al., 2008). It is said that chirp signal is the most robust code for medical ultrasound image (Misaridis & Jensen, 2005). THI can acquire higher spatial resolution image and has been used in the commercial medical ultrasound system. A combination of coded excitation and THI (coded THI) has been investigated (Arshadi et al., 2007), (Hu et al., 2001), (Song et al., 2010), (Tanabe et al., 2010).

As a problem of THI, the frequency bandwidths of the fundamental and the harmonic components often overlap. The spectral overlap causes degradation of spatial resolution and the undesirable artifact. For the solution to the problem, only the harmonic component is extracted by pulse inversion (PI) method. However, if reflectors in the region of interest (ROI) move even a little, the fundamental components of echos are not cancelled completely. The intensity of the extracted harmonic components is still much smaller than the intensity of the residual fundamental component. Hence, the residual fundamental component has a bad effect on THI.

In sections II through IV, THI, coded excitation, and the combination of them are explained. In section V, we propose a new method which can extract broader bandwidth of the harmonic component for coded THI. The feasibility of the method is evaluated with experiments and simulations, and the expected performance in term of axial resolution and SNR has been verified.

2. Tissue harmonic imaging

THI has become a more common option for B-mode scanning. THI makes use of the nonlinearity of the sound propagation in the medium. The equation of a sound velocity c is expressed as

$$c = c_0 + \frac{1}{\rho_0 c_0}\left(\frac{B}{2A} + 1\right)p, \tag{1}$$

where c_0 is a sound velocity at atmospheric pressure, ρ_0 is an atmospheric density, B/A is a nonlinear parameter, and p is a sound pressure. The sound velocity increases at high acoustic pressures, and decreases at negative high acoustic pressures, and thus, the signal is distorted, as shown in Fig. 1(a). The harmonic components generate gradually, so that THI can obtain further region of interest. Additionally, The beamwidth of the harmonic component is narrower than that of the fundamental component. Therefore, THI can suppress sidelobe artifacts. However, there is frequency dependent attenuation (FDA) in human body, thus, the harmonic components attenuate more greatly than the fundamental components. Therefore, it is said that the intensity of the harmonic component depends on the propagation distance and the excitation intensity.

The amplitude of the harmonic component is much smaller than that of the fundamental component, thus, THI suffers from the poor SNR, resulting in limited penetrating depth.

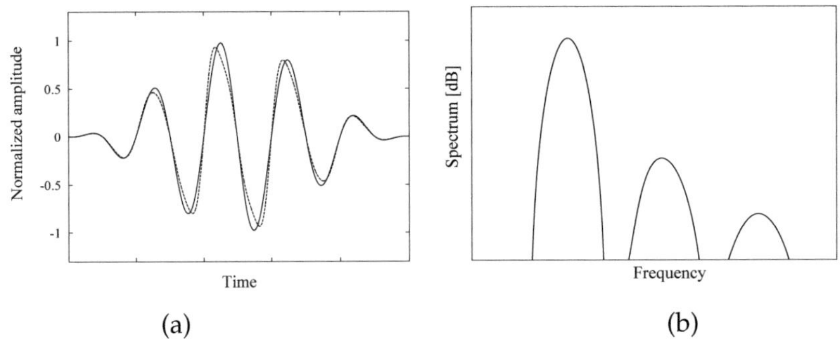

Fig. 1. THI. (a) Initial signal (solid line) and distorted signal (dash line). (b) Frequency spectrum of distorted signal.

3. Coded excitation

Next, let me explain coded excitation with linear chirp signal. The linear chirp signal is defined as a signal which frequency changes linearly, as described below

$$s(t) = \sin[2\pi(f_0 + \frac{B}{2T}t)t], \text{ for } 0 \le t \le T, \quad (2)$$

where f_0 is a starting frequency, B is a frequency bandwidth, and T is a time duration. An example of the linear chirp signal and its frequency spectrum are shown in Figs. 2 (b) and 2 (c). To decode the signal, auto-correlation function (ACF) is calculated as

$$\text{ACF}(\tau) = \int_{-\infty}^{\infty} s(t)s(t-\tau)dt, \quad (3)$$

where τ is a time shift. The ACF and its envelope are shown in Fig. 2(d). The half-bandwidth of the decoded signal is $1/B$ [s]. The SNR improvement is determined by the product of the duration T [s] and the bandwidth B [Hz] of the signal; it is called time-bandwidth product (TBP). An unmodulated pulse of duration T [s] at a carrier frequency f_c $(= f_0 + B/2)$ [Hz] has a frequency bandwidth $B = 1/T$ [Hz] around f_c [Hz]. The SNR of the decoded signal is

TB times higher than the unmodulated pulse. An advantage of chirp signal is to design the frequency bandwidth within the system properties.

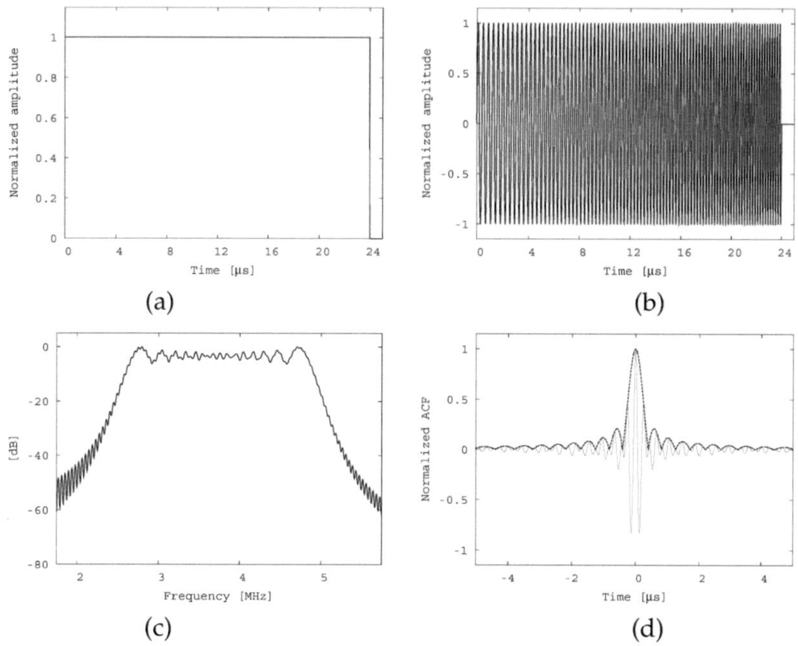

Fig. 2. Chirp signal with rectangular window. Time duration is 24 μs, and frequency is 2.5−5 MHz. (a) Window shape, (b) time domain, (c) frequency spectrum, and (d) ACF (solid line) and its envelope (dashed line).

As shown in Fig. 2(d), the rectangular window causes a range sidelobe. The range sidelobe has a bad effect on imaging. For suppression of the sidelobe, the signal is weighted by a window function. For example, the Hanning window $w_1(t)$ is expressed as

$$w_1(t) = 0.5 - 0.5\cos(2\pi t/T) \text{ for } 0 \leq t \leq T. \tag{4}$$

Figure 3 describes a Hanning weighted chirp signal. As shown in Fig. 3(d), the ACF of the Hanning window doesn't cause a range sidelobe. However, the half pulse-width is wider than that of the rectangular window as shown in Figs. 2(d) and 3(d).
It is said that there is a trade-off between the range sidelobe level and the half pulse-width. As a derived form of the Hanning window, the Hanning window is applied at starting and ending parts of the signal below

$$w_2(t) = \begin{cases} 0.5 - 0.5\cos(\pi t/(dT)) & (0 \leq t \leq dT) \\ 1 & (dT \leq t \leq (1-d)T) \\ 0.5 - 0.5\cos(\pi(t-T)/(dT)) & ((1-d)T \leq t \leq T), \end{cases} \tag{5}$$

where, d is the starting and the ending ratio. Figure 4 describes a chirp signal with the window in which d is 0.3.

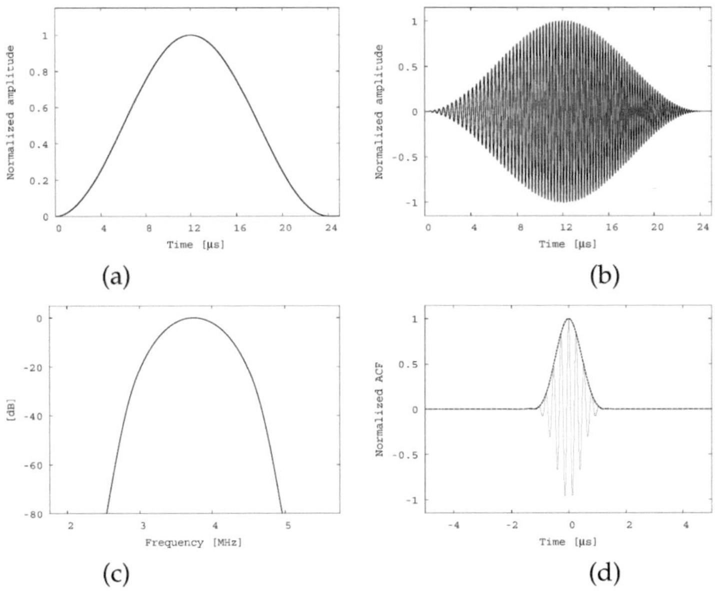

Fig. 3. Chirp signal with Hanning window. Time duration is 24 μs, and frequency is 2.5–5 MHz. (a) Window shape, (b) time domain, (c) frequency spectrum, and (d) ACF (solid line) and its envelope (dashed line).

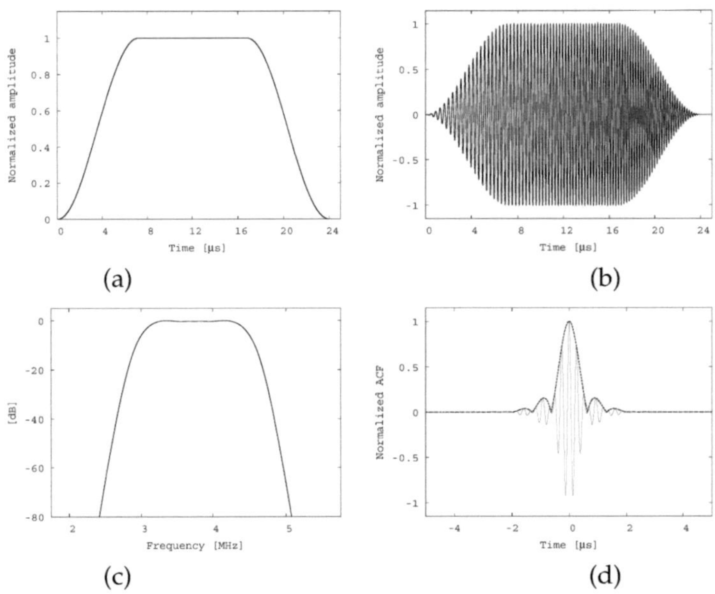

Fig. 4. Chirp signal with partial Hanning window (d=0.3). Time duration is 24 μs, and frequency is 2.5–5 MHz. (a) Window shape, (b) time domain, (c) frequency spectrum, and (d) ACF (solid line) and its envelope (dashed line).

The window shapes and the ACFs with various d are shown in Figs. 5(a) and 5(b).

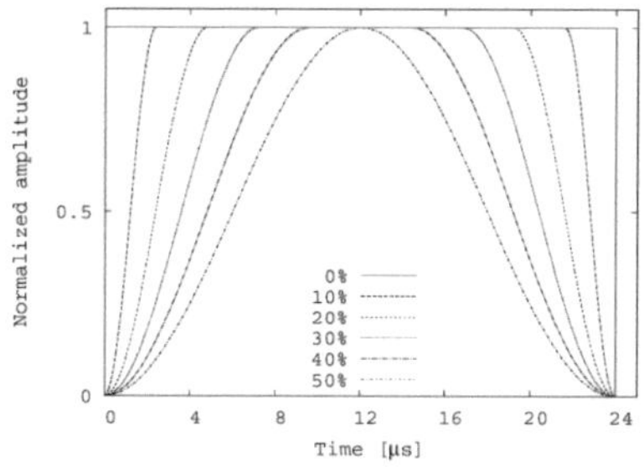

(a)

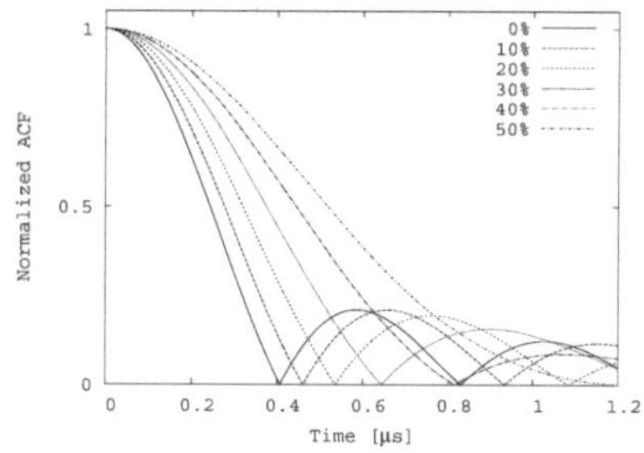

(b)

Fig. 5. (a) Window shapes and (b) envelopes of ACFs with various d. Time duration is 24 μs, and frequency is 2.5–5 MHz.

It is said that the window shape has an influence on the spatial resolution and the sidelobe level and that there is a trade-off between the spatial resolution and the sidelobe level.
In actual use, after transmission of $s(t)$, an echo signal $r(t)$ is received. To decode the signal, the cross-correlation function (CCF) is calculated as

$$\mathrm{CCF}(\tau) = \int_0^{\infty} r(t)s(t-\tau)dt. \tag{6}$$

4. Coded tissue harmonic imaging and spectral overlap consideration

To obtain both sufficient SNR and spatial resolution, a method which combines THI and coded excitation, has been proposed. When a chirp signal is transmitted into the medium, the obtained echo has harmonic components. The harmonic component of the chirp is also chirp because chirp maintains their coded phase relationship in the harmonic domain (Misaridis & Jensen, 2005). Therefore, the harmonic component can be compressed with a matched filter. The template signal used in the matched filter for the harmonic component is designed as the same time duration, and twice as bandwidth as the fundamental component of the chirp as

$$m(t) = \sin[2\pi(2f_0 + \frac{B}{T}t)t]. \text{ for } 0 \leq t \leq T \tag{7}$$

If the harmonic and the fundamental components are not overlapped in frequency domain, the harmonic component can be isolated by bandpass filtering (BF) as shown in Fig. 6(a). However, if the harmonic component overlaps the fundamental component in frequency domain due to the frequency broadness of the transmitted signal, the overlapped part of the harmonic component cannot be extracted. Therefore, in the BF, the extracted bandwidth has to be narrower, and thus, the image quality becomes poor, as shown in Fig. 6(b).
For avoiding the spectral overlap in THI, pulse inversion (PI) method has been used. The PI transmits two phase-inverted pulses, as shown in Fig. 7. By simply summing two echo signals, the harmonic component is doubled, and the fundamental component is cancelled, as shown in Fig. 8. However, if the PI is used for fast moving target such as cardiac valves, phase decorrelation occurs and the cancellation of the fundamental component cannot be done.

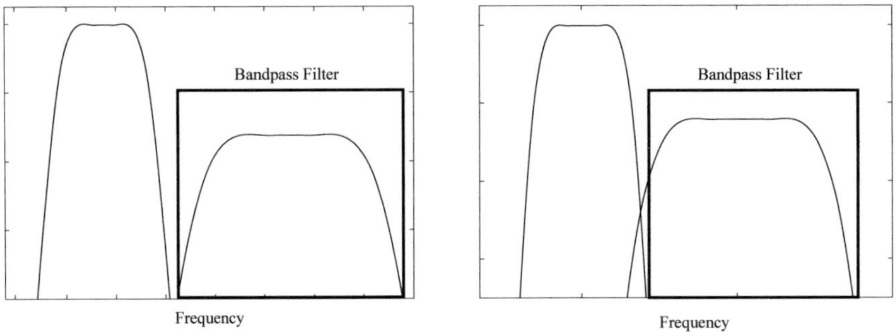

(a) (b)

Fig. 6. Bandpass filter (a) when overlap doesn't occur and (b) occurs.

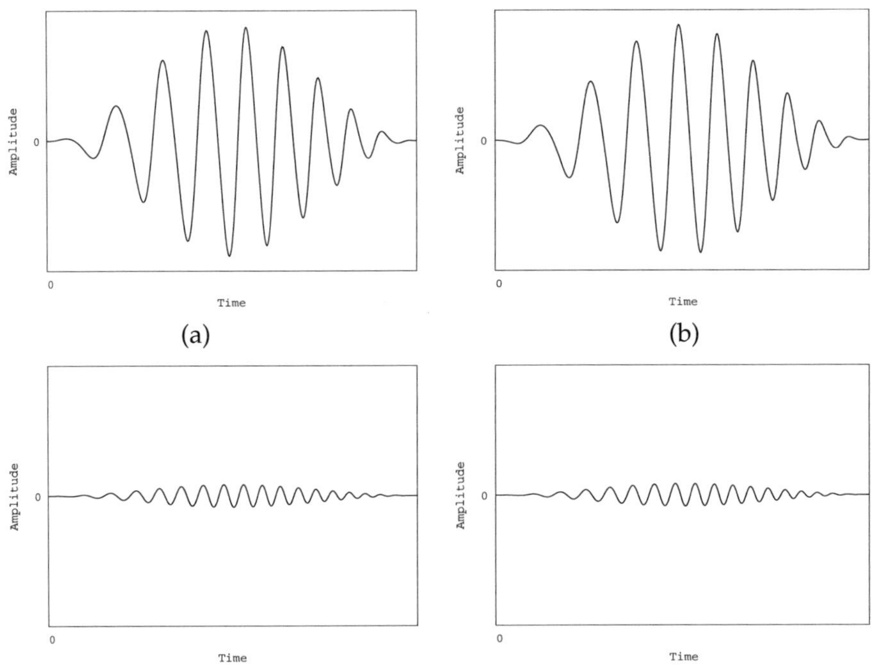

(a) (b) (c) (d)

Fig. 7. (a) (b) Transmitted signals of pulse inversion and (c) (d) harmonic components of received signals.

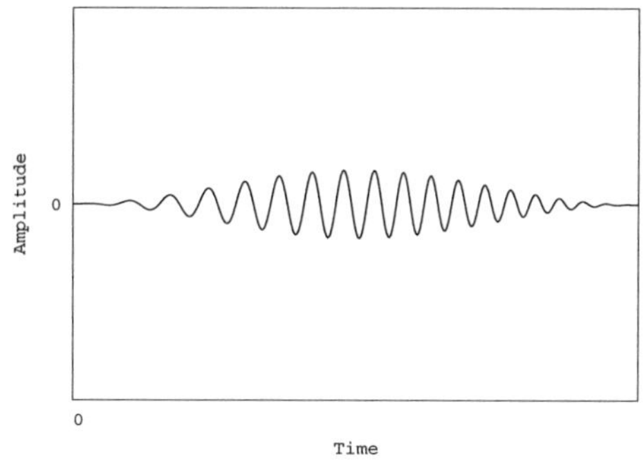

Fig. 8. Sum of received signals of pulse inversion.

In coded THI, there still remains the problem of the spectral overlap, which exists in THI. The matched filter is designed for the harmonic component. There is a cross-correlation between the fundamental frequencies of received echo and the second harmonic matched filter. As a result, an undesirable peak occurs at different time from the time of arrival.
By suppressing the bandwidth to avoid the spectral overlap, the problem does not occur as shown in Fig. 6(b), but the spatial resolution becomes worse. As mentioned above, we can of course also apply the PI, but the method is susceptible to the target motion.
In this study, a novel harmonic isolation method is proposed, and the impact of spectral overlap is examined through simulations and experiments.

5. Method

5.1 Principle

In this section, we explain the proposed method. The method uses multi chirp signals. The spectrum of the each signal is designed for not overlapping between the fundamental and harmonic components. The each chirp signal is transmitted separately, and only the harmonic component of the echo signal can be extracted by the bandpass filter simply. Consequently, decoding with the isolated harmonic components, high spatial resolution signal with high SNR can be obtained.

5.2 Coding process

When the number of excitations is defined as N, the ith chirp signal $s_i(t)$ $(i = 1,2,...,N)$ is expressed as

$$s_i(t) = \alpha(t)\sin\{2\pi[f_i + \frac{B}{2T}\cdot t]\cdot t\}, \quad (0 \le t \le T/N), \tag{8}$$

$$f_i = f_0 + \frac{B(i-1)}{N}, \tag{9}$$

where $\alpha(t)$ is the amplitude modulation, f_i is the ith starting frequency, B/N is the bandwidth of each shot, T/N is the time duration of each shot.

5.3 Matched filter and decoding process

After transmission, N echo signals are received. The harmonic component of the each echo signal is separated from the fundamental component. Therefore, it is easy to isolate the harmonic component by bandpass filtering.
For decoding with the harmonic components, the each matched filter $m_i(t)$ has a same time duration and a twice frequency bandwidth as the transmitted signal.

$$m_i(t) = \alpha(t) \sin 2\pi[2f_i + \frac{B}{T}t]t, \quad (0 \leq t \leq T/N). \tag{10}$$

The echo signals $r_i(t)_{i=1,2,...,N}$ are decoded bellow

$$CCF(\tau) = \sum_{i=1}^{N}[\int_0^{\infty} r_i(t)m_i(t-\tau)dt]. \tag{11}$$

The TBP of the decoded signal is assumed as TB below

$$(T/N \times N) \times (B/N \times N) = TB. \tag{12}$$

6. Experiments and simulations

6.1 Experimental procedure

To evaluate the proposed method, *in vitro* experiments are conducted. The stainless steel block is placed in a water tank. The signal is transmitted by a transducer (KB-AEROTECH MLB50DL, the center frequency is 5 MHz). Figure 9 describes the experimental circumstance. In the proposed method, N is 2, the frequencies of the proposal are 2.5−3.7 MHz and 3.6−5 MHz, the time duration 13.5 μs, each 3 μs of the start and the end of the signal is half of the Hanning window ($d = 3/13.5$)..
For comparison, conventional coded THI method is also used. The frequency of the conventional type is 2.5−5 MHz, time duration 24 μs, and each 3 μs of start and end of the signal is half of the Hanning window ($d = 0.125$). The time duration of conventional coded THI is adjusted as sum of two signals of the proposed method. Figures 10, 11(a) and (b) describe the transmitted signals.

6.2 Axial resolution

The received echo signals are shown in Figs. 12(a), 13(a) and 13(b). As shown in Fig. 12(b), in conventional coded THI, the harmonic component is overlapped with the fundamental component at −30 dB. While, as shown in Fig. 14, in proposal, the each harmonic component is overlapped with the fundamental component at approximately −55 dB and −60 dB. Therefore, it is obvious that the proposed method can obtain the harmonic component more easily than the conventional method.
Subsequently, envelopes of the CCFs are shown in Figs. 15 and 16. In Figs. 15 and 16, the solid and the dashed lines describe the CCF using the fundamental and the harmonic components, respectively. Fig. 15 (b) is a part at 86−90 μs of Fig. 15(a). As shown in Fig. 15(b), it is shown that the CCF of the harmonic component is narrower than that of the fundamental component. However, in conventional coded THI, it is shown that the CCF with the harmonic component has an artifact at approximately 110 μs, as shown in Fig. 15(a). The artifact is the

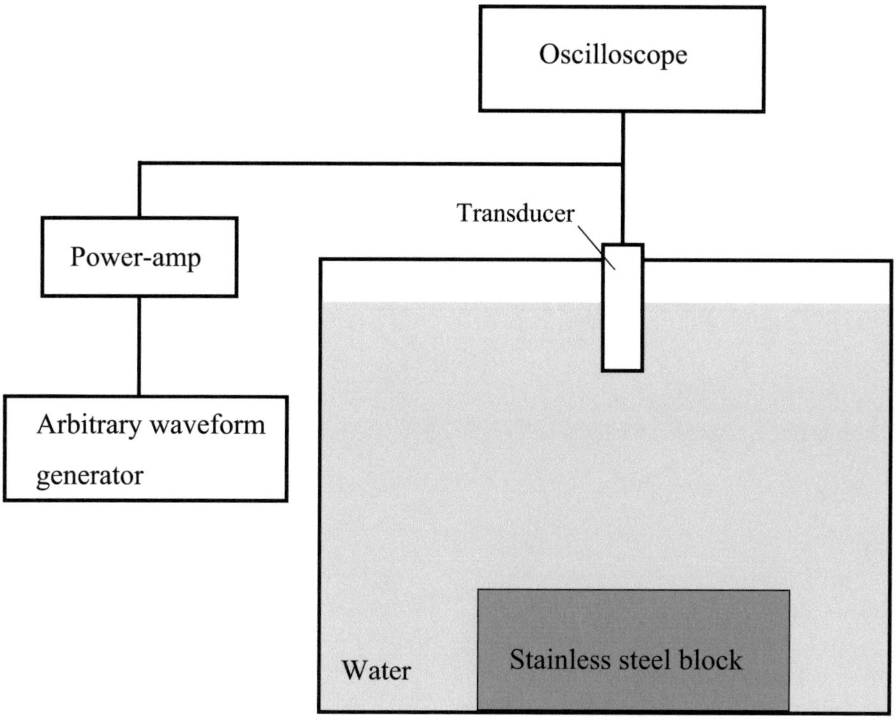

Fig. 9. Experimental circumstance

cross-correlation between the fundamental component of the echo signal and the harmonic matched filter. The CCF of the proposal, there is no artifact such as the conventional THI, and the CCFs of the fundamental and the harmonic components have the same axial resolution as that of the conventional THI.

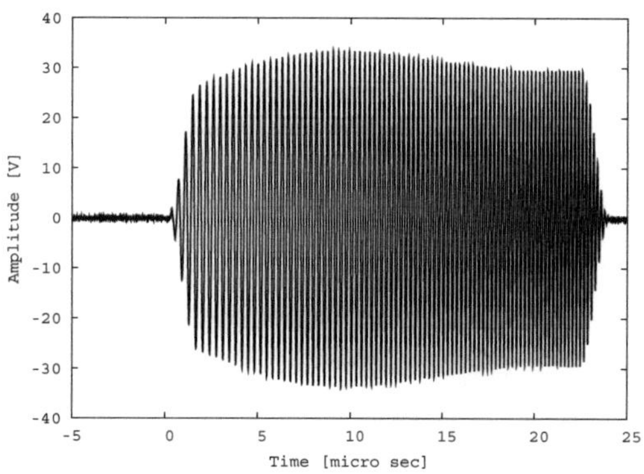

Fig. 10. Transmitted signal of conventional coded THI.

6.3 SNR

To examine the SNR of the proposed method, the decibel representations of the envelopes of the CCFs in conventional coded THI are shown in Figs. 17(a) and (b), and those of

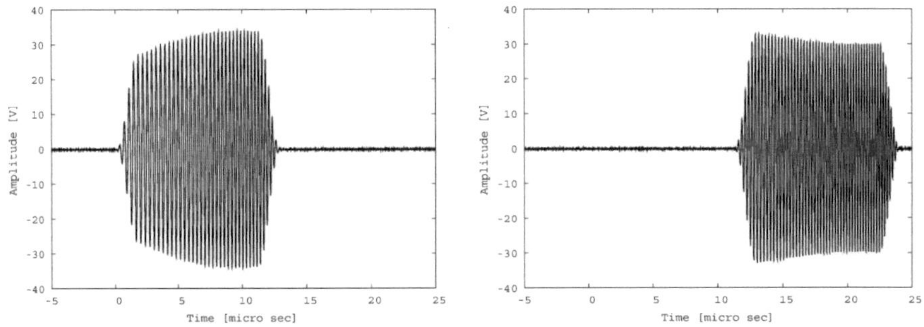

(a) (b)

Fig. 11. Transmitted signals of proposed coded THI. (a)1st and (b)2nd shots.

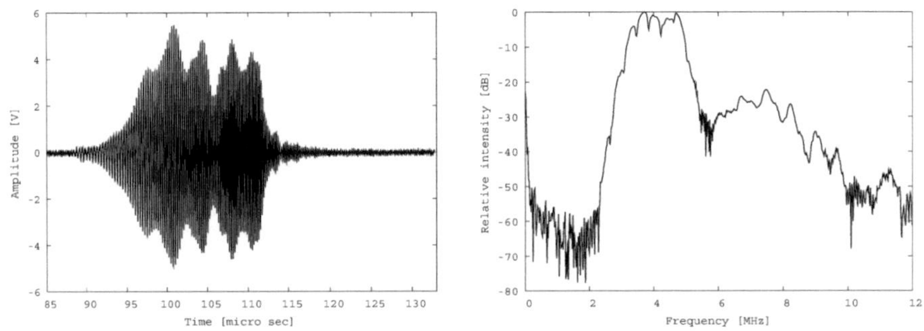

(a) (b)

Fig. 12. Echo signal of conventional coded THI in (a)time domain and (b)frequency domain.

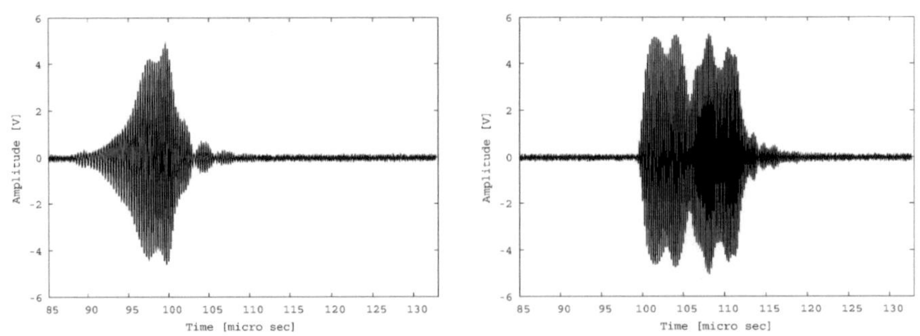

(a) (b)

Fig. 13. Echo signals of proposed coded THI in time domain. (a)1st and (b)2nd shots.

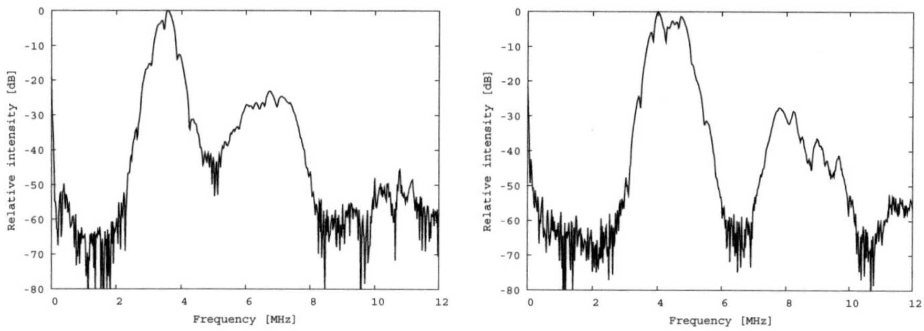

(a) (b)

Fig. 14. Echo signals of proposed coded THI in frequency domain. (a)1st and (b)2nd shots.

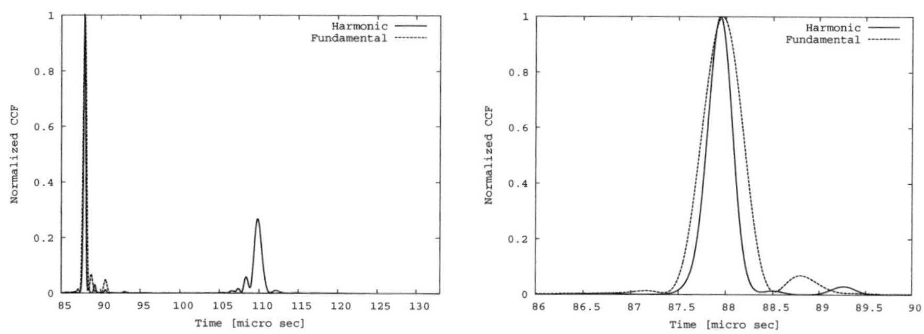

(a) (b)

Fig. 15. Envelope of CCF of conventional coded THI at (a)85-135 μs and (b)86-90 μs.

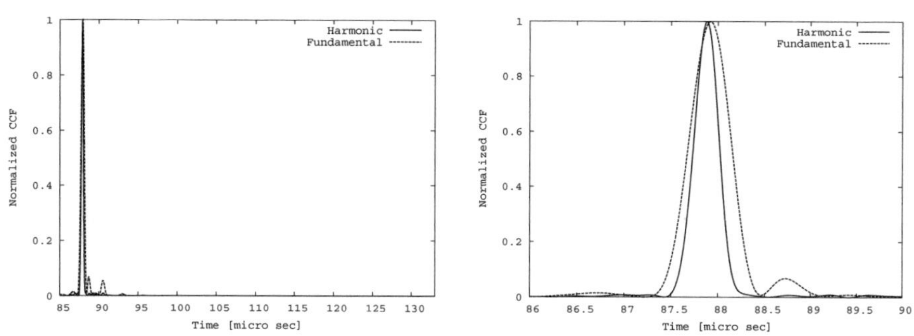

(a) (b)

Fig. 16. Envelope of CCF of proposed coded THI at (a)85-135 μs and (b)86-90 μs.

proposed method are shown in Figs. 18(a) and (b). As compared with conventional coded THI, excepting the artifact at approximately 110 μs, it is shown that the proposed method can obtain almost the same SNR.

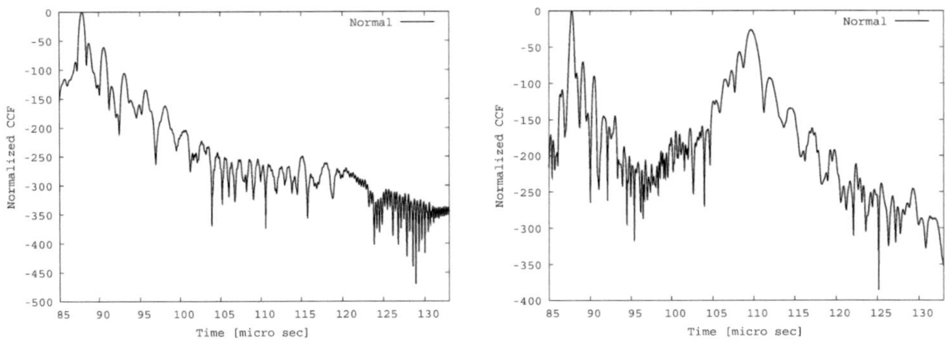

(a) (b)

Fig. 17. SNR of conventional coded THI. CCF with (a)fundamental and (b)harmonic components.

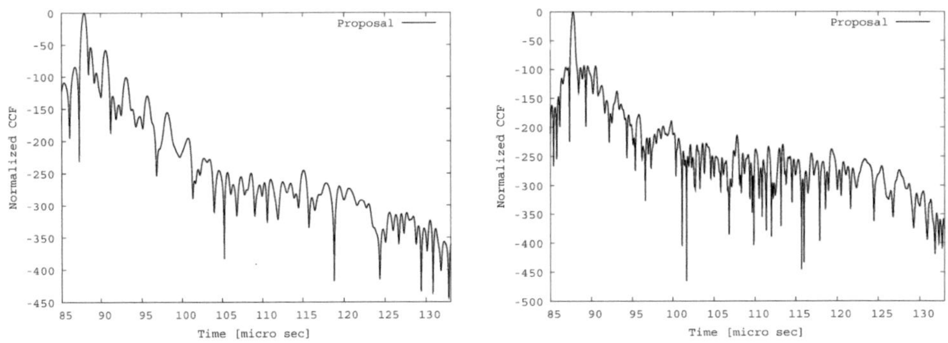

(a) (b)

Fig. 18. SNR of proposed coded THI. CCF with (a)fundamental and (b)harmonic components.

6.4 Tissue motion effects

The robustness of the proposal method against tissue motion is evaluated through FEM simulator PZFlex (Weidlinger Associates, Inc.). In a water tank, a point sound source is excited, and monitored from 6 cm away. In proposal, the number of shots N is 2, the each time duration is 20 μs, and the each frequency is 2–3.8, and 3.2–5 MHz, separately. For comparison, the pulse inversion method is also evaluated. In the PI method, the each transmitted signal is 2–5 MHz and 20 μs. Time difference ξ between two shots is caused by tissue motion. In this study, the Doppler shift is ignored, and the time difference ξ is given as time shift artificially.

The received signals are shown in Figs. 19 and 20. When ξ=0 μs, as shown in Figs. 21(a),the fundamental components are cancelled completely, and the CCF can be conducted,

as shown in Figs. 21(a) and (b). When ξ=0.05 μs, as shown in Figs. 22(a), the fundamental components are not cancelled and and the spectral overlap occurs. As described in Fig. 22(b), the cross-correlation between the fundamental component and the harmonic matched filter occurs.
Figured 23 and 24 show the results of the proposed method. When ξ=0 μs, as shown in Fig. 23(b), the half pulse-width is the same as that of the PI. When ξ=0.05 μs, as shown in Fig. 24(b), the half-width of CCF is wider than that when ξ=0 μs, however, the cross-correlation like the PI does not occur.

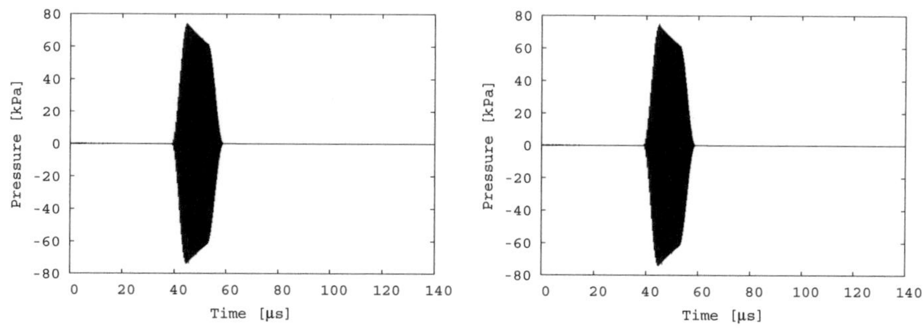

(a) (b)

Fig. 19. Received signals of conventional coded THI with PI. (a)1st and (b)2nd shots.

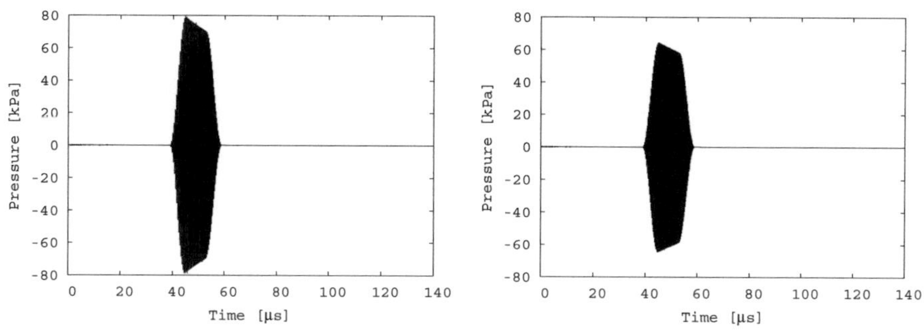

(a) (b)

Fig. 20. Received signals of proposed coded THI. (a)1st and (b)2nd shots.

7. Conclusion

In this study, we proposed a new method which can avoid the occurrence of the spectral overlap. From the experimental results, it was shown that the proposed method can extract harmonic component. In simulations, it was shown that the proposed method can suppress the tissue motion effects compared with the PI.
This study is assumed that the imaging target has the static aspect. Although the Doppler shift was ignored in this study, the proposed method is still valid if the target moves at the constant speed. In future work, we will consider a situation that the target moves at an accelerating pace.

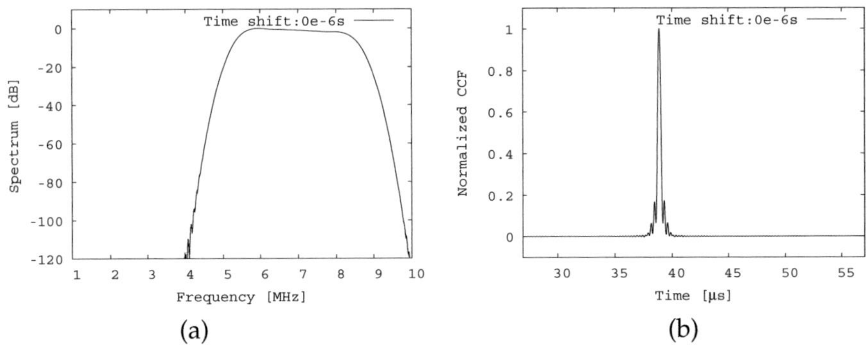

Fig. 21. Received signals of conventional coded THI with PI when $\xi = 0\mu s$. (a) Frequency spectrum and (b) CCF.

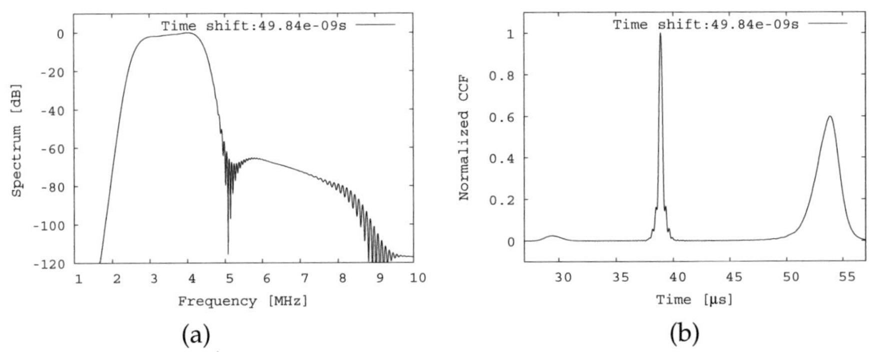

Fig. 22. Received signals of conventional coded THI with PI when $\xi = 0.05\mu s$. (a) Frequency spectrum and (b) CCF.

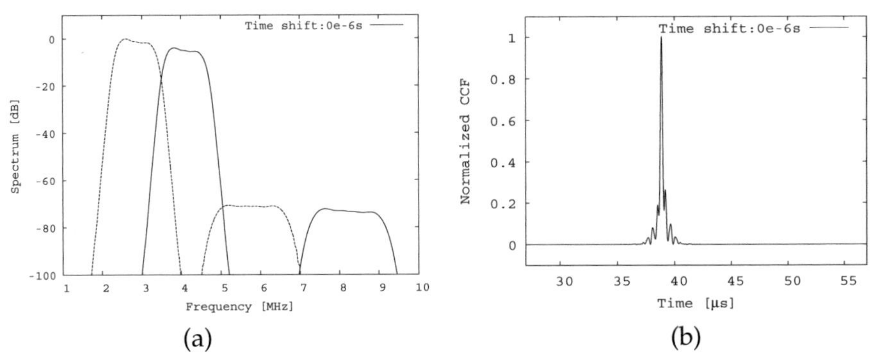

Fig. 23. Received signals of proposed coded THI when $\xi = 0\mu s$. (a) Frequency spectrum and (b) CCF.

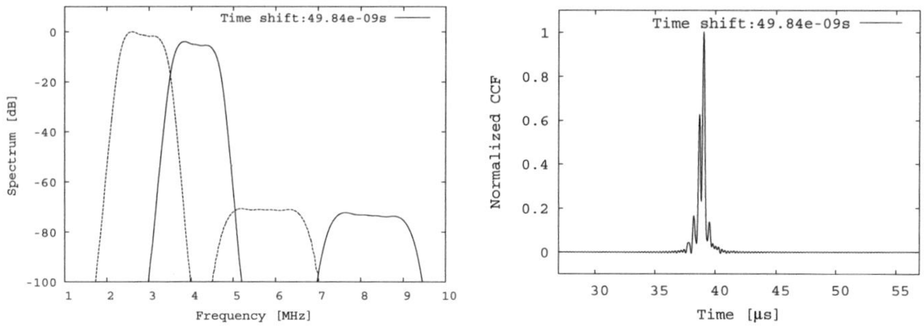

(a) (b)

Fig. 24. Received signals of proposed coded THI when $\xi = 0.05\mu$s. (a) Frequency spectrum and (b) CCF.

8. Acknowledgment

This work was partially supported by Grants-in-Aid for Scientific Research (B) (21300191) and Japan Society for the Promotion of Science.

9. References

Arshadi, R., Yu, A. C. H., & Cobbold, R. S. C. (2007). Coded Excitation Methods for Ultrasound Harmonic Imaging, *Canadian Acoustics*, Vol. 35 (No. 2), pp.35-46

Chiao, R. Y. & Hao X. (2005). Coded Excitation for Diagnostic Ultrasound: A System Developer's Perspective, *IEEE Transactions on Ultrasonics, Ferroelectrics and Frequency Control*, Vol. 52, pp.160-170

Hu, Z., Moriya, T., & Tanahashi, Y. (2001). Imaging System for Intravascular Ultrasonography Using Pulse Compression Technique, *Japanese Journal of Applied Physics*, Vol. 40, pp.3896

Kim, D. Y., Lee, J. C., Kwon, S. J., Song & T. K. (2001). Ultrasound Second Harmonic Imaging with a Weighted Chirp Signal, *Proceedings of IEEE Ultrasonics Symposium*, Atlanta, pp.1477-1480

Li, Y & Zagzebski, J. A. (2000). Computer Model for Harmonic Ultrasound Imaging, *IEEE Transactions on Ultrasonics, Ferroelectrics and Frequency Control*, Vol. 47 (No. 50), pp.1259-1272

Misaridis, T. & Jensen, J. A. (2005). Use of Modulated Excitation Signals in Medical Ulltrasound. *IEEE Transactions on Ultrasonics, Ferroelectrics and Frequency Control*, Vol. 52, pp.177-219

Song, J., Kim, S., Sohn, H., Song & T., Yoo, Y. M. (2010). Coded Excitation for Ultrasound Tissue Harmonic Imaging, *Ultrasonics*, Vol. 50, pp.613-619

Tanabe, M., Okubo, K., Tagawa & N., Moriya, T. (2008). Inline Transmitter/Receiver System Using $Pb(Zn_{1/3}Nb_{2/3})O_3-PbTiO_3$ Single Crystal and Poly(Vinylidene Fluoride) for Harmonic Pulse Compression Imaging, *Japanese Journal of Applied Physics*, Vol. 47, pp.4149-4154

Tanabe, M., Yamamura, T., Okubo, K. & Tagawa, N. (2010). Medical Ultrasound Imaging Using Pulse Compression Technique Based on Split and Merge Strategy, *Japanese Journal of Applied Physics*, Vol. 49, pp.07HF15·1-07HF15·5

7

Ultrasonic Measurement and Imaging with Lateral Modulation – Echo, Tissue Motion and Elasticity

Chikayoshi Sumi
Sophia University
Japan

1. Introduction

It is remarkable that the pathological state of human soft tissues highly correlates with static and low-frequency mechanical properties, particularly shear elasticity (e.g., Sumi, 2005d). Accordingly, we have been developing ultrasonic (US)-strain-measurement-based one-dimensional (1D) (Sumi et al., 1993, 1995a, 2010f; Sumi, 1999b, 2005d, 2008a, 2010d; Sumi & Matsuzawa, 2007b), 2D (Sumi et al., 1993, 1995a; Sumi, 1999c, 2005d, 2006b, 2007g, 2008a, 2008c, 2010d) and 3D (Sumi, 1999c, 2005d, 2006b, 2007g, 2010d) shear or Young modulus reconstruction/imaging techniques as differential diagnostic tools for deseases of various *in vivo* tissues, such as the breast (Sumi, 1999a, 2005b, 2005d; Sumi & Matsuzawa 2007b; Sumi et al., 1995b(strain), 1996, 1997, 1999b, 2000b) and liver (Sumi et al., 2001a, 2001b; Sumi, 2005d), i.e., cancerous deseases etc. Other soft tissues such as heart or blood vessel are also our targets, i.e., myocardinal infraction, atherosclerosis etc. After the first report of the differential type inverse problem of shear modulus by Sumi (1993, 1995a), immediately the results obtained on agar phantoms [e.g., Sumi et al., 1994a(strain & shear modulus), 1994b, 1995d], *in vivo* breasts (e.g., Sumi et al., 1995b, 1996, 1997; Sumi, 1999a, 1999b) and *in vivo* liver (e.g., Sumi et al., 2000a, 2001a, 2001b; Sumi 2005d) were reported. For such *in vivo* tissues, a suitable combination of simple, minimally invasive therapy techniques such as chemotherapy, cryotherapy, and thermal therapy (e.g., Sumi, 2005d; Sumi et al., 2001a) etc with our reconstruction techniques would lead to an innovative, new clinical strategy that would enable differential diagnosis followed by immediate treatment so that overall medical expenses could be substantially reduced (Sumi, 2005d). This is because our developed techniques allow non-invasive confirming of a treatment effectiveness in real-time, i.e., a degeneration. Our early reports on the interstitial rf/micro wave thermal coagulation thrapy are Sumi et al., 2000a, 2001b; Sumi, 2005d, etc.

In the respective 1D, 2D and 3D techniques, a 1D (axial) displacement field, and 2D and 3D displacement vector fields generated by compression, vibration, heart motion, radiation force etc are measured to obtain 1D (axial) strain, and 2D and 3D strain tensor fields by partial differentiation. Many other researchers are also developing shear modulus reconstruction methods (e.g., Kallel & Bertrand, 1996; Plewes et al., 2000; Doyley et al., 2005) based on various displacement/strain measurement methods, e.g., conventional 1D Doppler method (Wilson & Robinson, 1982) and 1D autocorrelation method (1D AM) (Kasai et al.,

1985; Loupas et al., 1995) for blood flow measurement, and 1D (Ophir et al., 1991) or multidimensional (Yagi & Nakayama, 1988; Bohs & Trahey, 1991) crosscorrelation method (CCM). Now, various tissue motion and elasticity measurement/imaging have been performed over the world (see also references in Sumi et al., 2008i). In our case, other low frequency mechanical properties or quantities can also be reconstrcuted or measured, e.g., Poisson's ratio or Bulk modulus (Sumi, 2006b), density or inertia (Sumi, 2006b,2010d), viscoelasticity (e.g., Sumi, 2005d; Sumi et al., 2005a) and mechanical source (e.g., Sumi & Suekane, 2009e). Fluid such as blood is also our target (Sumi & Suekane, 2009e). These methods will also be used for a non-destructive evaluation, e.g., food engineering etc.

Previosuly, we reported a multidimensional phase matching method (Sumi et al., 1995d; Sumi, 1999a, 2008b) together with three novel methods of measuring *a multidimensional displacement vector* using a US signal phase, i.e., the multidimensional cross-spectrum phase gradient method (MCSPGM) (Sumi et al., 1995d; Sumi, 1999a, 2008b), multidimensional autocorrelation method (MAM) (Sumi, 2002c, 2005c, 2008b) and multidimensional Doppler method (MDM) (Sumi, 2002c, 2005c, 2008b). These methods can be applied to the measurement of the tissue strain tensor for above-mentioned shear modulus reconstruction (breast, liver, heart etc.), blood flow vector, sonar data, and other target motions. That is, the multidimensional phase matching allows coping with the decorrelation generated by out-of-motion from a beam or a 2D frame. Although the CCM requires the numerical interpolation of the crosscorrelation function using cosine, parabolic functions, etc to yield analogue displacement vector data, our developed multidimensional methods do not require such interpolation. That is, these methods require only sampled echo data and then do not suffer any artifact errors due to such interpolation. Specifically, in MCSPGM (Sumi et al., 1995d; Sumi, 1999a, 2008b), a local displacement vector is estimated using the local echo phase characteristics, i.e., from the gradient of the phase of the local cross-spectrum evaluated from the local region echo data. In contrast, the other two methods use an instantaneous US phase (Sumi, 2002c, 2005c, 2008b). By performing the multidimensional phase matching using a coarsely measured displacement data by a multidimensional cross-correlation method (MCCM) (Sumi et al., 1995d; Sumi, 1999a, 2008b) or MCSPGM using sampled echo data spatially thinned out (Sumi, 2005d, 2008b), all the methods enable *simultaneous* axial, lateral and elevational displacement measurements. The multidimensional phase matching method can cope with the decorrelation of local echo data and aliasing that occurs due to a large displacement, i.e., by searching for corresponding local echo data. Significantly, this phase matching method improves the measurement accuracies of multidimensional methods. As shown by simulations (Sumi, 2008b), the accuracies of the multidimensional displacement vector measurement methods are comparable; however, MAM and MDM require less computational time (particularly, MDM) than MCSPGM.

Generally, when using such displacement vector measurement methods, the measurement accuracy of lateral displacement was lower than that of axial displacement (Sumi et al, 1995d; Sumi, 1999a, 1999c, 2005c, 2008b; Sumi & Sato, 2007c; Sumi & Ebisawa, 2009a). Even if the target dominantly moves or becomes deformed in the lateral direction, our simultaneous measurements using the multidimensional phase matching result in the accurate measurement of axial displacement (Sumi, 2007f; Sumi et al., 1995b, 1995c). The multidimensional phase matching method also enabled us the high accuracy manual axial strain measurement (e.g., for breast, Sumi, 2005b, 2005d; Sumi & Matsuzawa, 2007b; Sumi et al., 1995b, 1996, 1997, 1999b, 2000b; liver, Sumi et al., 2001a, 2005d; others). By Sumi (1995b), the manual strain measurement was made possible by using multidimensional rf-echo

phase matching (cf. the first reports of shear modulus reconstrcution on *in vivo* beast, Sumi et al., 1996 and 1997; liver, Sumi et al., 2001b). Over the world, such an axial strain measurement/imaging by a manual axial compression using a US transducer has been clinically used. The modality is called as *Elastography* as named by Ophir (Ophir et al., 1991; Cespedes et al., 1993; Garra et al., 1997). Although the mesurement accuracy is significantly lower, some convetional 1D displacement measurement methods are also used instead of the multidimensional methods (e.g., Sumi 1999c; Sumi & Ebisawa, 2009a), i.e., ones originally used only for an axial displacement measurement along the axial direction. (e.g., Loupas at al., 1995; AM by Yamakawa & Shiina, 2001).
In our case, the measuement of axial strains generated by the axial compression or an arbitrary mechanical source are used for a multidimensional imaging of 1D reconstrcution (Sumi et al., 1993, 1995a, 2010f; Sumi, 1999c, 2005d, 2008a, 2010d; Sumi & Matsuzawa, 2007b). On the basis of the calculation of an axial strain ratio, several 1D reconstrcution methods were developed by Sumi. When the measurement accuracy of the axial strain is low, e.g., during thermal treatment (Sumi, 2005d; Sumi et al., 2001a), being dependent of the accuracy at each position, our developed *spatially-variant regularization* is performed for the strain measurement (Sumi & Sato, 2008c) or shear modulus reconstrcution (Sumi, 2008e; Sumi & Itoh, 2010e), i.e., an application of our developd implicit-integration (Sumi, 1998). That is, the measurement and reconstruction are stabilized to cope with the echo noise and strain measurement noise, respectively. For a focal lesion, by properly setting a reference region of shear modulus for the 1D reconsrcution, the 1D reconstruction allows yielding a higher contrast-to-noise ratio (CNR) than the axial strain (Sumi, 2005d; Sumi & Matsuzawa, 2007b; Sumi et al., 2010f). That is, the reference region should be set in the stress-concentrated or stress weak region in front of or behind the target stiff or soft lesion such that the reference region extends in the direction orthogonal to that of the dominant tissue deformation (Sumi, 2005b; Sumi & Matsuzawa, 2007b; Sumi et al., 1995d, 2010f). In addition, a mechanical source should be realized such that the target tissue deforms dominantly in a direction that extends in the direction of much shear-modulus varying (e.g. Sumi et al., 2010f). For the 1D strain measurement/imaging and 1D reconstruction, strain in the dominat deformation direction generated should be measured (e.g. Sumi & Ebisawa, 2009a). Moreover, for the practical imaging of 1D reconstruction, although human perception with respect to gray (negative or positive) scales and color scales must also be considered together with actual tissue shear modulus distributions, optimal displaying could be achieved by determining if the relative shear modulus or the inverse of the relative shear modulus should be imaged on the basis of their CNRs calculated using a stationary statistics of measured strains in the focal lesion and the surrounding region (Sumi et al., 2010f). Although the techniques for shear modulus reconstrcution methods including strain tensor calculations, multidimensional shear modulus reconstructions and the regularizations mentioned (Sumi, 1998, 2005d, 2006b, 2007g, 2008a, 2008e; Sumi & Sato, 2008c; Sumi & Itoh, 2010e) cannot be reviewed in detail in this chapter due to the limitation of the space, the important multidimensional phase matching is reviewed later (section 2.1).
However, if the lateral and elevational displacements can be measured with the same degree of an accuracy as that of the axial displacement, manual strain measurement and shear modulus reconstruction can be performed without considering the direction of the beam and target motion or mechanical source with the position (Sumi, 1999c, 2002a, 2002b, 2008a; Sumi et al., 2007e, 2008f, 2008i). That is, for an arbitrary mechanical source, 3D or 2D measurement/reconstruction with only attachment of the US transducer enables such

measurement and reconstruction. Clinically, such a measurement will enable the evaluation of the elasticity of more various tissues, e.g., under normal motion such as the heart, arm and leg muscles (during exercise) and even for the deep ROIs such as liver tissues, which are inaccessible from the body surface and normally deformed by heart motion or pulsation. Various possible configurations will increase the applications of the tissue motion measurement and mechanical property reconstrcutions.

For the blood flow vector measurement, a high accuracy displacement vector measurement had been performed (Jensen, 1998, 2001; Anderson, 1998, 2000) using a lateral oscillating method obtained by using Fraunhofer approximation (Steinberg, 1976; Goodman, 1996) together with some conventional 1D displacement measurement methods in respective axial and lateral directions, i.e., ones are originally used only for an axial displacement measurement along the axial direction. The measurement of blood flow in vessels running parallel to the surface of the body had been achieved. The method enabled the measurement of the lateral displacement/velocity that was more accurate than the use of the change in bandwidth (Newhouse, 1987).

The method falls in a category of the lateral modulation (LM) approach Sumi called (Sumi, 2002c, 2005c, 2005d). The LM was resolved by Sumi as the more simple beamforming that uses a coherent superimposition of steered, crossed beams (Sumi, 2002a, 2008a, 2008b; Sumi et al., 2008f, 2008i).

In the field of strain tensor measurement, the LM approach was applied first by Sumi (Sumi, 2004). For our tissue shear modulus reconstruction, to realize comparable high measurement accuracies of axial, lateral and elevational displacements, lateral and elevational modulation frequencies had to be significantly increased (Sumi, 2004, 2005c) compared with that observed in the reported application to the blood flow vector (Jensen, 1998, 2001; Anderson, 1998, 2000) and other tissue strain tensor (Liebgott et al., 2005) measurements (modulation frequency, 2.5 vs 1 mm^{-1}). This is because the strain tensor is obtained by differentiating the measured displacement vector components using a differential filter (i.e., a kind of high pass filter), the displacement vector must be measured with a considerable high accuracy. Deeply situated tissues must also be considered (e.g., liver). By Sumi (2005c, 2008b), a spherical focusing was obtained as a suitable focusing. Moreover, to increase the measurement accuracy, only a digital processing was used for obtaining plural multidimensional analytic signals (Sumi, 2002c, 2005c, 2008b). Moreover, it was confirmed that our developed LM methods are useful for imaging of the spatial difstribution of US reflectivity, i.e., echo imaging (Sumi, 2008a; Sumi et al., 2008f, 2008i). That is, a high resolution can be achieved in lateral and elevational directions as almost the same as that in the axial direction. Thus, it is expected that LM will lead to a next-generation US diagnosis equipped with various new modes such as displacement/velocity vector, strain tensor measrements and thier applications.

Although the LM methods developed by other groups (Jensen, 1998, 2001; Anderson, 1998, 2000; Liebgott, 2005) yield band-unlimited, modulated spectra by using infinite-length apodization functions (e.g., ringing-expressed by sinc functions), our developed lateral Gaussian envelope cosine modulation (LGECM) method realizes band-limited, modulated spectra, i.e., by using a finite length (not ringing) apodization function (Sumi, 2005c, 2008b). This does not cause aliasing. Moreover, for the blood flow vector measurement (Jensen, 1998, 2001; Anderson, 1998, 2000) and other strain tensor measuement (Liebgott et al., 2005), the respective measurements of axial and lateral displacements are performed using a conventional 1D displacement measurement method by realizing point spread functions

(PSF's) oscillating only in the lateral direction and only in the axial direction through a demodulation. Although we also developed a new accurate demodulation method only using digital signal processing (Sumi, 2010g), all the measurements suffer from the decorrelation of echo signals due to displacement orthogonal to the oscillation direction (Sumi, 2008b; Sumi & Shimizu, 2011). However, the highest accuracy in measuring target motions can be achieved by combined use (Sumi, 2002c, 2005c, 2008a, 2008b; Sumi et al., 2008f, 2008i) of the LM approach and our developed displacement vector measurement methods that enable *simultaneous* axial and lateral displacement measurements (Sumi et al., 1995d, 2002c; Sumi, 1999a, 2008b, 2005c). Not only our developed measurement increases the measurement accuracy of lateral displacements but also that of axial displacement (Sumi, 2005c, 2008b).

Our developed LM can be performed by superimposition of the simultaneously or successively transmitted/received, plural steered beams or frames with different steering angles obtained with the multiple transmission method (MTM, Sumi, 2002a, 2005d; Fox, 1978; Techavipoo, 2004). Alternatively, LM can also be realized from a set of received echo data (Sumi, 2008b; Sumi et al, 2008f, 2008i) using not a classical synthetic aperture but our previously developed multidirectional synthetic aperture method (MDSAM, e.g., Sumi, 2002a, 2005d; Tanter, 2002). That is, the aperture is synthesized in multidirections after receiving US signals. Because MDSAM requires less data acquisition time than MTM using successive US beam transmissions, if the transmitted US energies are sufficient, the beamforming suffers the less tissue motion artifact. To obtain high intensity transmitted US signals, a virtual source can be used (Sumi et al., 2010h). However, if tissue motion artifacts do not occur, MTM yields more accurate measurements. With this type of beamforming, multiple transducers can also be used (Sumi, 2008b; Sumi et al, 2008f, 2008i), e.g., when dealing with heart motion due to the existence of the obstacles such as bones. On the evaluations of statitics of measured strain tensor components and reconstructed relative shear modulus in a stiff inclusion of an agar phantom, accurate measurements and reconstructions were obtained (e.g., see Table I in Sumi, 2008f; Table VIII in Sumi, 2008i).

Alternatively, with MTM (Fox, 1978; Sumi, 2002a, 2005d; Techavipoo, 2004) and MDSAM (Sumi, 2002a, 2008b; Tanter, 2002), only the most accurately measured axial displacements from the respective beams obtained was used to obtain a displacement vector (i.e., there is no superimposition of beams). Although 1D measurement methods can also be used (Fox, 1978; Sumi, 2002a, 2005d; Tanter, 2002; Techavipoo, 2004) in place of the multidimensional measurement methods (Sumi, 2002a, 2008b), the same decorrelation of local echo signals (mentioned above) occurs due to target displacement in a direction orthogonal to the beams (Sumi et al., 1995d; Sumi, 2008b). Thus, the 1D measurement methods will result in a lower measurement accuracy than the corresponding multidimensional measurement methods, i.e., the 1D cross-spectrum phase gradient method (1D CSPGM) (Sumi et al., 1995d; Sumi, 1999a), conventional 1D AM (Kasai et al., 1985; Loupas et al., 1995), 1D DM (Sumi, 2008b), and 1D CCM (Ophir et al., 1991). Thus, not conventional 1D axial displacement measurement methods (e.g., 1D AM) but multidimensional displacement vector measurement methods should be used. Also for these beamformings, if necessary, separate plural transducers are also used simultaneously or successively.

However, under conditions in which motion artifacts do not occur, our previous comparison (Sumi, 2008b) of LM (or coherent superimposition) and non-superimposition methods by geometrical evaluations clarifies that the LM has the potential to yield more accurate measurements of axial and lateral displacements with less computational time.

However, for practical beamforming applications, the echo SNRs from steered beams must also be considered, i.e., an overly large steered angle makes the echo SNR low (Sumi et al., 2008i).
Moreover, LGECM method was improved using parabolic functions or Hanning windows instead of Gaussian functions in the apodization function. Hereafter, the new methods are respectively referred to as the parabolic modulation (PAM) method or Hanning modulation (HAM) method (Sumi, 2008a; Sumi et al., 2008i). Particularly, PAM enables decreases in effective aperture length (i.e., channels) and yield more accurate displacement vector measurements than LGECM. Although the Fourier transform of a parabolic function results in ringing effects, the new modulation yields no ringing effects in the spectra. PAM also yields a high spatial resolution in the reflectivity (echo) imaging with a high echo signal-to-noise ratio (SNR). Thus, we stop using the Fraunhofer approximation for LM. PAM is obtained on the basis of the *a priori* knowledge of the differences in the focusing scheme and shape between the parabolic function, Hanning window and Gaussian function, and the effects on the decays of the US signals during the propagation. That is, the US energy of the feet is lost during the US propagation and the main lobe contributes to echo signals, the mountains in the apodization functions should have a large full width at half maximum (FWHM) and short feet. Thus, we suceeded in a breakway from the Fraunhofer approximation (Sumi et al., 2006a).
Usually, for US imaging, US beam-forming parameters such as frequency, bandwidth, pulse shape, effective aperture size, and apodization function are designed and set appropriately. In addition, US transducer parameters such as the size and materials of the US array element used are also set appropriately. In determining such settings, the US properties of the target are also be considered (e.g., attenuation and scattering). Thus, all parameters are set appropriately for the consideration of a system that involves the US properties of the target. Previously, we proposed to set such parameters in order to realize the required PSF for LM on the basis of optimization theory by using the minimum norm least-squares estimation method (Sumi et al., 2006a; Sumi, 2007d, 2010a). The better envelope shape of the PSF than that of the PA is searched for on the basis of the knowledge of the ideal shape of PSF, i.e., having a large FWHM and short feet (e.g., Sumi et al., 2010c). Nonlinear optimization is also effective to yield such a proper PSF (Sumi et al., 2009c). Although conventional US beam-forming parameters are usually set on the basis of the experience of an engineer, our proposed method realizes the best possible beam-former using optimally determined parameters. Thus, spatial resolution and echo SNR are improved.
Although the optimized parameter can also be used, in this chapeter, PAM and LGECM are performed because they can be analytically obtained (Sumi et al., 2008i). As mentioned above, it was confirmed through simulations that when echo SNR is high (SNR $\approx$ 20 dB), MAM yields a higher accuracy measurement than MDM and vice versa (Sumi, 2008b). Here, the 2D demonstrations are shown on agar phantom that was statically compressed dominantly in a lateral direction (Sumi et al., 2008f), displacement of which cannot be accurately measured by a conventional beamforming. In addition, 2D shear modulus reconstrcutions are also shown together with strain tensor measurements.
In this chapeter, after reviewing our developed phase matching, PAM and LGECM, and MAM and MDM (section 2), the images and measurements obtained on an agar phantom are shown (section 3). Comparisons of the spatial resolution of the US images are made and the accuracies of the measured displacement vectors and elasticity (i.e., strain, shear modulus) are determined. Finally, discussions and future problems are provided with conclusions.

2. Brief reviews

2.1 Phase matching

To cope with the occurrence of decorrelation due to target motion and echo noise, we proposed the iterative phase matching method (Sumi et al., 1995d, 1999a, 2008b), i.e., the iterative search method for corresponding local region echo data. The search can be realized in spatial and spatial frequency domains using the estimate of the displacement vector obtained by a displacement vector measurement method or using *a priori* data of compression/stretching etc., i.e., by shifting echo data in a spatial domain or by multiplying a complex exponential by echo data in a spatial frequency domain using the estimate. First, this search method was used to increase the measurement accuracy of MCSPGM (e.g., Sumi et al., 1995d; Sumi, 1999a) using the estimate obtained by MCSPGM or MCCM. Here, we note that, strict echo compression/stretching can also be realized in the phase matching by setting a corresponding echo data in the local region using measured displacements and strains (Sumi, 2008b), whereas the effectiveness of the local echo compression/stretching is reported by Srinivasan et al. (2002). In the first phase matching, the estimate obtained at the adjacent point can be used to reduce the number of iterations of phase matching.

This phase matching method can also be used for MAM and MDM to increase measurement accuracy (Sumi, 2008b). That is, for MAM, this method enables the increase in the accuracy of instantaneous phase change and instantaneous spatial frequencies by improving the correlation of the local complex correlation function, whereas for MDM, this method enables the increase in their accuracy by increasing that of the temporal derivative in the Taylor expansion of the instantaneous phase of the complex signal. During the iterative phase matching, the moving-average width decreases as the local region size of MCSPGM decreases (Sumi, 1999a). This enables the increase in spatial resolution. Moreover, this increases the accuracy of strain measurement because the estimation accuracies of the instantaneous phase change and instantaneous spatial frequencies are improved due to their being not constant. If there exists no noise in echo data, the moving averaging is not needed and only phase matching should be performed. LM increases the convergence speed of the phase matching (Sumi, 2008b).

Thus, various applications of the actual axial strain measurements have been reported using axial (Cespedes et al., 1993; Garra et al., 1997) and multidimensional (Sumi et al., 1995b) displacement measurements, e.g., diagnosis of cancers of human *in vivo* breasts (Cespedes et al., 1993; Sumi et al., 1995b; Garra et al., 1997) and monitoring various low-invasive treatments such as interstitial rf/micro wave coagulation therapies of an *in vivo* liver carcinoma (Sumi et al., 2000a, 2001a, 2001b, 2005a, Sumi, 2002b, 2005d, 2007a). By Sumi (1995b), the manual strain measurement was made possible by using multidimensional rf-echo phase matching (Sumi et al., 1995d). These were achieved without any regularizations nor LMs.

However, reports of actual shear modulus reconstruction using measured strain tensor distributions are few with the exception of our reports (e.g., Sumi, 2007a, 2008a, 2008e; Sumi & Sato, 2008c; Sumi & Itoh, 2010e using the regularizations for strain measurement or shear modulus reconstrcution; Sumi, 2008a; Sumi et al., 2008f, 2008i using LM) and the reconstruction using a measured axial displacement distribution (e.g., Doyley et al., 2005 using another regularization for Young modulus). Specifically, we reported 2D direct shear modulus reconstruction using regularized strain tensor measurement (Sumi & Sato, 2008c; Sumi & Itoh, 2009b) as well as regularized direct 1D shear modulus reconstruction (Sumi, 2008e; Sumi & Itoh, 2010e; Sumi, 2007a) using raw strain tensor measurement. These reconstructions were stably performed for agar phantoms by using our developed regularization, i.e., *spatially variant regularization* being dependent of the accuracies at each position of the measured strain tensor components. Because the measurement accuracy depends on the direction of the displacement, according to the accuracies of the respective displacements, they are also properly regularized, i.e., referred to as *displacement component-dependent regularization* or *directional-dependent regularization* (Sumi & Sato, 2008c; Sumi & Itoh, 2009b). As briefly reviewed in section 1, various 1D reconstructions using the axial strain were also obtained by Sumi for human *in vivo* tissues when the targets become deformed in the axial and lateral directions, respectively. By Sumi, in addition to the report (2008e), the regularizations were also performed (2005d; 2007a) for the strain measurement or shear modulus reconstrcution before, during and after the *in vivo* thermal coagulation treatment. However, simulations revealed that the 1D reconstrcutions such as strain ratio, implicit-integration etc lead to the inaccurate value of reconstrcution and geometrical artifact even if there exists no noise in the axial strain data used (Sumi, 2005d; Sumi & Matsuzawa, 2007b). Moreover, when the target deforms in the lateral direction, the 1D reconstruction further decreases the accuracy in reconstrcution (Sumi, 2007f). Moreover, for the 2D reconstruction, the use of only the regularizations still yields an inaccurate reconstruction (Sumi & Sato, 2008c; Sumi & Itoh, 2009b). Thus, LM was also used later (Sumi, 2008a; Sumi et al., 2008f, 2008i).

2.2 Complex signals with different single-octant and different single-quadrant spectra

Both the multidimensional autocorrelation method (MAM) and multidimensional Doppler method (MDM) use the instantaneous US signal phase (Sumi, 2002c, 2005c, 2008b). To measure a three-dimensional (3D) displacement vector (u_x,u_y,u_z), three or four 3D complex signals with different single-octant spectra (Fig. 1a reported by Sumi, 2008b) that extend analytic signals are calculated for respective echo data r_1(x,y,z) and r_2(x,y,z) obtained before and after a pulse repetition interval Δt, i.e., r_{c1i}(x,y,z) and r_{c2i}(x,y,z) [i = 1,..,3 or 1,..,4]. The multidimensional complex signal having single-orthant spectra was introduced by Hahn (1992) [1D complex signal phase and instantaneous frequency are specifically described in a literature by Bracewell (1986)].

Each 3D complex signal obtained has three instantaneous spatial frequencies, i.e., US frequency fx, lateral frequency fy and elevational frequency fz. Hereafter, (fx,fy,fz) is referred to as a frequency vector. When lateral and elevational modulations are performed, fy and fz are respectively the lateral and elevational modulation frequencies, whereas when lateral and elevational modulations are not performed (i.e., beam-steering is not performed), fy and fz are respectively yielded by synthesizing the lateral (Sumi 2002a, 2002c; Chen et al., 2004) and elevational phases (but, the frequencies are low and then the measurement accuracy is lower than that of LM [Sumi et al., 2010g; Sumi et al., 2010i; 2006c; Sumi & Shimizu, 20011]). Thus, as described next, an equation regarding with the unknown displacement vector (u_x,u_y,u_z) is derived from each pair of complex signals r_{1ci}(x,y,z) and r_{2ci}(x,y,z) having a same frequency vector (fx,fy,fz) [i = 1,..,3 or 1,..,4], and then the displacement vector (u_x,u_y,u_z) can be obtained by simultaneously solving the three or four independent equations having the independent vectors (fx,fy,fz) as the coefficients. The three equations can be arbitrary chosen from the four equations. To mitigate the calculation errors of the instantaneous phases and frequencies, the least-squares method can also be used to solve all the four equations simultaneously.

Measuring a 2D displacement vector requires calculating two 2D complex signals with different single-quadrant spectra (Hahn, 1992) (Fig. 1b reported by Sumi, 2008i) and then solving two correspondingly derived simultaneous equations.

2.3 LCMs (Lateral Cosine Modulation Methods) using PAM, HAM and LGECM and optimizations

For respective PAM (Sumi, 2007d, 2008a, Sumi et al., 2008f, 2008i) and LGECM (Sumi, 2005c, 2008a, 2008b; Sumi et al., 2008f, 2008i) using a one-dimensional (1D) linear array-type transducer (lateral direction, y), the following apodization functions are used for the transmission or reception of US, i.e.,

$$\frac{1}{2\lambda x}\{\exp[-\frac{(2\pi)^2(\frac{y}{\lambda x}+f_y+f_a)^2(\frac{\sigma_y}{a})^2}{2}]+\exp[-\frac{(2\pi)^2(\frac{y}{\lambda x}-f_y-f_a)^2(\frac{\sigma_y}{a})^2}{2}]\} \tag{1}$$

and

$$\frac{1}{2\lambda x}\{[-\frac{4}{9}(\frac{\sigma_y}{a})^2\pi^2\left(\frac{y}{\lambda x}+f_y+f_a\right)^2+1]+[-\frac{4}{9}(\frac{\sigma_y}{a})^2\pi^2\left(\frac{y}{\lambda x}-f_y-f_a\right)^2+1]\}. \tag{2}$$

The apodization functions are superimpositions of two Gaussian functions and two parabolic functions. The apodization obtained for 20, 30, 60 and 100 mm depths are shown in Fig. 2 in the report by Sumi (2008b). HAM is also described by Sumi (2008i). These apodization functions are obtained using the Fraunhofer approximation such that the transmitted US energy used are same when realizing the Gaussian-type lateral PSF at a depth x for US with a wavelength λ, i.e.,

$$\exp(-\frac{y^2}{2\sigma_y^2})\cos(2\pi f_y y). \tag{3}$$

Here, f_y is the lateral modulation frequency and σ y corresponds to the lateral beam width for LGECM. f_a and a are parameters introduced to regulate lateral modulation frequency and bandwidth, respectively. For comparisons of FWHM and feet length, the Guassian and parabolic functions that have the same area are shown in Fig. 1c in the report by Sumi et al. (2008i).

The apodization functions for two-dimensional (2D) modulation (i.e., modulations in two directions y and z) using a 2D array-type transducer are also obtained for PAM and LGECM in a similar fashion (Sumi, 2005c; Sumi et al., 2008f, 2008i). According to the type of transducer (e.g., convex), other arbitrary orthogonal coordinates can also be used. When steered beams cannot be transmitted symmetrically in a lateral direction due to the existence of the obstacles such as a bone (for heart, liver etc), the original coordinate can be rotated such that the steered beams become laterally symmetric. However, our developed MCSPGM, MAM and MDM can yield measurement results even if the coordinate is not set in such a way, and the measurement accuracy in a displacement vector will be increased by the fact that the measurement accuracy of a lateral displacement can be significantly improved (Sumi, 2010g; 2010i). Such a rotation also allows the use of our developed demodulation method with one of conventional 1D displacement measurement methods.

When carrying out PAM, HAM or LGECM, Methods 1 and 2 developed for transmission/reception focussing are used (Sumi, 2005c, 2007d, 2008a, 2008b; Sumi et al., 2008i, 2008f). The Methods used for LCM are also reviewed in this section. Both Methods 1 and 2 yield twofold lateral modulation frequency (Sumi, 2004, 2008b) compared with a method that performs only a receiving modulation, i.e., the method using a non-steered plane wave for a transmission with a rectangular window, Bingham window, Hanning window or Gaussian function as the apodization function (Jensen et al., 1998; Anderson, 1998. Also both Methods 1 and 2 enable decreases in effective aperture length (i.e., channels). When using LGECM method together with Method 1, the following PSF would be realized, i.e.,

$$\exp\left(-\frac{y^2}{2(\sigma_y/\sqrt{2})^2}\right)\cos\left[2\pi\left(2f_y\right)y\right]. \tag{4}$$

Different from Method 2, Method 1 also enables an increase in lateral bandwidth compared with the method that performs only a receiving modulation. For both methods, a low-frequency envelope signal must also be removed. By Basarab (2007), a twofold frequency sine modulation (i.e., not LCM) is carried out. However, the modulation is not appropriate for US imaging and measurement of displacement. This can be easily understood by assuming the existence of a point reflection target in the region of interest (ROI).

Method 1: (i) When a point of interest is dealt with, twofold frequency modulation can be performed using the same lateral modulation apodization (i.e., PAM) and spherical focusing in transmitting/receiving beam-forming as in conventional beam-forming (Sumi, 2004, 2008b). For 2D displacement vector measurement, two steered beams are used, whereas for 3D displacement vector measurement, three or four steered beams are used. These beams can be simulataneously transmitted. Alternatively, they can be superimposed after transmitting and receiving the respective beams successively. To obtain the steered beams, mechanical scans can also be performed. Plural transducers can also be used. When a finite ROI is dealt with, multiple transmitting modulations may also be useful for so-called multiple transmitting focusing. (ii) When performing a twofold frequency modulation over a finite ROI, the classical synthesis of an aperture (i.e., a monostatic or multistatic synthetic aperture) can also be carried out. However, if the target motion is rapid, a motional artifact may occur due to the low US energy transmitted from an element. In such a case, low-SNR echo modulation may be achieved. To increase the echo SNR, virtual sources can be used (e.g., Sumi and Uga, 2010h).

By performing a modulation using (i) or (ii), LGECM theoretically yields $\sqrt{2}$ times as wide a lateral bandwidth as that yielded by a method that performs only a receiving modulation (theoretically, the beam width becomes $\sigma y/\sqrt{2}$). Similarly, when performing other modulations such as PAM and HAM, an increase in lateral bandwidth is also achieved. Thus, using the same effective aperture width (i.e., the same number of channels), Method 1 realizes twofold lateral modulation frequency and a wide lateral bandwidth. The same lateral modulation frequency and lateral bandwidth can also be obtained by using a small effective aperture width (i.e., fewer channels).

Method 2: When dealing with a finite ROI, transmissions of steered two laterally wide plane waves that are realized simultaneously or successively with the same steering angles as those used in the receiving modulation can also be performed, of which apodizations are also properly performed. Although Method 2 cannot increase the lateral bandwidth, it is useful because the measurement accuracies of MCSPGM, MAM, and MDM are more sensitive to US and modulation frequencies than the axial and lateral bandwidths, particularly when measuring a rigid motion (Sumi, 2008b). Method 2 realizes a more rapid echo modulation than Method 1. Thus, Method 2 is also robust against tissue motion during echo data acquisition. Similarly to Method 1, plural transducers can be used.

The combinations of PAM, HAM, and LGECM with Methods 1 and 2 are examined in reports by Sumi, 2007d, 2008a; Sumi et al., 2008i by simulations and agar phantom experiments. For all the combinations, by increasing the lateral modulation frequency (i.e., steering angles) to some extent, the echo SNR decreases due to improper beam-forming. For instance, when using a transducer for an agar phantom as that used in section 3, a modulation with the same frequency as that of US has a low echo SNR. The highest effective modulation frequency is determined by the US frequency and the transducer (e.g., element size). For the combinations, the echo SNRs were evaluated using the US echos, PSF values (see appendicies in reports by Sumi et al., 2008f, 2008i), or PSF energy (i.e., within a bandwidth). When using MAM for the phantom, the modulations at half the US frequency enabled accurate measurements of displacement vectors and elasticity, i.e., strain tensor and shear modulus. In addition, Methods 1 and 2 (i.e., twofold frequency modulations) yielded higher echo SNRs than the method that performs only receiving modulation, even if the same modulation frequency was realized by using a large effective aperture size and large steering angles.

Specifically, the order of echo SNRs obtained was PAM > LGECM when using Method 1 (Sumi, 2007d, 2008a; Sumi et al., 2008i). Moreover, PAM yields a wider lateral bandwidth than LGECM for the same effective aperture size. HAM yields almost the same results as LGECM, although the effective aperture size can be substantially decreased. As revealed in reports by Sumi, 2007d, 2008a, 2008b; Sumi et al., 2008i, compared with spherical focusing (Sumi, 2004), the use of plane waves decreases the achievable modulation frequency (Sumi, 2008b) and the echo SNR (Sumi, 2007d, 2008a; Sumi et al., 2008i). In addition, the use of plane waves also makes it difficult to deal with a deeply situated ROI. Thus, Method 1 yielded higher echo SNRs than Method 2 that uses two plane waves for transmission of US. However, in Method 2, the order of echo SNRs was inverted, i.e., LGECM > PAM (Sumi, 2007d, 2008a; Sumi et al., 2008i). This can be understood by considering the shapes of the apodization functions. The shape of the parabolic function is more similar to the rectangular function than to the Gaussian function (i.e., the Gaussian function has long feet, whereas the parabolic function has a wide main lobe).

To obtain a higher quality US image (i.e., an image with a high echo SNR and high or uniform spatial resolution) and to realize more accurate measurements of blood vector flow and elasticity, we have also conducted the determination of optimal beam-forming parameters as mentioned in section 1 (e.g., Sumi et al, 2006a, 2009c, 2010c; Sumi, 2007d, 2010a). For the optimization, the beam property of one element must be obtained in advance, analytically, numerically, or experimentally, as a function of the parameters. Because the synthesized US beam can be considered as a linear-weighted superimposition of the beams transmitted widely or received at the respective elements with suitable delays for focusing, we obtain simultaneous linear equations involving the unknown apodization function vector $\mathbf{x}$, a matrix $\mathbf{A}$ comprising the US beam values transmitted to an ROI from the respective elements of the US array, and a vector $\mathbf{b}$ comprising the designed PSF values in the ROI (i.e., $\mathbf{Ax} = \mathbf{b}$). However, because the independence of the rows of matrix $\mathbf{A}$ is low, the vector $\mathbf{x}$ must be determined stably by obtaining the inverse of $\mathbf{A}$ using singular-value decomposition (SVD: Sumi, 2008d), a weighted minimum-norm least-squares solution (WMNLSQ: Sumi, 2007d, 2010a), regularization (Sumi, 2007d, 2010a) or nonlinear optimization (Sumi et al., 2009c). As far, a new analytic function that is expressed using a direct current and a power function divided has been obtained as the better PSF (Sumi et al., 2008g, 2009d, 2010c). The uses of the optimally determined apodization functions are beyond the scope of this paper.

2.4 MAM and MDM

Both the multidimensional autocorrelation method (MAM) and multidimensional Doppler method (MDM) use the instantaneous US signal phase (Sumi, 2002c, 2005c, 2008b). To measure a three-dimensional (3D) displacement vector (u_x,u_y,u_z), three or four 3D complex signals with different single-octant spectra that extend 1D analytic signal are calculated for echo data obtained before and after a pulse repetition interval Δt . The displacement vector (u_x,u_y,u_z) is obtained by solving the simultaneous equations (i.e., four or three independent equations) derived from the complex signals.
In MAM, an equation holds for the phase θ of each autocorrelation signal obtained from a pair of complex signals, i.e.,

$$\theta(0,0,0)+\frac{\partial}{\partial x}\theta(x,y,z)u_x+\frac{\partial}{\partial y}\theta(x,y,z)u_y+\frac{\partial}{\partial z}\theta(x,y,z)u_z=0. \tag{5}$$

Here, $\theta(0,0,0)$ equals the phase of the temporally or spatially moving-averaged lag one autocorrelation of the slow-time-axis signal sampled at the pulse repetition interval Δt [i.e., $\theta(0,0,0)$ is the moving-averaged instantaneous phase change that occurs during the pulse repetition interval Δt]. Moreover, $\partial/\partial x\ \theta$, $\partial/\partial y\ \theta$, and $\partial/\partial z\ \theta$ are the instantaneous spatial frequencies of the 3D echo signal, i.e., the US frequency fx (instantaneous frequency of the fast-time-axis signal sampled at the sampling interval of the AD converter), lateral frequency fy, and elevational frequency fz. The instantaneous spatial frequencies are estimated from the moving-averaged phase with spatial lags (x,y,z) by finite-difference approximation or differentiation using a differential filter with a cutoff frequency.
In MDM, an equation holds for the phase θ of each complex signal, i.e.,

$$\frac{\partial}{\partial t}\theta(x,y,z)\Delta t+\frac{\partial}{\partial x}\theta(x,y,z)u_x+\frac{\partial}{\partial y}\theta(x,y,z)u_y+\frac{\partial}{\partial z}\theta(x,y,z)u_z=0. \tag{6}$$

Here, $\partial/\partial t\ \theta\Delta t$ is the temporally or spatially moving-averaged instantaneous phase change that occurred during the pulse repetition interval Δt , and $\partial/\partial x\ \theta$, $\partial/\partial y\ \theta$ and $\partial/\partial z\ \theta$ are the instantaneous spatial frequencies of the 3D echo signal. The spatial and temporal derivatives can be obtained from the temporally or spatially moving-averaged instantaneous phase using the finite-difference approximation or a differential filter. $\partial/\partial t\ \theta\Delta t$ can also be obtained as the phase of the autocorrelation signal. Large displacements are dealt with by combining MCSPGM or MCCM.
When measuring a 2D displacement vector, two 2D complex signals with different single quadrant spectra are calculated, and the correspondingly derived simultaneous equations (i.e., two independent equations) are solved.

For respective MAM and MDM, by assuming a rigid motion locally, eqs. (5) and (6) can also be made simultaneously in the local region windowed to measure the motion as a local displacement vector (Sumi, 2002c, 2008b). The method obtained falls in a category of a block matching method such as MCSPGM and MCCM etc, these are respectively referred to as MAMb and MDMb (Sumi, 2002c, 2010g). However, through the simulations, their accuracies are significantly lower than those of the corresponding original methods. Then, these are not used now.

By Sumi (2008b), it was clarified by simulations that, for rigid motions, the order of the measurement accuracies of the displacement vectors is MAM > MDM for a high echo SNR and MDM > MAM for a low echo SNR. On deformed agar phantoms, when lateral modulations were not carried out, the order of the measurement accuracies of axial strains were the same as that for the high echo SNR (Sumi & Ebisawa, 2009a), whereas when using LGECM with Method 1, that of strain tensors was also same (Sumi et al., 2008i). Thus, although decorrelation noise generated due to target deformation also increased echo noise in the sense that pre- and post-deformation echo data were used, the laterally modulated echo data obtained by LGECM had a high SNR (Sumi, 2008b). Thus, in section 3, after showing, for the samely, laterally deformed agar phantom as that of previous reports (Sumi, 2008a, Sumi et al., 2008f, 2008i), US images and the corresponding 2D spectra laterally modulated with a half US frequency by PAM as well as LGECM using Methods 1 and 2, the measurement accuracies of MAM and MDM are also compared with each other.

3. Agar phantom experiments using PAM and LGECM with MAM and MDM

We have made a target agar phantom [40 (axial) × 96 (lateral) × 40 (elavational) mm^3] having a central circular cylindrical inclusion (diameter, 10 mm; depth, 19 mm) with a shear modulus different from that of the surrounding region, and shear moduli of 2.63 and 0.80 × 10^6 N/m^2 in the inclusion and surrounding regions, respectively (Sumi, 2008a, Sumi et al., 2008f, 2008i). Thus, the relative shear modulus was 3.29. Manually, the phantom was compressed by 2.0 mm in the lateral direction. The contact surfaces of the transducer and phantom were separated by immersing them in water in a tank, and a sponge was put under the phantom to allow the phantom to elongate in the axial direction by lateral uniform compression from the right-hand side using a large plate as in Case 1 in the experiments by Sumi (2007f). The left surface was fixed to a wall. A rectangular ROI 13.7 (axial, x) × 13.2 (lateral, y) mm^2 was centered on the inclusion (depths from 12.2 to 25.9 mm). For SA, Compaq Workstation DS20E (833 MHz) was used.

3.1 US imaging

Fig. 1 shows B-mode images for the ROI obtained by square detection for (a) nonmodulation (i.e., conventional beam-forming), (b) PAM with Method 1, (c) PAM with Method 2, (d) LGECMM with Method 1, and (e) LGECMM with Methos 2. The nominal frequency of US used was 7.5 MHz. The lateral modulation frequency was half the nominal frequency, i.e., 3.75 MHz [wavelengths, 0.408 vs axial 0.204 mm]. The lateral waves can be confirmed in Figs. 1(b) to 1(e). As shown, the lateral bandwidth of Fig. 1(b) is the largest. This can be confirmed by the lateral speckle sizes and specular echos (i.e., circled ones). Their lateral bandwidths can be more clearly compared in their 2D spectra in Figs. 2(a) to 2(e).

3.2 Elasticity measurement/imaging

Next, 2D shear modulus reconstructions (Sumi, 2005d) were performed together with 2D strain tensor measurements using the laterally modulated echo data obtained on the agar phantom (Figs. 1 and 2). For the 2D displacement vector measurement, MAM and MDM (Sumi, 2002c, 2005c, 2008b) were used (moving-average window size, 0.54 × 0.55 mm^2). For the coarse measurement, to prevent MAM and MDM from being subjected to aliasing in the evaluation of instantaneous phase due to the large lateral displacement (maximum, 2 mm), a 2D CCM was used (local window size, 0.54 × 2.15 mm^2). The local region size used was decreased when using MAM and MDM (Sumi et al., 1995d; Sumi, 1999a). After displacement vector measurements, 2D strain tensor components were obtained using a differential filter with a cutoff frequency of 0.89 mm^{-1}. For the 2D reconstruction, the method using a typical Poisson's ratio (0.5) was used under a 2D stress condition with regularization (Sumi, 2005d). Because the phantom was deformed primarily in the lateral direction, the reference region was set on the right borderline of the ROI. In addition, regularized 1D reconstruction (Sumi, 2005d, Sumi et al., 2007b) was also carried out using the principal lateral strain ε yy.

Table 1 shows the means and standard deviations obtained in a central square region having 5.5-mm-long sides in the inclusion for axial, lateral, and shear strains. By comparing the accuracies obtained by MAM and MDM, the order of echo SNRs is clarified to be the same as that reported by Sumi (2007d, 2008a, 2008i), i.e., inherent to the used beam-formings. This result arises because decorrelation noise generated due to the target deformation increases echo noise monotonically in the sense that pre- and post-deformation echo data are used. As the echo SNR decreases, the measurement errors in MAM and MDM increase. For instance, the SDs of the lateral strain ε yy measured by MAM are 0.28 (PAM with Method 1), 0.34 (LGECM and Method 1), 0.50 (LGECM and Method 2), and 0.72 (PAM and Method 2). In

	Strains			Shear	moduli
Methods	Axial (ϵ_{xx})	Lateral (ϵ_{yy})	Shear (ϵ_{xy})	2D	1D (Ratio of ϵ_{yy})
Parabolic -Method 1, MAM	0.01	-0.20	0.07	3.28	1.95
	(0.10)	(0.28)	(0.22)	(0.35)	(0.12)
MDM	0.01	-0.18	0.09	3.23	1.94
	(0.11)	(0.35)	(0.34)	(0.35)	(0.15)
-Method 2, MAM	0.005	-0.20	0.01	2.34	1.45
	(0.28)	(0.72)	(0.66)	(0.18)	(0.05)
MDM	0.003	-0.20	0.02	2.34	1.64
	(0.27)	(0.69)	(0.64)	(0.18)	(0.08)
Gaussian -Method 1, MAM	0.01	-0.22	0.06	3.14	1.85
	(0.13)	(0.34)	(0.24)	(0.32)	(0.13)
MDM	0.004	-0.22	0.08	3.17	1.89
	(0.14)	(0.36)	(0.30)	(0.33)	(0.15)
-Method 2, MAM	0.002	-0.21	0.03	2.60	1.94
	(0.21)	(0.50)	(0.44)	(0.22)	(0.12)
MDM	0.002	-0.22	0.04	2.63	1.69
	(0.21)	(0.45)	(0.45)	(0.22)	(0.09)

Table 1. For lateral modulation echo data obtained on agar phantom using listed methods, means and standard deviations (SDs in parentheses) evaluated for two-dimensional (2D) strain tensor measurement and 2D shear modulus reconstruction in central 5.5-mm-side square region of stiff inclusion (relative modulus 3.29). Results for 1D reconstructions obtained using lateral strain ratio are also shown.

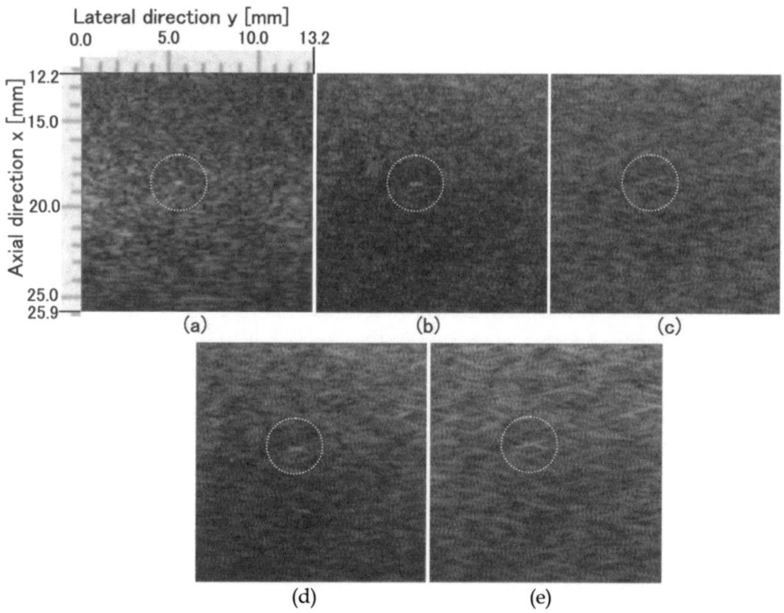

Fig. 1. B-mode images obtained using (a) no modulation; lateral cosine modulation (LCM), i.e., PAM with (b) Method 1 and (c) Method 2; LGECMM with (d) Method 1 and (e) Method 2. The specular echos from the same position are circled in the respective images.

the same manner, the order of the measurement accuracies of MAM and MDM became the same as that obtained in simulations for the rigid motion case (Sumi, 2008b). Specifically, for the lowest echo SNR obtained by PAM and Method 2, the order of accuracies of strain measurements is MDM > MAM, although large differences were not detected between their SDs; for instance, for lateral strain MDM became the same as that obtained in simulations for the rigid motion case: ε yy, 0.69 vs 0.72. For other modulations, the order of measurement accuracies is almost always MAM > MDM. In this case (Sumi, 2008b), the echo SNR obtained by PAM and Method 2 is low; that obtained by PAM and Method 1 is the highest of all. For the highest echo SNR, large differences were detected between the SDs; for example, for lateral strain ε yy, 0.28 vs 0.35.

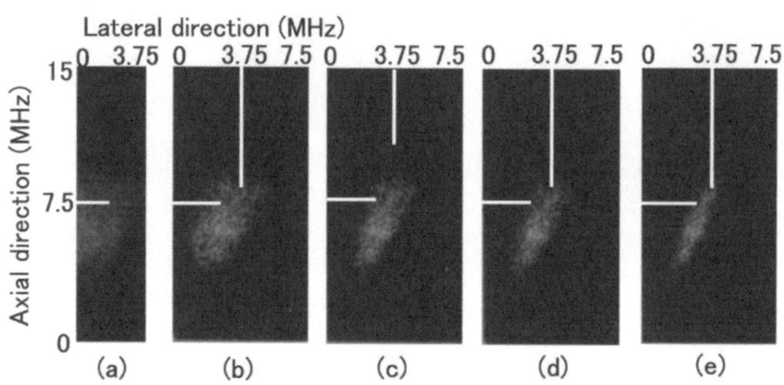

Fig. 2. 2D spectra for the ROI obtained from laterally modulated rf-echos corresponding to Figs. 1(a) to (e), i.e., (a) no modulation; lateral cosine modulation (LCM), i.e., PAM with (b) Method 1 and (c) Method 2; LGECMM with (d) Method 1 and (e) Method 2.

For visual comparison of the measurement accuracies, in Figs. 3 and 4 for the respective highest and lowest echo SNRs (i.e., PAM and Method 1, and PAM and Method 2), the lateral, axial, and shear strains ε yy, ε xx and ε xy measured using (a) MAM and (b) MDM are shown in a linear gray scale together with lateral and axial displacements dy and dx. As shown, for the highest echo SNR, both displacements dy and dx were stably measured by MAM [in Fig. 3(a)] and a circular stiff inclusion could be detected from the stably measured lateral and axial strain images. In the lateral strain image, the upper borderline of the inclusion was estimated to be quite soft. At the upper borderline of the inclusion, the inclusion and the surrounding region might be separated. However, in Figs. 3(b), 4(a), and 4(b), the effects due to the low echo SNRs and inherent to the displacement vector measurement methods can be visually confirmed in terms of the measured displacements and strains, particularly, in the lateral strain ε yy at the boundary of the circular stiff inclusion.

Next, 2D lateral shear modulus reconstructions are shown for all the combinations of PAM, LGECM, Methods 1 and 2, and MAM and MDM. The means and SDs of relative shear moduli obtained in the stiff inclusion are also summarized in Table 1, and for the highest and lowest echo SNRs, the log-gray-scaled reconstruction images are also shown in Figs. 3(a), 3(b), 4(a) and 4(b). For the highest echo SNR as well as other echo SNRs, the stiff circular region can be stably detected (LGECM data not shown). However, although for the highest echo SNR, the relative shear modulus was accurately reconstructed (the evaluated mean relative shear modulus, 3.28; SD, 0.35), the effects of strain measurement errors on the shear modulus reconstructions were confirmed, particularly from the mean shear moduli evaluated in the inclusion (Table 1). With increasing strain measurement error, the mean shear modulus decreased, i.e., for MAM, 3.28 (PAM and Method 1), 3.14 (LGECM and Method 1), 2.60 (LGECM and Method 2), 2.34 (PAM and Method 2); however, marked differences between the results obtained by MAM and MDM were not confirmed in this experiment, probably because of the proper smoothing achieved by the regularization (Sumi, 2005d).

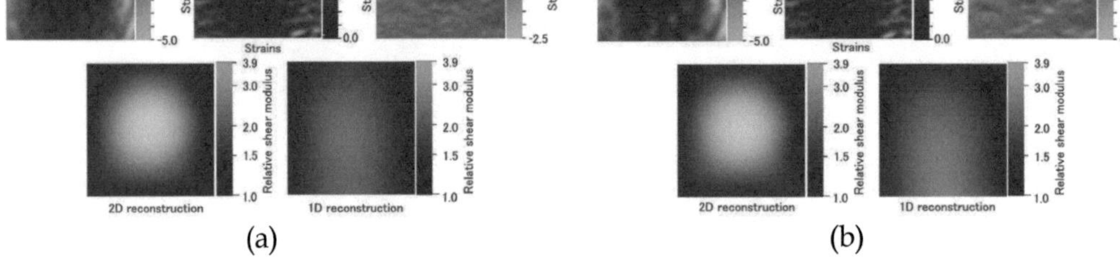

(a) (b)

Fig. 3. For the highest echo SNR obtained using PAM with Method 1 (lateral modulation frequency, 3.75 MHz vs US freq., 7.5 MHz), measured by (a) MAM and (b) MDM, i.e., lateral and axial displacements dy and dx, lateral, axial and shear strains ε yy, ε xx and ε xy, 2D shear modulus reconstruction and lateral 1D shear modulus reconstruction.

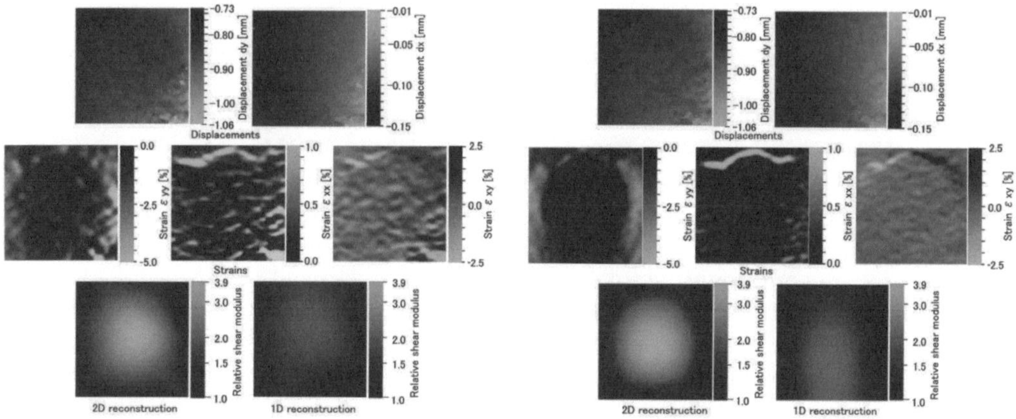

(a) (b)

Fig. 4. For the lowest echo SNR obtained using PAM with Method 2 (lateral modulation frequency, 3.75 MHz), measured by (a) MAM and (b) MDM. See captions of Fig. 3.

Furthermore, because the target phantom was deformed primarily in the lateral direction (Sumi, 2007f), the lateral 1D reconstruction might yield a useful shear modulus reconstruction, as was the case with the axial 1D reconstruction where the target was deformed primarily in the axial direction (Sumi, 2005d, 2007f). However, even for the highest echo SNR, as shown, the shape of the inclusion is not a circle. The phantom was not deformed horizontally, i.e., not accurately, in the lateral direction. The strains generated were small in the neighborhood of the lower borderline of the ROI. For the highest echo SNR, the mean relative shear modulus of the inclusion was 1.95 (SD, 0.12). This value lower than the original value is also affected by an artifact of the 1D reconstruction, i.e., the dynamic range of stiffness is estimated to be smaller than the original (Sumi, 2005d). For all the combinations, the means and SDs are shown in Table 1. Almost the same effects caused by strain measurement errors were confirmed as were confirmed in the 2D reconstructions.

4. Discussions and conclusions

In this report, we reviewed our several trials, searching for the best lateral modulation (i.e., coherent superimposition of echo signals) for US imaging with a high lateral resolution and accurate measurement of displacement vectors such as blood vector flow, a tissue displacement vector, a strain tensor, a strain rate tensor and an acceleration vector. PAM and HAM were introduced after LGECM to increase the echo SNR and lateral spatial resolution and decrease the effective aperture size. Such modulations were obtained on the basis of our knowledge about US propagation. The energy of the foot is lost during US propagation, and the main lobe contributes to the echo signals.

In the agar phantom experiment, PAM yielded a high echo SNR and a high lateral spatial resolution. Moreover, we compared the combinations of modulation methods and displacement vector measurement methods. Although for PAM, Method 1 yielded a more accurate 2D displacement vector/2D strain tensor than Method 2, in practical applications for *in vivo* tissues, rapid target motion will significantly affect the accuracy of Method 1. Because, a monostatic SA was used in this study, the echo SNR must be lower than that obtained when a conventional beam-former is used. In future studies, the limitations of Method 2 will also be clarified such as obtaining of a high echo SNR in shorter time. A multistatic SA will also be reported. However, because large differences were not confirmed between MAM and MDM in this experiment, the echo data obtained by the monostatic SA had a rather high SNRs (Sumi, 2008b). If we can obtain a higher echo SNR, MAM will be more useful than MDM. Because MDM requires less calculation time than MAM (Sumi, 2008b), MDM may be better suited for 2D measurements of complex 3D blood flow and tissue motion and the 3D or 2D monitoring of various thermal treatments (Sumi, 2005d). Multiple transmitting modulations will also be performed. In future studies, the strain measurement accuracies of MAM and MDM will be clarified theoretically or through simulations or phantom experiments.

By using lateral deformation in the agar phantom experiment, we also obtained a meaningful result. The LCMs enable the attachment only of a US transducer to the target body in order to measure blood vector flow, the tissue strain tensor, and shear modulus reconstruction. In the axial strain measurement and 1D shear modulus reconstruction using the strain ratio (e.g., Sumi, 2005d, 2007f; Sumi & Matsuzawa, 2007b), the target must be compressed or elongated in the axial direction. Otherwise, the principle strain must be measured by setting the US beam in the direction of the target motion in successive scans (Sumi, 2010g). However, the LCMs enable freehand measurement and reconstruction in addition to dealing with uncontrollable target motion due to heart motion or pulsation and with deeply situated tissue that cannot be accessed from the body surface (e.g., liver and heart), although for the 2D measurements, a proper frame must be used to remove the out-of-motion from the frame. Recently, in addition to the reconstruction method used in this chapter [Method F referred to as in report by Sumi (2010d)], we have developed a shear modulus reconstruction method E from Methods F [Sumi et al., 1993, 1995a; Sumi, 1999c, 2005d, 2010d] and A to C [Sumi, 2006b, 2007g], which also enables the use of a quasi-reference shear modulus (quasi-reference value, e.g., unity) in order to obtain an accurate and unique shear modulus reconstruction in that the reconstruction has no geometrical artifacts, although the reconstruction has not absolute but relative shear modulus values (i.e., it depends on the quasi-reference value of shear modulus used) [Sumi, 2010d]. The use of a quasi-reference shear modulus enables us to deal with such deeply situated tissues. In Method F, when taking the logarithm of the shear modulus, an absolute or relative shear modulus reconstruction had been obtained as in this chapter; when not taking the logarithm and using a quasi-reference shear modulus, similarly an absolute or relative shear modulus reconstruction can also be obtained (Sumi et al., 1995a; Sumi, 2005d). Hereafter, all such relative reconstructions are referred to as those obtained by Method E (Sumi, 2010d).

In the experiment, accurate strain tensor measurements and shear modulus reconstructions were achieved, because we used the shear modulus reconstruction method F using a 2D stress assumption (Sumi, 2005d) and realized such a stress condition approximately. Thus, strictly speaking, the use of 2D US array will enable perfect measurement and reconstruction regardless of the direction of the dominant target motion. For tissue elasticity measurements, 3D shear modulus reconstruction should be performed with 3D displacement vector measurement. We have already developed six useful 3D shear modulus reconstruction methods, Methods F (Sumi et al., 1995a; Sumi, 1999c, 2005d, 2010d), A (Sumi, 2006b), B (Sumi, 2006b; 2007g), C (Sumi, 2007g), D (Sumi, 2008a, 2010d) and E (Sumi, 1999c, 2005d, 2010d), in which a finite difference method or a finite element method is properly used. Such 3D reconstruction can also be carried out in real-time as low-dimensional reconstruction (e.g., Sumi & Matsuzawa, 2007b) by setting a narrow 3D ROI even if a personal computer (PC) is used. The comparison of the methods will be reported elsewhere.

In this chapter, although we applied regularization only to the shear modulus reconstruction (Method F: Sumi, 2005d), its application to the displacement vector measurement, i.e., displacement component-dependent regularization or directional-dependent regularization (Sumi & Sato, 2008c; Sumi & Itoh, 2009b) will also be effective in stabilizing the strain tensor measurements by MAM, MDM, and MCSPGM in addition to shear modulus reconstruction. In both regularizations, the measured or theoretically predicted strain tensor variances are used to set the regularization parameters (Sumi & Sato, 2008c; Sumi, 2007a, 2008e; Sumi & Itoh, 2009b, 2010e). With such regularizations, a spatially varying regularization is also realized. As a result, the reconstructed shape of shear modulus inhomogeneity will be more improved.

We also referred to the determination of beam-forming parameters using optimization theory. Although we reported the use of analytic functions such as a parabolic function for PSF envelope, the better PSF has been obtained (Sumi et al., 2008g, 2009d, 2010c). The best PSF will also be sought in the same manner as the design of filters and windows. From the viewpoint of spatial resolution, PSF will be designed in the spatial and frequency domains. For echo SNR, knowledge of US propagation and decay is also required. By RanganathanIn & Walker (2003) and Guenther & Walker (2007), for conventional US imaging of a cyst, the contrast resolution is optimized by using a least squares estimation. In our case, target US properties such as a frequency-dependent attenuation will also be used in the determination of PSFs. Such a method of determination will be reported elsewhere together with the simultaneous determination of multiple parameters. Nonlinear optimization will also be used to determine a US element size and materials. Such an optimally realized PSF or laterally modulated PSF should also be used in US harmonic imaging and measurements as well as in radar (sumi, 2007d). These determinations may also reveal a new aspect of superresolution imaging by inverse filtering (Sumi et al., 2006a, 2008d, 2009c). For instance, in US imaging, a spatial resolution of less than 3mm is currently required to overcome the clinical limitations in conventional digital US imaging equipment (Sumi et al., 2008f; Sumi, 2010a).

Thus, an accurate real-time 3D US imaging, 3D tissue motion measurements (3D blood flow vector, tissue strain tensor, strain tensor rate etc.) and 3D shear modulus and viscoelasticity reconstructions (Sumi, 2005d, 2007d; Sumi et al., 2005a, 2008f, 2008i, 2009e) using a 2D US array will also be achieved. That is, the optimal determination of a 1D apodization function achieved can be easily extended to 2D functions (Sumi, 2008b). LCM makes it possible to attach an US transducer to the target body in order to achieve the measurements and reconstructions without considering the direction of the target motion. That is, being different from the 2D measurement, the LCM permits complete freehand measurements and reconstructions.

Optimal beamforming (LCM, etc.) can also enable the use of effective high intensity focused ultrasound (HIFU) with a high lateral resolution (Sumi, 2007d). Although the pulse shape and length of US must be considered technically, a proper high intensity US can also be used as a radiation force (ARF) [Bercoff et al., 2004; Dahl et al., 2007] for the imaging of shear waves or treatments. The use of a suitable receiver for HIFU and ARF will also be effective for diagnosis, monitoring and treatment (Sumi, 2002a, 2007d). The evaluation of the newly developed PSFs will also be performed by reconstruction of the mechanical source (e.g., Sumi et al., 2009e) or thermal source (e.g., Sumi et al., 2010b) using the proposed differential-type inverse methods. Thus, beamforming parameter determinations will also be used to develop a spatially uniform efficient and accurate treatment. A perfect minimum invasive treatment will be also realized. Efforts will also be made to determine the high-frequency components in an apodization function for a very near field. A various *in vivo/in situ* microscope can also be realized using LM (e.g., skin: Sumi, 2008h; other applications such as a cultured cardiac cell: Sumi, 2009e; thermal properties: Sumi, 2010b).

In this chapter, we also reviewed MDSAM, MTM and thier applications (Sumi, 2002a, 2005d, 2008b). When small steering angles must be used, non-superimposition methods are more accurate than LCM (Sumi, 2008b). However, when realizing the modulation at half the US frequency as in the agar phantom experiment, the accuracies are almost the same (Sumi et al., 2008i). If we can achieve a higher lateral modulation frequency by realizing a more appropriate US transducer, LCM becomes more accurate than the non-superimposition methods. Moreover, such methods has the same problem as Method 1, and further requires accurate interpolations of the measured displacements at proper coordinates to evaluate the strain tensor.

By Sumi (2010g), a new more simple beamforming method was reported, i.e., ASTA referred to as by abbreviation of "a single steering angle." In conjunction, we also developed a new displacement vector measurement methods and lateral displacement measurement methods (Sumi, 2010g). For non-steered scanning, by rotating a coordinate when performing a beamforming or after obtaining a beam, a lateral frequncy can also be obtained. This is a version of ASTA. Thus, for instance, for the original and another version of ASTA, the application of MAM or MDM to an orthant spectra divided in a frequency domain also yields an accurate displacement vetor measurement (Sumi, 2010g; Sumi et al., 2010i). Also low frequency spectra can be disregared to increase a measurement accuracy of displacement (Sumi, 2010g; Sumi et al., 2010i). Although these methods are beyond the scope of this chapter, we briefly mention the problems of LM that can be coped with by ASTA (Sumi, 2010g), i.e.,

1. For a measurement in a 2D or 3D ROI, when a classical synthetic aperture (SA) is used, the US intensity transmitted from an element is small, which may yield low SNR echo data.
2. Alternatively, when crossed beams are superimposed, although a large US intensity can be obtained, time differences between the transmission of the beams can cause measurement errors, if the displacement occurs during these time differences.
3. If plural beams which have different paths are used, the inhomogeneity of tissue properties affects beamforming. Specifically, propagation speed affects focusing (i.e., the beam-crossing position), whereas attenuation and scattering lead to different frequencies of the crossed beams for the applications of 1D displacement measurement methods.
4. At the minimum, more time is required to complete a beamforming than that required with ASTA. Occasionally, more time is also required to complete a displacement calculation than is required with ASTA.
5. If obstacles such as bone exist in a superficial region, a deeply situated tissue cannot be dealt with, because a larger physical aperture is required than for conventional beamforming.

In contrast, with ASTA, although used for a displacement vector measurement, the number of available methods may be limited, and being dependent on the measurement method, only a lateral displacement measurement can be performed, and any of the above concerns, (1) to (5), will not become a problem, and a simple beamforming increases the number of applications of displacement measurement.

Because the highest quality and accuracy of imaging, measurement, and treatment should be spatially uniform, an optimization will also be performed under conditions in which transducers have physically finite effective aperture widths and various shapes. Thus, efforts to develop next-generation US diagnosis/treatment systems using proper beamforming and various methods of computational imaging are currently underway.

5. References

Anderson, M. E. (1998). Multi-dimensional velocity estimation with ultrasound using spatial quadrature. *IEEE Trans. Ultrason. Ferroelect. Freq. Contr.*, Vol. 45, No. 3, May 1998, pp. 852-861.

Anderson, M. E. (2000). A heterodyning demodulation technique for spatial quadrature. In: *Proceedings of the 2000 IEEE Ultrasonics Symposium*, p. 1487-1490, San-Juan, Oct 2000.

Basarab, A.; Gueth, P.; Liebgott, H.; Delachartre, P. (2007). Two-dimensional least-squares estimation for motion tracking in ultrasound elastography. In: *Proceedings of the 29th Ann. Int. Conf. IEEE Eng. Med. Biol. Soc.*, pp. 2155-2158, Lyon, Aug 2007.

Bercoff, J., Tanter, M., & Fink, M. (2004). Supersonic shear imaging: a new technique for soft tissue elasticitymapping. *IEEE Trans. Ultrason. Ferroelect. Freq. Contr.*, Vol. 51, No. 4, April 2004, pp. 396–409.

Bracewell, R. N. (1986). The Fourier transform and its applications. McGraw-Hill, New York

Bohs, L. N. & Trahey, G. E. (1991). A novel method for angle independent ultrasonic imaging of blood flow and tissue motion. *IEEE Trans. on Biomed. Eng.*, Vol. 38, No. 3, Mar 1991, pp. 280-286.

Cespedes, I.; Ophir, J.; Ponnekanti, H. & Maklad, N. F. (1993). Elastography: elasticity imaging using ultrasound with application to muscle and breast *in vivo* ultrasound imaging. *Ultrason. Imag.*, Vol. 15, No. 2, Apr 1993, pp. 73-88.

Chen, X.; Zohdy, M. J.; Emelianov, S. Y. & O'Donnell, M. (2004). Lateral speckle tracking using synthetic lateral phase. *IEEE Trans. Ultrason. Ferroelect. Freq. Contr.*, Vol. 51, No. 5, May 2005, pp. 540-550.

Dahl, J. J., Pinton, G. F., Palmeri, M. L., Agrawal, V., Nightingale, K. R., & Trahey, G. E. (2007). A parallel tracking method for acoustic radiation force impulse imaging. *IEEE Trans. Ultrason. Ferroelect. Freq. Contr.*, Vol. 54, No. 2, Feb 2007, pp. 301–311.

Doyley, M. M.; Srinivasa, S.; Pendergrass, S. A.; Wu, Z. & Ophir, J. (2005). Comparative evaluation of strain-based and model-based modulus elastography. *Ultrasound Med. Biol.*, Vol. 31, No. 6, Jun 2005, pp. 787-802.

Fox, M. D. (1978). Multiple crossed-beam ultrasound Doppler velocimetry. *IEEE Trans. on Sonics and Ultrasonics*, Vol. 25, No. 5, Sep 1978, pp. 281-286.

Garra, B. S., Cespedes, E. I. & Ophir, J. (1997). Elastography of breast lesions: initial clinical results. *Radiology*, Vol. 202, No. 1, Jan 1997, pp. 79–86.

Goodman, J. W. (1996). *Introduction to Fourier optics* (2nd ed). McGRAW-HILL COMPANIES, INC, New York.

Guenther, D. A. & Walker, W. F. (2007). Optimal apodization design for medical ultrasound using constrained least squares—part I: theory. *IEEE Trans. Ultrason. Ferroelect. Freq. Contr.*, Vol. 54, No. 2, Feb 2007, pp. 332–341.

Hahn, S. L. (1992). Multidimensional complex signals with single-orthant spectra. *Proc. IEEE*, Vol. 80, No. 8, Aug 1992, pp. 1287-1300.

Jensen, J. A. & Munk, P.(1998). A new method for estimation of velocity vectors. *IEEE Trans. Ultrason. Ferroelect. Freq. Contr.*, Vol. 45, No. 3, May 1998, pp. 837-851.

Jensen, J A. (2001). A new estimator for vector velocity estimation. *IEEE Trans. Ultrason. Ferroelect. Freq. Contr.*, Vol. 48, No. 4, Jul 2001, pp. 886-894.

Kallel, F. & Bertrand, M. (1996). Tissue elasticity reconstruction using linear perturbation method. *IEEE Trans. on Med. Imag.*, Vol. 15, No. 3, Jun 1996, pp. 299-313.

Kasai, C.; Namekawa, K.; Koyano, A. & Omoto, R. (1985). Real-time two-dimensional blood flow imaging using an autocorrelation technique. *IEEE Trans. on Sonics Ultrason.*, Vol. 32, No. 3, May 1985, pp. 458-464.

Liebgott, H.; Fromageau, J.; Wilhjelm, J. E.; Vray, D. & Delachartre, P. (2005). Beamforming scheme for 2D displacement estimation in ultrasound imaging. *EURASIP Journal on Applied Signal Processing*, Vol. 8, 2005, pp. 1212-1220.

Loupas, T.; Pomers, J.T. & Gill R.W. (1995). An axial velocity estimator for ultrasound blood flow imaging, based on a full evaluation of the Doppler equation by means of a two-dimensional autocorrelation method approach. IEEE Trans. Ultrasound Ferroelect., Freq. Contr., Vol. 42., No 4, Jully 1995, pp. 672-688.

Newhouse, V. L.; Censor, D.; Vontz, T.; Cisneros, J. A. & Goldberg, B. B. (1987). Ultrasound Doppler probing of flows transverse with respect to beam axis. *IEEE Trans. on Biomed. Eng.*, Vol. 34, No. 10, Oct 1987, pp. 779-789.

Ophir, J., Cespedes, I., Ponnekanti, H., Yazdi, Y. & Li, X. (1991). Elastography: a quantitative method for measuring the elasticity of biological tissues. *Ultrason Imaging*, Vol. 13, No. 2, Apr 1991, pp. 111-134.

Plewes, D. B.; Bishop, J.; Samani, A. & Sciarretta, J. (2000). Visualization and quantification of breast cancer biomechanical properties with magnetic resonance elastography. *Phys. Med. Biol.*, Vol. 45, No. 6, Jun 2000, pp. 1591-1610.

Ranganathan, K. & Walker, W. F. (2003). A novel beamformer design method for medical ultrasound—part I: theory. *IEEE Trans. Ultrason. Ferroelect. Freq. Contr.*, Vol. 50, No. 1, Jan 2003, pp. 15–24.

Srinivasan, S.; Kallel, F.; Souchon, R. & Ophir, J. (2002). Analysis of an adaptive strain estimation technique in Elastography. *Ultrasonic imaging*, Vol. 24, No. 2, Apr 2002, pp. 109-118.

Steinberg, B. D. (1976). *Principles of aperture & array system design*. John Wiley & Sons, Inc., New York.

Sumi, C.; Suzuki, A. & Nakayama, K. (1993). Estimation of shear modulus distribution in soft tissue from strain measurement. *Jpn. J. Med. Electr. Biol. Eng.*, Vol. 31(suppl.), p. 390, Koufu, May 1993 (in Japanese).

Sumi, C.; Suzuki, A.; Nakayama, K. (1994a). Estimation of shear modulus distribution in soft tissue from strain measurement. *Jpn. J. Med. Electr. Biol. Eng.*, Vol. 32(suppl.), p. 122, Takamatsu, May 1994.

Sumi, C.; Suzuki, A. & Nakayama, K. (1994b). Phantom experiment on reconstruction of shear modulus distribution in soft tissue from strain measurement. *Ultrasound in Medicine and Biology*, Vol. 20(Suppl 1: Proceedings of the *7th Congress of World Federation for Ultrasound in Medicine and Biology*), p. 14-4, Sapporo, July 1994.

Sumi, C.; Suzuki, A. & Nakayama, K. (1995a). Estimation of shear modulus distribution in soft tissue from strain distribution. *IEEE Trans. on Biomed. Eng.*, Vol. 42, No. 2, Feb 1995, pp. 193-202.

Sumi, C.; Suzuki, A.; Nakayama, K. & Kubota, K. (1995b). Estimation of stiffness distribution in soft tissue from displacement vector measurement. *Jpn. J. Med. Ultrasonics*, Vol. 22(suppl I), pp. 44, May 1995 (in Japanese).

Sumi, C.; Suzuki, A. & Nakayama, K. (1995c). Estimation of hardness distribution in soft tissue from strain ratio. *Jpn. J. Med. Ultrasonics*, Vol. 22(suppl II), p. 258, Nov 1995 (in Japanese).

Sumi, C.; Suzuki, A. & Nakayama, K. (1995d). Phantom experiment on estimation of shear modulus distribution in soft tissue from ultrasonic measurement of displacement vector field. *IEICE Trans. on Fundamental*, Vol. E78-A, No. 12, Dec 1995, pp. 1655-1664.

Sumi, C.; Suzuki, A. & Nakayama, K. (1996). Estimation of static elasticity distribution in living tissues from ultrasonic measurement of strain distributions. *Jpn. J. Med. Electr. Biol. Eng.*, Vol. 34(suppl.), p. 107, Osaka, May 1996 (in Japanese).

Sumi, C.; Nakayama, K.; Kubota, M. (1997). Tissue elasticity imaging based on ultrasonic strain measurement. *Jpn. J. Med. Electr. Biol. Eng.*, Vol. 35(suppl.), p. 171, Nagano, Apr 1997 (in Japanese).

Sumi, C. & Nakayama, K. (1998). A robust numerical solution to reconstruct a globally relative shear modulus distribution from strain measurements. *IEEE Trans. on Med. Imag.*, Vol. 17, No. 3, Jun 1998, pp. 419-428.

Sumi, C. (1999a). Fine elasticity imaging on utilizing the iterative rf-echo phase matching method. *IEEE Trans. Ultrason. Ferroelect. Freq. Contr.*, Vol. 46, No. 1, Jan 1999, pp. 158-166.

Sumi, C.; Shibata, K. & Kubota, M. (1999b). Shear modulus imaging of breast tissues. *Tech. Report of Jpn. Soc. of Ultrason. in Med.*, Vol. BT98, No. 4, pp. 28-31, Tokyo, Mar 1999 (in Japanese).

Sumi, C. (1999c). Toward 3-D reconstruction/imaging shear modulus distribution in living soft tissues. In: *Proceedings of Autumn Meeting Acoust. Soc. Japan*, pp. 1201–1202, Shimane, Sep 1999 (in Japanese).

Sumi, C., Ichiki, Y., Kanai, H. (2000a). Feasibility of monitoring thermal therapy by ultrasonic strain measurement-based shear modulus reconstruction. *Jpn. J. Med. Elect. And Biol. Eng.*, Vol. 38(suppl. I), p. 284, May 2000 (in Japanease).

Sumi, C., Nakayama, K. & Kubota, M. (2000b). An effective ultrasonic strain measurement-based shear modulus reconstruction technique for superficial tissues - Demonstration on in vitro pork ribs and in vivo human breast tissues. *Phys. in Med. Biol.*, Vol. 45, No. 6, June 2000, pp. 1511-1520.

Sumi, C.; Takegahara, S. & Kanai, H. (2001a). Feasibility of shear modulus imaging technique for monitoring the effectiveness of the interstitial RF electromagnetic wave thermal therapy. In: *Proceedings of SPIE*, Vol. 4247, pp. 151-157, San Jose, Jan 2001.

Sumi, C & Kojima, R. (2001b). Quantitative evaluation of effectiveness of thermal therapy through shear modulus reconstruction on utilization of interstitial RF electromagnetic wave thermal applicator system. Vol. BT2000, pp. 21-28, Mar 2001 (in Japanese).

Sumi, C. (2002a). Displacement measurement method and apparatus, strain measurement method and apparatus, elasticity and viscoelasticity constants measurement apparatus, and the elasticity and viscoelasticity constants measurement apparatus based treatment apparatus. Japanese Patent 4260523, Apr 30, 2009 (application Apr

25, 2002); US Patent US 7,775,980 B2, Aug 17, 2010 (application 10/326,526, Dec 23, 2002).

Sumi, C. (2002b). Realization of combined diagnosis/treatment style by ultrasonic strain measurement-based mechanical properties imaging technique - examples with applications on the interstitial rf-electromagnetic wave thermal therapy. *Abstracts of First International Conference of Ultrasonic Measurement and Imaging of Tissue Elasticity*, p. 23, Niagara-Falls, October 2002.

Sumi, C. (2002c). Digital measurement method of tissue displacement vector from instantaneous phase of ultrasonic echo signal. *Technical report of Japn. Soc. of Ultrason. in Med.*, Vol. 102, No. 4, pp. 37-40, Fukuoka, December 2002.

Sumi, C. (2004). Improvement of measurement accuracy of displacement vector by lateral modulation. In: *Proceedings of the 2004 Autumn Meeting of the Acoustical Society of Japan*, pp. 1353–1354, September 2004 (in Japanese).

Sumi, C.; Kubota, M.; Wakabayashi, G.; & Tanabe, M. (2005a). Usefulness of ultrasonic strain measurement-based mechanical properties imaging technique: Toward realization of short-time diagnosis/treatment, In: *Research and Development in Breast Ultrasound* eds by Ueno, E., Shiina, T., Kubota, M. & Sawai, K., pp. 16-43, Springer, New York.

Sumi, C. (2005b). Real-time reconstruction of shear modulus distribution by calculating strain ratio. In: *Proceedings of 27th Ann. Int. Conf. of IEEE Eng. in Med. Biol. Soc.*, CD-ROM, Shnaghai, September 2005.

Sumi, C. (2005c). Multidimensional displacement vector measurement methods utilizing instantaneous phase. In: *Proceedings of 27th Int. Conf. of IEEE Eng. of Med. and Biol. Soc.*, CD-ROM, Shanghai, September 2005.

Sumi, C. (2005d). Usefulness of ultrasonic strain measurement-based shear modulus reconstruction for diagnosis and thermal treatment. *IEEE Trans. Ultrason. Ferroelect. Freq. Contr.*, Vol. 52, No. 10, Oct 2005, pp. 1670-1689.

Sumi, C. & Noro, T. (2006a). Lateral Gaussian envelope cosine modulation method (LGECMM) (4th report)—a breakaway from Fraunhofer approximation, In: *Proceedings of the Autumn Meeting of the Acoustical Society of Japan*, pp. 1035–1036, Sep 2006.

Sumi, C. (2006b). Reconstructions of shear modulus, Poisson's ratio and density using approximate mean normal stress $\lambda\varepsilon_{\alpha\alpha}$ as unknown. *IEEE Trans. Ultrason. Ferroelect. Freq. Contr.*, Vol. 53, No. 12, Dec 2006, pp. 2416-2434.

Sumi, C.; Kikuchi, D.; Shimada, Y.; Nojiri, S. (2006c). Comparison of multidimensional shear modules reconstruction methods through simulations and phantom experiments. Abstract of fifth International Conference of Ultrasonic Measurement and Imaging of Tissue Elasticity, p. 139, Utah, October 2006.

Sumi, C. (2007a). Spatially variant regularization for tissue strain measurement and shear modulus reconstruction. *Journal of Medical Ultrasound*, Vol. 34, No. 3, Sep 2007, pp. 125-131.

Sumi, C. & Matsuzawa, H. (2007b). Shear modulus reconstruction by ultrasonically measured strain ratio. *Journal of Medical Ultrasonics*, Vol. 34, No. 4, Dec 2007, pp. 171-188.

Sumi, C. & Sato, K. (2007c). Evaluation of variances of ultrasonically measured strain tensor components. *Acoustical Science and Technology*, Vol. 28, No. 5, Sep 2007, pp. 352-356.

Sumi, C. (2007d). Beamforming for realizing designed point spread function, In: *Proceedings of IEEE Ultrasonics Symposium*, pp. 1557–1562, New York, Oct 2007.

Sumi, C.; Tanuma, A.; Itoh, T. & Takahashi, D. (2007e) Effectiveness of regularization and lateral modulation on multidimensional shear modulus reconstruction in displacement vector measurement.. In: *Proceedings of the sixth International Conference on the Ultrasonic Measurement and Imaging of Tissue Elasticity*, Santa Fe, p. 90, Oct 2007.

Sumi, C. (2007f). Ultrasonic axial strain measurement for lateral tissue deformation. *Ultrasound Med. Biol.*, Vol. 33, No. 11, Nov 2007, pp. 1830-1837.

Sumi, C. (2007g). Effective shear modulus reconstruction obtained with approximate mean normal stress remaining unknown. *IEEE Trans. Ultrason. Ferroelect. Freq. Contr.*, Vol. 54, No. 11, Nov 2007, pp. 2394-2403.

Sumi, C. (2008a). Increasing accuracy of tissue shear modulus reconstruction using ultrasonic strain tensor measurement - Regularization and lateral modulation," In: *Acoustical Im*aging (Vol. 29) ed by Akiyama I., pp. 59-69, Springer.

Sumi, C. (2008b). Displacement vector measurement using instantaneous ultrasound signal phase —Multidimensional autocorrelation and Doppler methods" *IEEE Trans. Ultrason. Ferroelect. Freq. Contr.*, Vol. 55, No. 1, Jan 2008, pp. 24-43.

Sumi, C. & Sato, K. (2008c). Regularization for ultrasonic measurements of tissue displacement vector and strain tensor. *IEEE Trans. Ultrason. Ferroelect. Freq. Contr.*, Vol. 55, No. 2, Feb 2008, pp. 787-799.

Sumi, C. (2008d). A case of apodization function using singular value decomposition: Determination of beamforming parameters by optimization. *Acoustical Science and Technology*, Vol. 29, No. 2, Mar 2008, pp. 185-187.

Sumi, C. (2008e). Regularization of tissue shear modulus reconstruction using strain variance. *IEEE Trans. Ultrason. Ferroelect. Freq. Contr.*, Vol. 55, No. 4, Apr 2008, pp. 297-307.

Sumi, C. & Tanuma, A. (2008f). Comparison of parabolic and Gaussian lateral cosine modulations in ultrasound imaging, displacement vector measurement, and elasticity measurement. *Jpn, J. Appl. Phys.*, Vol. 47, No. 5B, May 2008, pp. 4137-4144.

Sumi, C.; Komiya, Y. & Uga, S. (2008g). Proper point spread function for lateral modulation. In: *Proceedings of the 7th International Conference on Ultrasonic Measurement and Imaging of Tissue Elasticity*, Austin, Oct 2008 (6 pages).

Sumi, C. & Saijo, Y. (2008h). Shear modulus microscopy using displacement vector measurement, In: *Proceeding version of the seventh International Conference on the Ultrasonic Measurement and Imaging of Tissue Elasticity*, Austin, Oct 2008 (5 pages).

Sumi, C.; Noro, T.; Tanuma, A. (2008i). Effective lateral modulations with applications to shear modulus reconstruction using displacement vector measurement. *IEEE Trans. Ultrason. Ferroelect. Freq. Contr.*, Vol. 55, No. 12, Dec 2008, pp. 2607-2625.

Sumi, C. & Ebisawa, T. (2009a). Phantom experiments of axial strain measurements using multidimensional autocorrelation method, multidimensional Doppler method and direct strain measurement method. *Acoustical Science and Technology*, Vol. 30, No. 2, Mar 2009, pp. 117-123.

Sumi, C. & Itoh, T. (2009b). Spatially variant regularization of lateral displacement measurement using variance. *Ultrasonics*, Vol. 49, No. 4-5, May 2009, pp. 459-465.

Sumi, C.; Komiya, Y. & Uga, S. (2009c). A demonstration of optimal apodization determination for proper lateral modulation. *Jpn, J. Appl. Phys.*, Vol. 48, No. 7B, Jul 2009, 07GJ06 (10 pages).

Sumi, C.; Shimizu, K.; Takanashi, Y.; Tadokoro, Y. & Nozaki, Y. (2009d). 2nd report on proper point spread function for lateral modulation. In: *Proceedings of the 8th*

International Conference on Ultrasonic Measurement and Imaging of Tissue Elasticity, Vlissingen, Sep 2009 (3 pages).

Sumi, C. & Suekane S. (2009e). Reconstruction of a tissue shear modulus together with mechanical sources. *Therm. Med.*, Vol. 25, No. 4, Dec 2009, pp. 89-104.

Sumi, C. (2010a). Determination of lateral modulation apodization functions using a regularized, weighted least squares estimation. *Int. J. Biomed. Imag*, Mar 2010, ID635294 (7 pages).

Sumi, C.; Kanada, H. & Takanashi, Y. (2010b). Reconstructions of tissue thermal properties together with perfusion and thermal source. *Thermal Medicine*, Vol. 26, No. 1, Mar 2010, pp. 31–40.

Sumi, C.; Shimizu, K. & Matsui, N. (2010c). Proper analytic point spread function for lateral modulation. *Jpn J Appl Phys*, Vol. 49, No. 7B, Jul 2010, 07HF07 (2 pages).

Sumi, C. (2010d). Relative shear modulus reconstruction for visualization with no geometrical artifact. *Acoustical Science and Technology*, Vol. 31, No. 5, Sep 2010, pp. 347-359.

Sumi, C. & Itoh, T. (2010e). A limitation in use of spatially stationary strain variance estimate in regularization of shear modulus reconstruction. *Acoustical Science and Technology*, Vol. 31, No. 5, Sep 2010, pp. 360-367.

Sumi, C.; Takanashi, Y.; Shimizu, K. & Ishii, Y. (2010f). Determining if the relative shear modulus or the inverse of the relative shear modulus should be imaged using axial strain ratios on agar phantoms. *Ultrasound Med. Biol.*, Vol. 36, No. 9, Sep 2010, pp. 1481-1491.

Sumi, C. (2010g). Utilization of an ultrasound beam steering angle. *Reports in Medical Imaging*, Vol. 3, Sep 2010, pp. 61-81.

Sumi, C. & Uga, S. (2010h). Effective ultrasonic virtual sources which can be positioned independently of physical aperture focus positions. *Reports in Medical Imaging*, Vol. 3, Sep 2010, pp. 45-59.

Sumi, C., Shimizu, K., Takanashi, Y. (2010i). Increase in spatial resolution of lateral modulation imaging. In: *Proceeding version of the nineth International Conference on the Ultrasonic Measurement and Imaging of Tissue Elasticity*, Utah, Oct 2010 (in press).

Sumi, C. & Shimizu, K. (2011). Agar phantom experiment for comparison of measurement accuracy of tissue elasticity obtained by displacement vector measurement using lateral modulation with multidimensional autocorrelation and Doppler methods and corresponding one-dimensional methods. Jpn. J. Appl. Phys. (submitted).

Tanter, M.; Bercoff, J.; Sandrin, L. & Fink, M. (2002). Ultrafast compound imaging for 2-D motion vector estimation: application to transient Elastography. *IEEE Trans. Ultrason. Ferroelect. Freq. Contr.*, Vol. 49, No. 10, Oct 2002, pp. 1363–1374.

Techavipoo, U.; Chen, Q.; Varghese, T.; Zagzebski, J. A. (2004). Estimation of displacement vectors and strain tensors in elastography using angular isonifications. *IEEE Trans Med. Imag.*, Vol. 23, No. 12, Dec 2004, pp. 1479–1489.

Wilson, L. S. & Robinson, D. E. (1982). Ultrasonic measurement of small displacements and deformations of tissue. *Ultrason. Imaging*, Vol. 4, No. 1, Jan 1982, pp. 71-82.

Yagi, S. & Nakayama, K. (1988). Local displacement analysis of inhomogeneous soft tissue by spatial correlation of rf echo signals. In: *Proceedings of WFUMB Meeting*, p. 113, Washington DC, 1988.

Yamakawa, M. & Shiina, T. (2001). Strain estimation using the extended combined autocorrelation method. *Jpn. J. Appl. Phys.*, Vol. 40(Part 1), No. 5B, May 2001, pp. 3872–3876.

8

High Resolution Ultrasound Imaging of Melanocytic and Other Pigmented Lesions of the Skin

Laurent Machet, Mahtab Samimi, Gabriella Georgesco, Youssef Mourtada, Michaël Naouri, Jean Marc Grégoire, Frédéric Ossant, Frédéric Patat and Loïc Vaillant
Department of Dermatology, CHRU Tours,
UMRS Inserm U930, CNRS ERL 3106, Tours,
CIC-IT, CHRU Tours,
Université François Rabelais, Tours,
France

1. Introduction

For two main reasons, dermatology is one of the later medical disciplines to use imaging techniques: 1) skin lesions are readily visible to the naked eye or through a magnifying glass, allowing clinical diagnosis with no invasive examination, 2) skin lesions can easily be biopsied or removed for histological study. This approach has therefore remained the basis of clinicopathological diagnosis of skin diseases for a long time. There has also been a third factor, i.e. the technical factors limiting image resolution (1-12). It is often necessary to visualise sub-centimeter lesions or even smaller, as in the case when measuring the thickness of a melanoma, and this cannot be achieved using traditional 7-10 MHz ultrasound. However, such techniques are useful in dermatology, especially in detecting lymph node spread of melanoma (6,13,14).

Other techniques such as optical coherence tomography and confocal microscopy are now available, with better resolution than 20-100 MHz ultrasound. However, both are more expensive and more time-consuming than ultrasound. Moreover, in certain European countries (e.g. France and Germany) ultrasound examination of the skin is reimbursed by health insurance services.

High resolution ultrasound imaging systems enable ultrasound to differentiate structures of less than 100 microns on the beam axis (axial resolution) and 200 microns on the scan axis (resolution axis). This can be achieved by the use of ultrasound frequencies above 15 MHz. Several groups have been working to extend the limits of existing machines by increasing the frequency (11,12,15,16). Working in our group, Berson et al. proposed a new ultrasound device operating at 17 MHz (1).This device was compact and had a very handy probe with an acoustic window enclosed by a thin membrane, allowing easier exploration of skin tumours on the face where they are more frequent than on other sites of the skin. We currently use a device derived from this prototype (Dermcup 2020®, Atys Medica, St

Soucieu en Jarrest, France) (2). The frequency ranges from 20 to 50 MHz, allowing visualisation of the superficial layer of the skin (epidermis and dermis, and the upper part of hypodermis) (Fig. 1), where the majority of lesions and skin tumors are located.

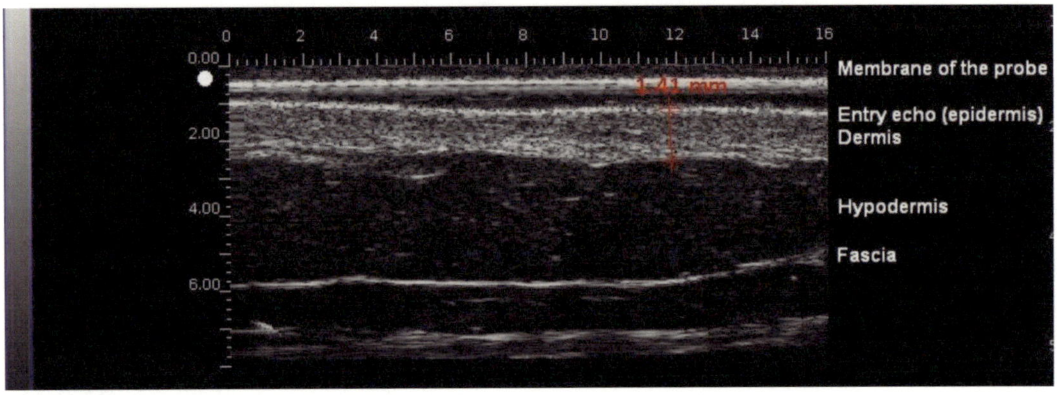

Fig. 1. Normal skin

Ultrasound imaging has been routinely used by dermatologists in our department for over ten years. The main indication is in the initial management of malignant tumors (including helping in the differential diagnosis and measurement of thickness). Moreover, ultrasound of the skin may be useful in the diagnosis of local recurrence and of locoregional melanoma , especially on certain very fibrous scars that are not easily accessible to palpation.

2. Ultrasound imaging of melanocytic lesions

Melanocytic lesions are often benign (melanocytic naevus) and affect many individuals. Melanoma is a highly malignant tumor, whose incidence has doubled every 20 to 30 years (1 to 2 new cases/10 000 inhabitants/year, representing a 1% probability of developing melanoma during a lifetime). The overall mortality rate is 20% and it is greater in the case of lesions thicker than 4 mm (50%). On the other hand, the overall survival of thin lesions (less than 0.5 mm thick) is excellent. The diagnosis of melanocytic lesions is initially clinical, frequently assisted by dermoscopy, and in the case of suspected malignancy, the second step is surgical removal and histology examination which remains the gold standard. Dermoscopy and ultrasound are both non-invasive techniques that can be combined to increase preoperative diagnostic accuracy in pigmented skin lesions (17). Dermoscopy has been proved to improve the sensitivity and the specificity of clinical examination. The goal is to remove all *in situ* or less than 0.5 mm thick melanomas and to reduce the unnecessary removal of benign melanocytic lesions. How can ultrasound imaging help in the management of such lesions?

2.1 Ultrasound imaging of naevi

The lesions are mainly hypoechoic, with many small echoes, symmetrical, and usually well delimited from the adjacent dermis (Fig. 2a). They are usually very thin in the case of junctional naevi (Fig. 2b) and thicker in the case of dermal naevi. However, the ultrasound image of clinically atypical naevi (which are often those that pose a problem of differential diagnosis) may be only slightly different from that observed in thin melanoma. Acoustic

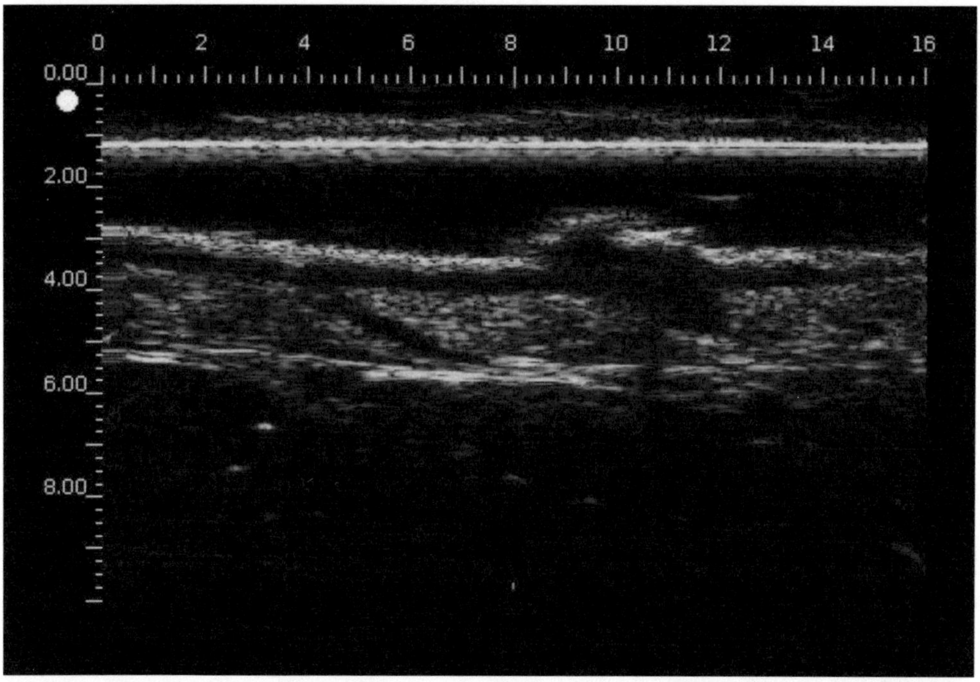

(a)

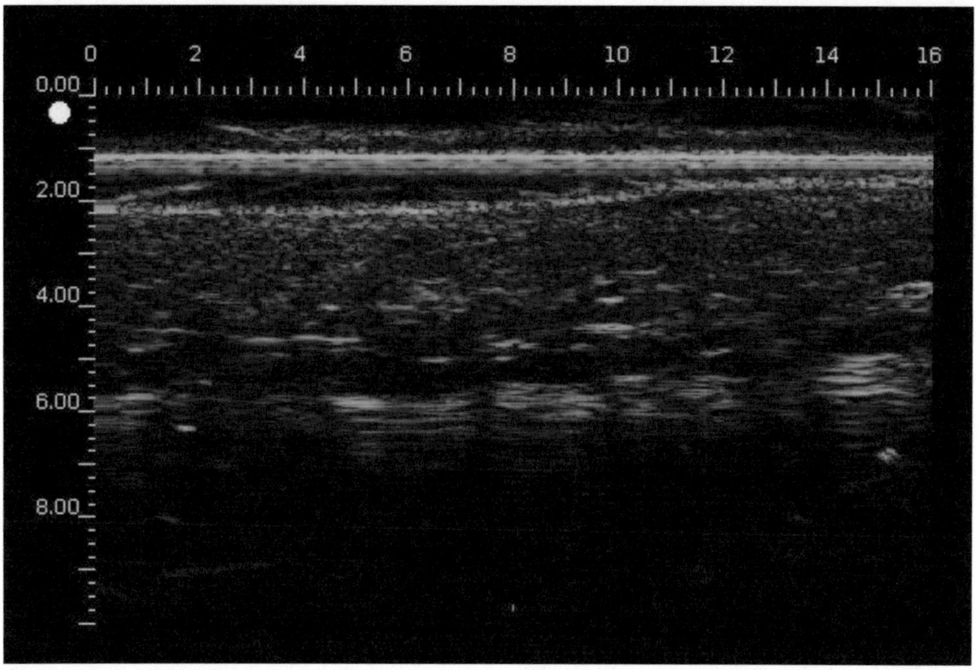

(b)

Fig. 2. a) echographic appearance of benign congenital melanocytic naevus; b) small acquired melanocytic naevus.

shadowing and retrolesional echogenicity may assist the diagnosis between benign naevus and melanoma (18) Quantitative discrimination of pigmented lesions seems possible using three-dimensional high-resolution ultrasound reflex transmission imaging (19). Blue naevi are also hypoechoic, and often have a dish shape or an ovoid shape (Fig.3a and 3b) (20).

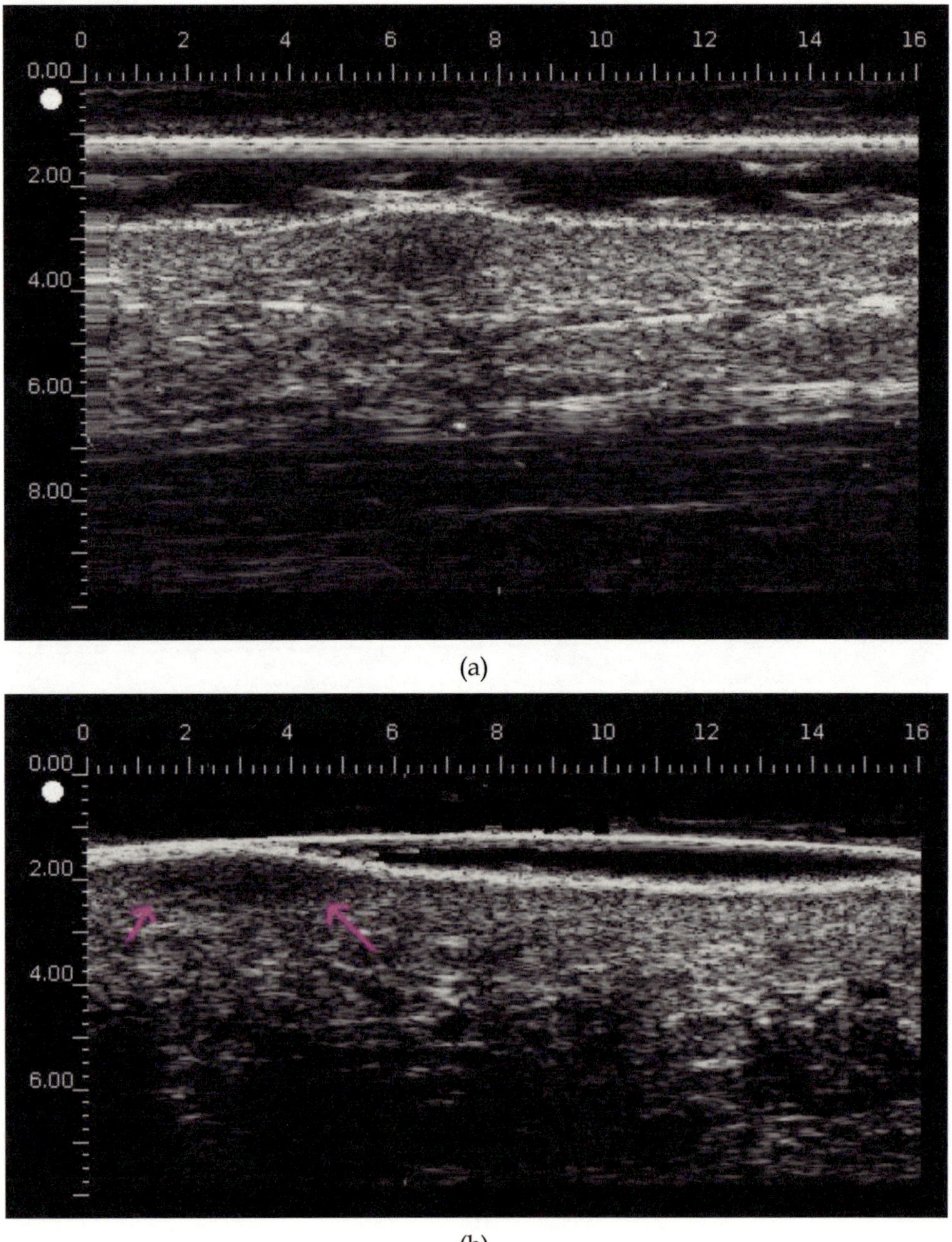

(a)

(b)

Fig. 3. a) Ovoid shaped benign blue naevus, b) dish shaped naevus

2.2 Ultrasound imaging of primary melanomas

The lesions are homogeneous and hypoechoic, often more so than benign naevi in our experience. Echo entry is usually clearly visible, but it is less visible in the case of ulcerated lesions. The lateral dermal component of superficial spreading melanoma is usually well delimited from the dermis, but the intra-epidermal part cannot be seen (Fig. 4) A thin melanoma with Breslow thickness below 0.5 mm may be hard to visualise on the face of an elderly person due to the Sub Epidermal NonEchogenic Band (SENEB). The vertical part of the lesion is easily shown within the dermis and to a lesser extent within the hypodermis (Fig. 5).

2.3 Ultrasound imaging of local or in transit recurrence and distant cutaneous metastasis:

Recurrences appear as hypoechoic nodules located within the dermis or the hypodermis. They are not well delimited and often infiltrate adjacent structures (Fig. 6). They are often visible or palpable, and may simulate a benign blue naevus. However, the shape of the lesion is different for a blue naevus and a recurrence of melanoma (20). Moreover, ultrasound examination is able to detect subclinical in transit recurrence in some cases.

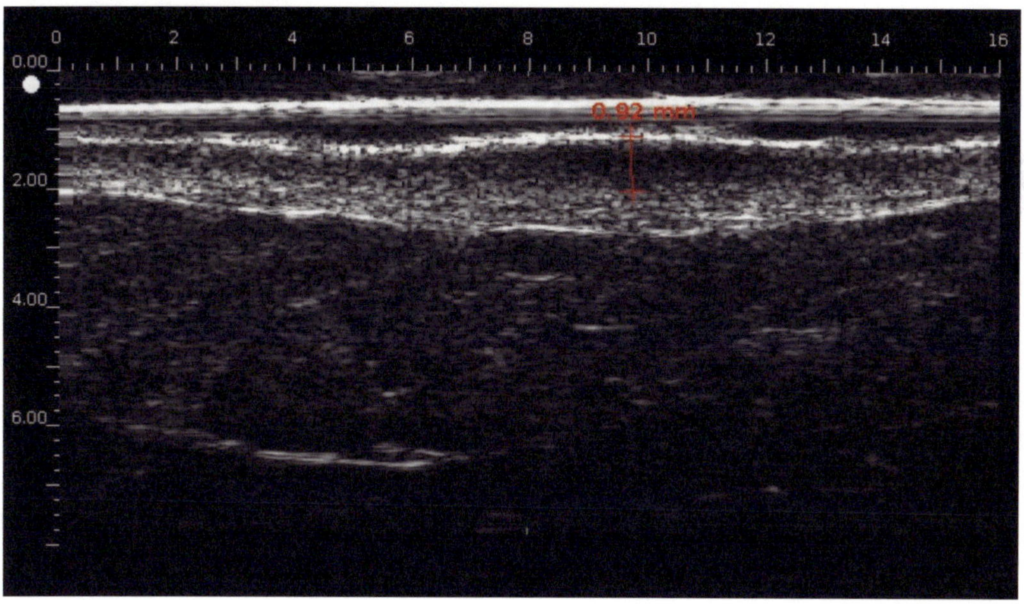

Fig. 4. Thin maligant melanoma.

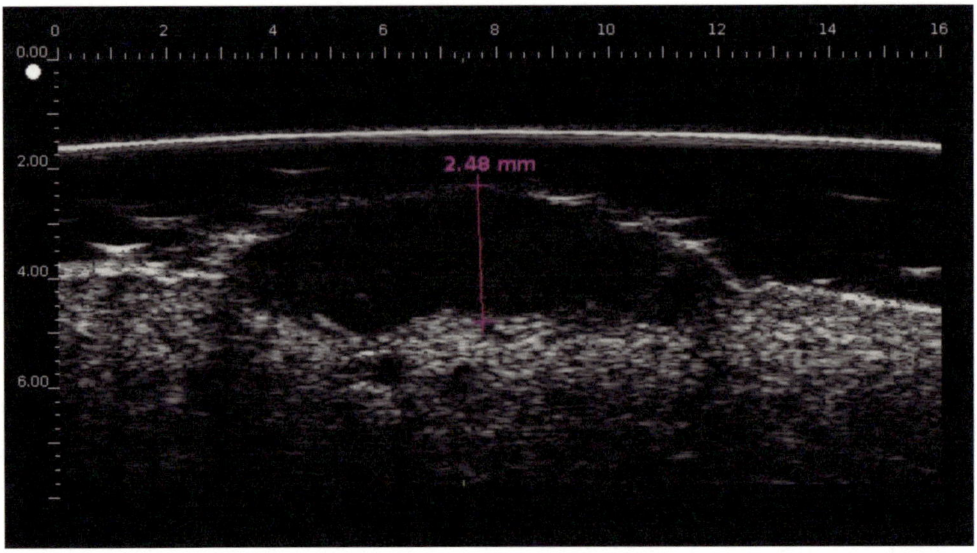

Fig. 5. Thick and ulcerated nodular malignant melanoma.

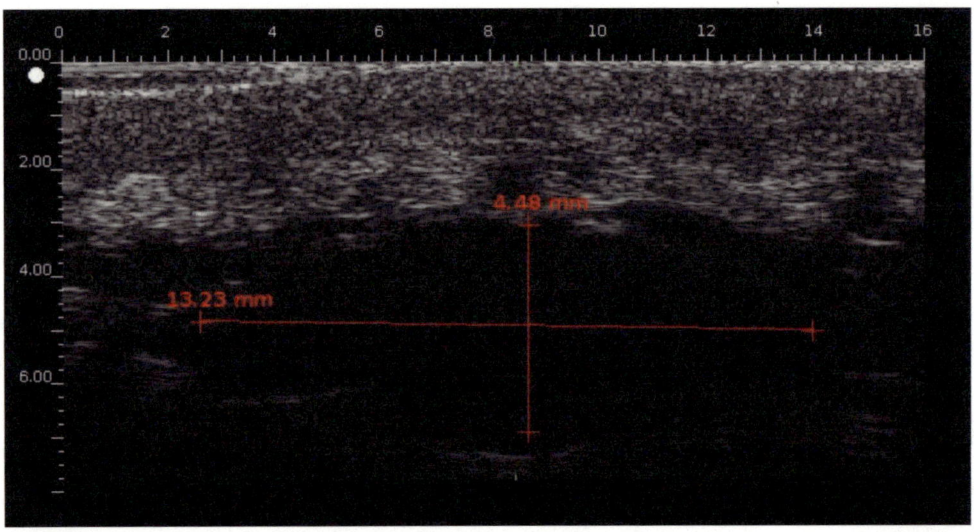

Fig. 6. In transit skin metastasis of malignant melanoma

2.4 Ultrasound measurement of thickness of melanocytic lesions:

The shape of a melanoma is often different from that of a benign naevus. However, the value of ultrasound imaging is mainly to measure the thickness of the lesion (3, 15,16,17, 21,23,24). Ultrasound thickness is well correlated with histological thickness (Fig. 7). This was recently demonstrated in a systematic review of the literature which identified 14 studies. Pearson's coefficient is generally good, ranging from 0.88 to 0.97 (21). However, there are some marked differences, as demonstrated in some cases using the graph of Bland and Altman (Fig. 8).This is particularly clear for thick melanomas, and in some particular locations (nail or plantar melanoma). Nevertheless, the width of surgical margins can be correctly determined from ultrasound thickness, allowing the patient to be operated on in a single operation in nearly 75% of cases (Table 1) (21).

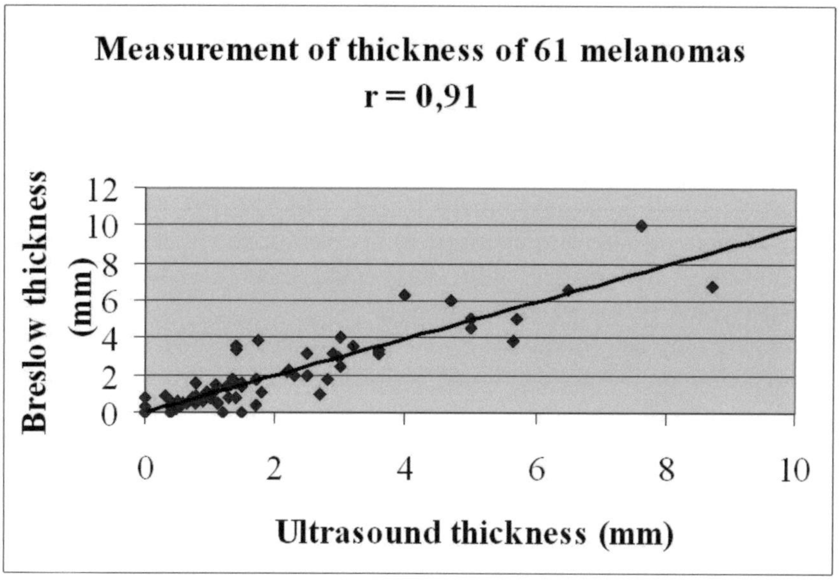

Fig. 7. Measurement of melanoma thickness with ultrasound (horizontal axis) as compared with histology, i.e. Breslow thickness (vertical axis), in a series of 61 melanomas treated in department.

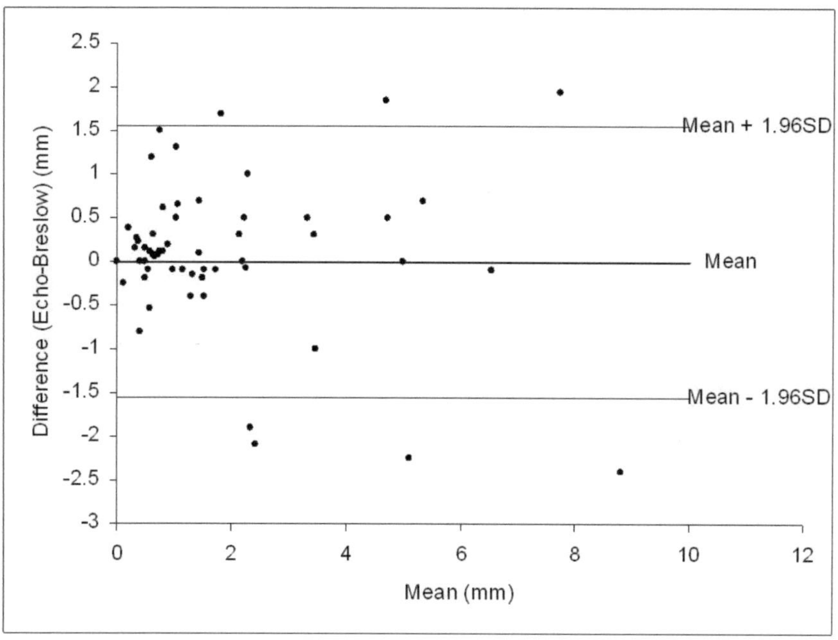

Fig. 8. Graph of Bland and Altman.

3. Differential diagnosis: ultrasound imaging of other frequent lesions

Ultrasound may assist the diagnosis of other pigmented or non pigmented tumors, as melanomas are sometimes achromic.

3.1 Basal Cell Carcinoma (BCC)

This is the most common skin cancer, most often located on areas of skin subjected to chronic sun exposure. The incidence is steadily increasing due to population aging and sun exposure habits. The pigmented variant of BCC may be confused with melanoma. In elderly subjects the tumor is mainly located on the face of. The first line of treatment is surgery, which allows complete excision and histological diagnosis. Radiotherapy or cryosurgery are therapeutic alternatives to surgery, with somewhat lower success rates (7% and 10% recurrence, respectively, versus 5% after surgery).

Ultrasound imaging may help in the diagnosis of BCC (25,26). The sonographic appearance is often stereotyped: overall anechoic tumor, including large focally dense echoes (Fig. 9). It is usually well delimited from the surrounding dermis.Ultrasound may also assist the detection of early recurrence, especially when surgical removal is incomplete or in cases treated with radiotherapy or cryosurgery. Ultrasound may also be used to help to determine the surgical margins or to delimitate the area treated with radiotherapy or cryosurgery (25, 27-32). This may decrease the rate of relapse.

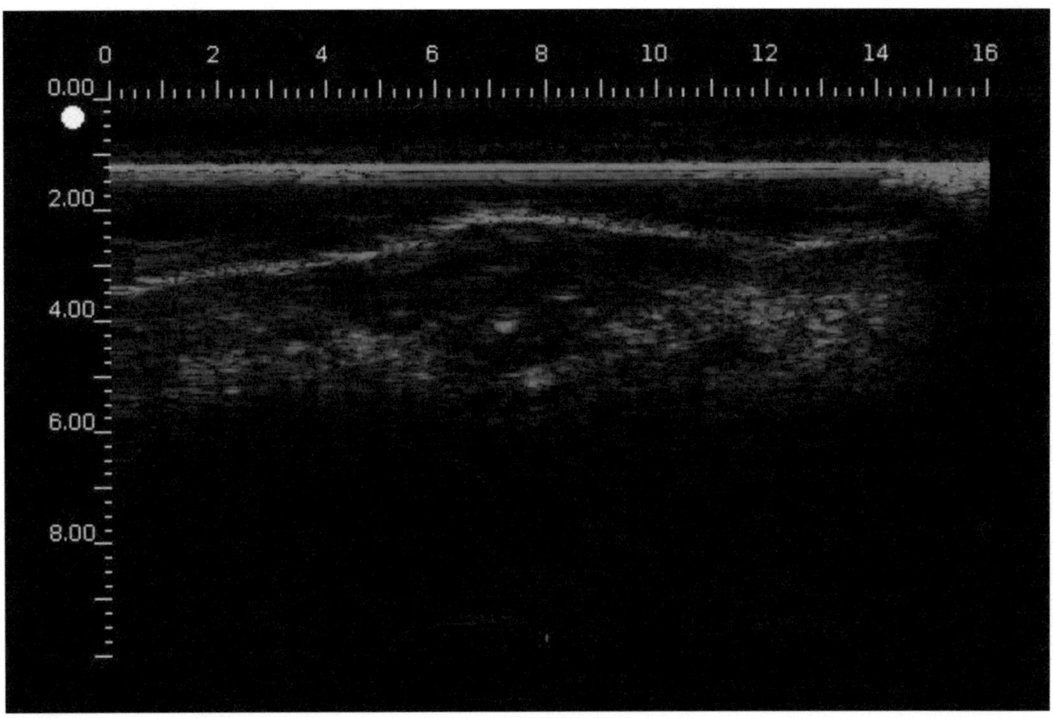

Fig. 9. Pigmented basal cell carcinoma showing some thick echoes within the tumor.

Epidermal cysts are limited, pushing the adjacent structures, and they have a heterogeneous structure, with both very echogenic and low echogenic areas (Fig. 10).

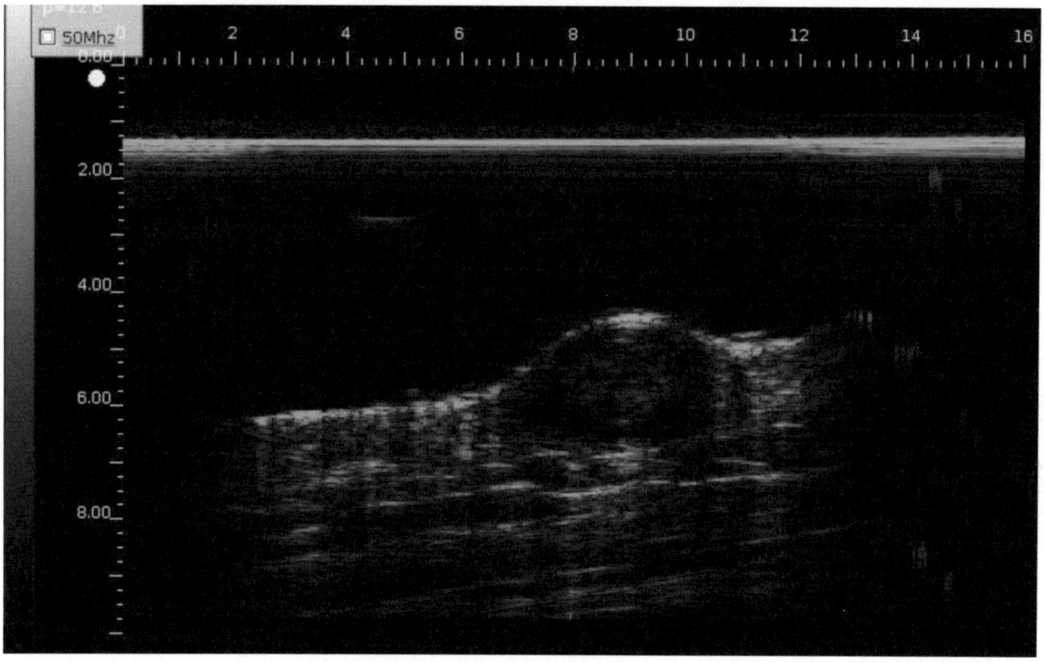

Fig. 10. Epidermal cysts showing a heterogeneous structure, with both very echogenic and low echogenic areas

Fibrous histiocytomas are fairly homogeneous, less echogenic than the normal dermis , with multiple small echoes, and their boundaries are poorly demarcated from the surrounding dermis (Fig. 11).

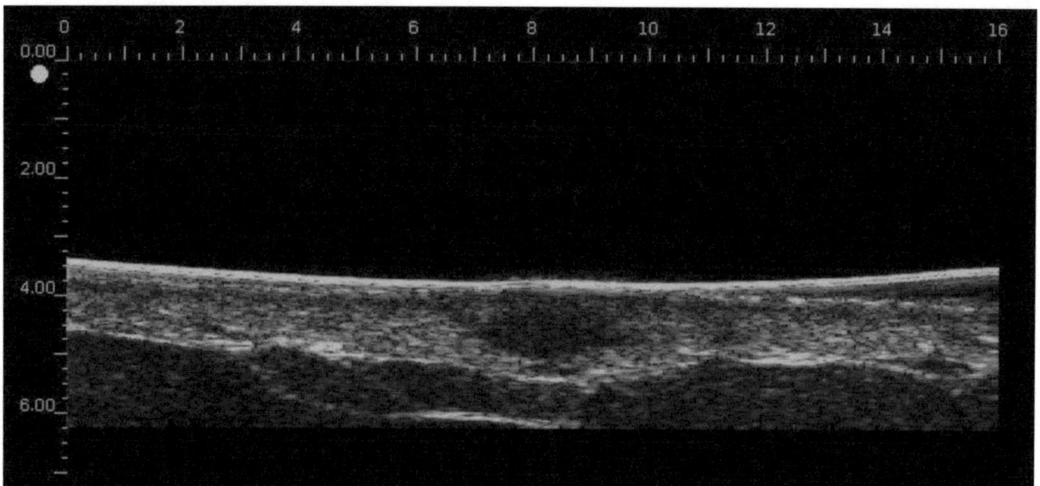

Fig. 11. Pigmented fibrous histiocytoma

Seborrheic keratoses are very well delimited, very superficial, as though laid on the skin, and may be misdiagnosed as melanoma. Ultrasound examination shows a dense echo input, under which there are very hypoechogenic lesions, in which one can sometimes see dense echoes (horny pseudocysts) (18) (Fig.12).

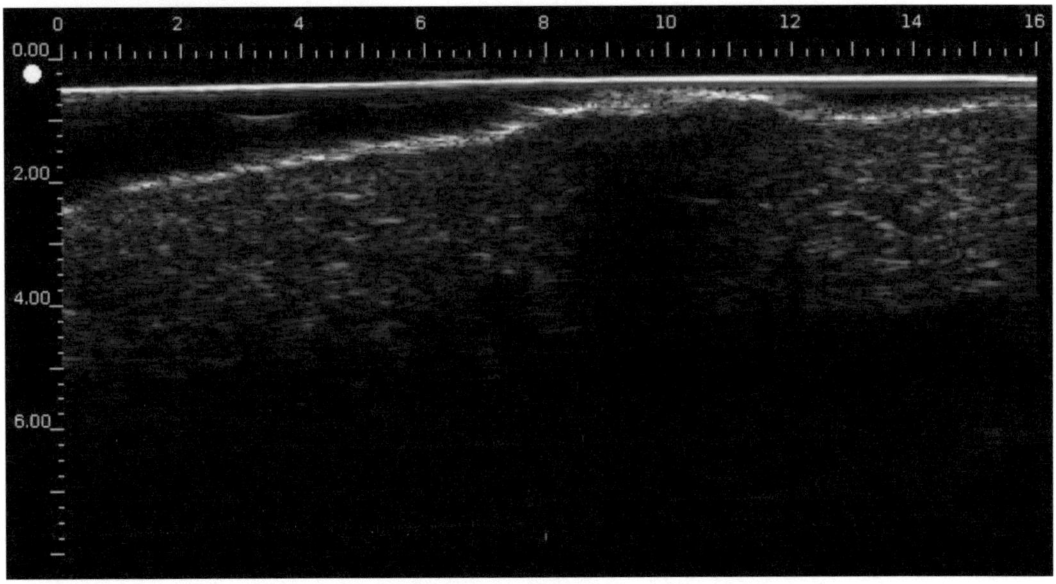

Fig. 12. Seborrheic keratosis with retrolesional acoustic shadowing

Acquired angiomas are sometimes a cause for concern especially in cases of inflammation or thrombosis, or sometimes in the differential diagnosis with amelanotic melanoma. They are fairly homogeneous lesions, less echogenic than the dermis, whose echogenicity is quite similar to that of the lip structure that is richly vascularized (Fig. 13).

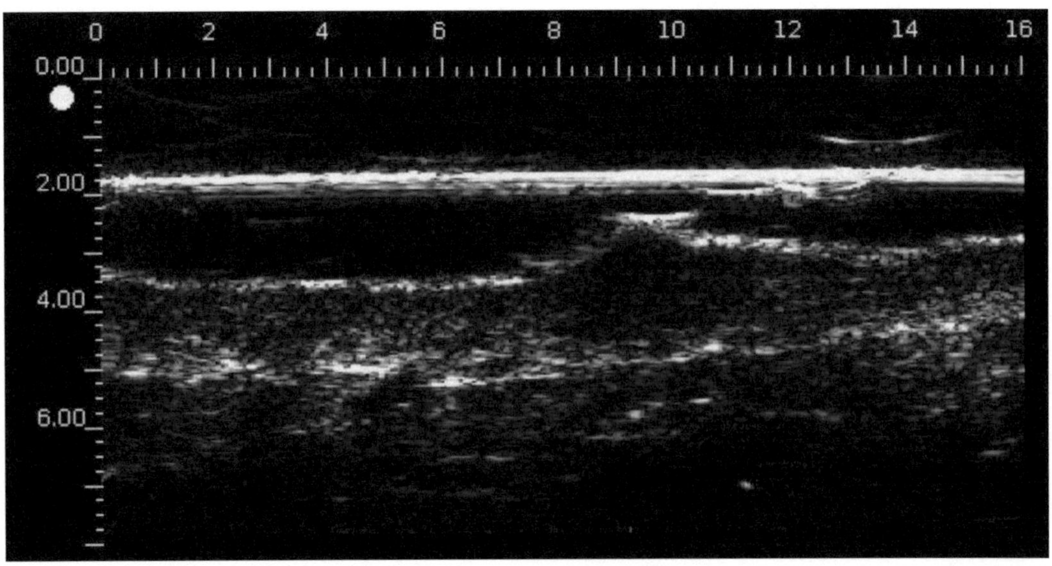

Fig. 13. Acquired hemangioma of the jaw.

4. Conclusion

Pathology examination remains the ultimate gold standard for diagnosis of skin tumors. However, it is not concievable to remove every skin lesion. Clinical examination (possibly assisted by dermoscopy) is often sufficient to determine whether a lesion has to be removed. However, ultrasound imaging provides additional information such as depth and lateral delimitation of the lesion, homegenous or heterogeneous structure, and hypo or hyperechoic appearance. These elements may of themselves be effective in terms of diagnostic accuracy and they are also valuable in the initial management or surveillance of patients.

5. References

[1] Berson M, Vaillant L, Patat F, Pourcelot L. High-resolution real-time ultrasonic scanner.Ultrasound Med Biol 1992;18:471-8.

[2] Berson M, Gregoire JM, Gens F, Rateau J, Jamet F, Vaillant L, Tranquart F,Pourcelot L. High frequency (20 MHz) ultrasonic devices: advantages and applications. Eur J Ultrasound 1999;10:53-63.

[3] Hoffmann K, Jung J, el Gammal S, Altmeyer P. Malignant melanoma in 20-MHz B scan sonography. Dermatology 1992;185:49-55.

[4] Fornage BD, McGavran MH, Duvic M, Waldron CA. Imaging of the skin with 20-MHz US. Radiology 1993;189:69-7.

[5] Harland CC, Bamber JC, Gusterson BA, Mortimer PS. High frequency, high resolution B-scan ultrasound in the assessment of skin tumours. Br J Dermatol 1993;128:525-32.

[6] Schmid-Wendtner MH, Burgdorf W. Ultrasound scanning in dermatology. Arch Dermatol 2005;141:217-24.

[7] Rallan C, Harland CC. Ultrasound in dermatology. Clin Exp Dermatol 2003 ;28 :632-638.

[8] Zymanska E, Nowicki A, Mlosek K, Litniewski J, Lewandowski M, Secomski W, Tymkiewicz R. Skin imaging with high frequency ultrasound - preliminary results. J Ultrasound 2000;12:9-16.

[9] Rallan D, Harland CC. Ultrasound in dermatology--basic principles and applications.Clin Exp Dermatol 2003;28:632-8.

[10] Rallan D, Harland CC. Skin imaging: is it clinically useful? Clin Exp Dermatol. 2004;29:453-9.

[11] Turnbull DH, Starkoski BG, Harasiewicz KA et al. A 40-100 MHz B-scan ultrasound backscatter microscope for skin imaging. Ultrasound Med Biol 1995;21:79-88.

[12] Vogt M, Opretzka J, Perrey C, Ermert H. Ultrasonic microscanning. Proc Inst Mech Eng H 2010;224:225-40.

[13] Machet L, Nemeth-Normand F, Giraudeau B, Perrinaud A, Tiguemounine J, AyoubJ, Alison D, Vaillant L, Lorette G. Is ultrasound lymph node examination superior to clinical examination in melanoma follow-up? A monocentre cohort study of 373 patients.Br J Dermatol 2005;152:66-70.

[14] Ulrich J, Voit C. Ultrasound in dermatology. Part II. Ultrasound of regional lymph node basins and subcutaneous tumours. Eur J Dermatol 2001;11:73-9.

[15] Guitera P, Li LX, Crotty Ket al. Melanoma histological Breslow thickness predicted by 75-MHz ultrasonography. Br J Dermatol 2008; 159: 364–9

[16] Gambichler T, Moussa G, Bahrenberg K et al. Preoperative ultrasonic assessment of thin melanocytic skin lesions using a 100-MHz ultrasound transducer: a comparative study. Dermatol Surg 2007; 33: 818–824.

[17] Krahn G, Gottlober P, Sander C, Peter RU. Dermatoscopy and high frequency sonography: two useful non-invasive methods to increase preoperative diagnostic accuracy in pigmented skin lesions. Pigment Cell Res 1998;11:151-4.
[18] Harland CC, Kale SG, Jackson P, Mortimer PS, Bamber JC. Differentiation of common benign pigmented skin lesions from melanoma by high-resolution ultrasound. Br J Dermatol 2000;143:281-9.
[19] Rallan D, Bush NL, Bamber JC, Harland CC. Quantitative discrimination of pigmented lesions using three-dimensional high-resolution ultrasound reflex transmission imaging. J Invest Dermatol 2007 ;27: 189-95.
[20] Samimi M, Perrinaud A, Naouri M, Maruani A, Perrodeau E, Vaillant L, Machet L. High resolution ultrasonography helps the differential diagnosis between blue naevi and cutaneous metastases of melanoma. Br J Dermatol 2010; 163: 550–56.
[21] Machet L, Belot V, Naouri M, Boka M, Mourtada Y, Perrinaud A, Giraudeau B, Laure B, Machet MC, Vaillant L. Preoperative measurement of thickness of cutaneous melanoma using high-resolution 20 mhz ultrasound imaging: feasibility and pitfalls to predict surgical margins. A prospective study of 31 cases and a systematic review of the litterature. Ultrasound Med Biol 2009;35:1411-20.
[22] Pellacani G, Seidenari S. Preoperative melanoma thickness determination by 20-MHz sonography and digital videomicroscopy in combination. Arch Dermatol 2003;139:293-8.
[23] Serrone L, Solivetti FM, Thorel MF, Eibenschutz L, Donati P, Catricala C. High frequency ultrasound in the preoperative staging of primary melanoma: a statistical analysis. Melanoma Res 2002;12:287-90.
[24] Lassau N, Spatz A, Avril MF, Tardivon A, Margulis A, Mamelle G, Vanel D, Leclere J. Value of high-frequency US for preoperative assessment of skin tumors. Radiographics 1997;17:1559-65.
[25] Vaillant L, Grognard C, Machet L, Cochelin N, Callens A, Berson M, Aboumrad J, Patat F, Lorette G. Imagerie ultrasonore haute résolution: utilité pour le traitement des carcinomes basocellulaires par cryochirurgie. Ann Dermatol Venereol 1998;125:500-504.
[26] Uhara H, Hayashi K, Koga H, S Toshiaki. Multiple hypersonographic spots in basal cell carcinoma. Dermatol Surg 2007; 33: 1215–9.
[27] Desai TD, Desai AD, Horowitz DC, Kartono F, Wahl T. The use of high-frequency ultrasound in the evaluation of superficial and nodular basal cell carcinomas. Dermatol Surg 2007;33:1220-7
[28] Mogensen M, Nürnberg BM, Forman JL, Thomsen JB, Thrane L, Jemec GB. In vivo thickness measurement of basal cell carcinoma and actinic keratosis with optical coherence tomography and 20-MHz ultrasound. Br J Dermatol 2009;160:1026-33.
[29] Marmur ES, Berkowitz EZ, Fuchs BS, Singer GK, Yoo JY. Use of high-frequency, high-resolution ultrasound before Mohs surgery. Dermatol Surg 2010;36:841-7.
[30] Jambusaria-Pahlajani A, Schmults CD, Miller CJ, Shin D, Williams J, Kurd SK, Gelfand JM. Test characteristics of high-resolution ultrasound in the preoperative assessment of margins of basal cell and squamous cell carcinoma in patients undergoing Mohs micrographic surgery. Dermatol Surg 2009;35:9-15
[31] Bobadilla F, Wortsman X, Muñoz C, Segovia L, Espinoza M, Jemec GB. Pre-surgical high resolution ultrasound of facial basal cell carcinoma: correlation with histology. Cancer Imaging 2008;8:163-72.
[32] Moore JV, Allan E. Pulsed ultrasound measurements of depth and regression of basal cell carcinomas after photodynamic therapy: relationship to probability of 1-year local control.Br J Dermatol 2003;149:1035-40.

Clinical Usefulness of Contrast-Enhanced Three-Dimensional Ultrasound Imaging with Sonazoid for Hepatic Tumor Lesions

Kazushi Numata[1], Wen Luo[1,2], Manabu Morimoto[1], Hiroyuki Fukuda[1], Naoto Sato[3] and Katsuaki Tanaka[1]
[1]Gastroenterological Center, Yokohama City University Medical Center, 4-57 Urafune-cho, Minami-ku, Yokohama, Kanagawa, 232-0024,
[2]Department of Ultrasound, Xijing Hospital, Fourth Military Medical University, 15th Changle Xi Road, Xi'an, ShaanXi, 710032,
[3]GE Healthcare Japan Corporation, 4-7-127, Asahigaoka, Hino, Tokyo 191-8503
[1,3]Japan
[2]China

1. Introduction

In the last few years, three-dimensional ultrasound (3D US) imaging has attracted the interest among medical imaging researchers, because of its unique ability to provide images in three orthogonal planes, and the imaging tool has been proven to be useful clinically in the fields of obstetrics, hepatology, cardiology, urology, and mastology (Badea et al., 2007; Benacerraf et al., 2006; Tutschek & Sahn, 2007; Taylor et al., 2005; Kotsianos-Hermle et al., 2009).

Multiplanar 3D US imaging is thought to provide more spatial information and allow easier anatomic assessment than the conventional two-dimensional ultrasound imaging. Contrast-enhanced three-dimensional ultrasound (CE 3D US) imaging is a new medical imaging technique that uses reflections of microbubbles to clearly depict blood vessels and allows the images to be displayed spatially at different visual angles. Although CE 3D US imaging has recently been evaluated as a tool for clinical diagnosis (Krenning et al., 2007; Yukisawa et al., 2007; Ohto et al., 2005; Wessels et al., 2004; Forsberg et al., 2004), only a few studies have investigated its usefulness in the assessment of hepatic tumors (Yukisawa et al., 2007; Ohto et al., 2005). Hepatic tumors, especially hepatocellular carcinoma (HCC), remain one of the most commonly encountered diseases worldwide (Bosch et al., 2004), and efficacious methods for the diagnosis and therapy of this disease, including CE 3D US imaging, need to be explored further (Camaggi et al., 2007; Kudo, 2007; Dietrich, 2002).

Sonazoid (Daiichi Sankyo, Tokyo, Japan) is a newly-developed second-generation ultrasound contrast agent that has been used clinically in Japan since January 2007 for the evaluation of liver tumors and for phase-inversion harmonic gray-scale sonography. Sonazoid consists of perfluorobutane surrounded by a phospholipid shell and has been reported, from previous studies, to be stable enough to allow image acquisition under ultrasound exposure for 5 to 10 minutes (Numata et al., 2008; Halpern et al., 2002).

Currently, automatically scanned CE 3D US with Sonazoid using the GE LOGIQ 7 ultrasound system (GE Healthcare, Milwaukee, WI, USA) is being used as a clinical diagnostic tool in Japan, especially for liver lesions (Luo et al., 2009a; Luo et al., 2009b; Luo et al., 2009c; Luo et al., 2010a; Luo et al., 2010b; Numata et al., 2010a; Numata et al., 2010b). With the use of coded harmonic angio (CHA) mode and high mechanical index (MI) contrast conditions, which reduce microbubbles in microvessels, but not in relatively large vessels, such as tumor vessels and portal veins, CE 3D US with Sonazoid facilitates detailed observation of tumor vessels. As compared to CE (two dimensional) US with Sonazoid, automatically scanned CE 3D US with Sonazoid allows the volume of interest to be viewed in three orthogonal planes, thereby more spatial information and facilitating easier anatomic assessment.

In this chapter, we present the methods used for acquisition and reconstruction of CE 3D US images obtained with Sonazoid, and also clinical usefulness of this diagnostic modality in the evaluation of hepatic tumor lesions, especially HCC lesions, using many figures to facilitate comprehension.

2. US equipment

The US scanning was performed with a commercially available ultrasound imaging system (LOGIQ 7; GE Healthcare, Milwaukee, WI) and a convex volume 4D3C-L probe with a frequency of 2.0-5.5 MHz.

3. Advantage of Sonazoid over Levovist as a contrast agent for CE 3D US

In our experience, Levovist is unstable, and therefore, not a suitable contrast agent for CE 3D US. As with Levovist, contrast-enhanced US with Sonazoid involves two phases of contrast enhancement: the vascular phase and the late (parenchyma-specific, delayed, post-vascular) phase. The drawback of the poor stability of Levovist is overcome with the high stability of Sonazoid and the microbubbles of Sonazoid have the advantage of allowing more prolonged imaging and providing stronger contrast effects; hence, more detailed observations are possible with Sonazoid than with Levovist.

4. CE 3D US at a high mechanical index (MI)

Sonazoid-enhanced US at a low MI using software for a low MI contrast mode (coded phase inversion mode: CPI mode) permits visualization of tumor vessels and tumor enhancement of liver lesions. However, not only relatively large vessels, such as tumor vessels and portal veins, but also microvessels within the liver parenchyma become rapidly filled with Sonazoid microbubbles under low MI conditions, which in turn, permits rapid enhancement of the tumor and of the liver parenchyma simultaneously. This phenomenon allows only a short time for detailed observation of the tumor vessels and tumor enhancement in the vascular phase of Sonazoid-enhanced US.

Sonazoid-enhanced US at a high MI using software for a high MI contrast mode (coded harmonic angio mode: CHA mode) allows observation of vessels in the early phase by eliminating microbubbles in the microvessels but not in the relatively large vessels, such as tumor vessels and portal veins (Numata et al., 2008), which permits a more prolonged of observation time of the tumor vessels, clear tumor enhancement, and also automatically scanned CE 3D US with Sonazoid.

5. Data acquisition

2D grey-scale US was carried out for identifying the tumor prior to the CE 3D US, and also for measurement of the tumor size.

Prior to the CE 3D US, 0.2 mL Sonazoid was injected as a bolus by hand through an antecubital vein, followed by injection of 2 mL of 5% glucose and then a infusion of glucose at 10 mL/min. The coded harmonic angio (CHA) mode with a mechanical index (MI, 0.5-0.9) of 8 to 13 frames per second was used for the CE US. The entire contrast procedure was divided into three phases: early phase, 15-50 s after injection of the contrast medium; middle phase, 80-120 s after injection of contrast medium; late phase, more than 5 minutes after injection of contrast medium.

For data acquisition, the ultrasound imaging system is equipped with two functions: the Static 3D function and the Autosweep 3D function. For both functions, the probe held by the sonographer automatically sweeps the region in the volume of interest (VOI), the size and position of which is already adjusted on the grey-scale US to contain the target tumor and the surrounding tissues. Static 3D enables easy volume scanning and rendering. However, it is difficult to control the complex acoustic power protocol required for high-MI contrast imaging, and this may cause unexpected bubble destructions in the middle and late phases. On the other hand, the AutoSweep 3D provides the acoustic power control needed for high-MI imaging, without unexpected bubble destructions. Therefore, in the early phase we performed two scanning procedures using the two functions, while in the two subsequent phases, only one procedure each was conducted, with the Autosweep 3D. The scanning angle can be selected in the range of 15° to 84°. We used angles in the range of 30°-70°, depending on the tumor size.

When we used the Static 3D for the data acquisition in the early phase, there were five levels of acquired image quality, Max, Hi 2, Hi 1, Mid 2, Mid 1, and Low. The Max level combined the highest density with the slowest speed, and the Low level combined the lowest density with the highest speed. Both the scanning time and image quality should be taken into consideration for proper image acquisition. The Mid 2 or Hi1 quality was selected for the patients, considering the short breath-holding duration. Accordingly, the time for one scanning session was 4.5 s to 26 s (mean 10 s). Therefore, the number of scanning sessions was 1 or 2 times during the early phase using the Static 3D function. The data acquired were stored as cineloops in the hard disk of the ultrasound imaging system.

When we used the Autosweep 3D for data acquisition in each of the three phases, there were four levels of acquired image quality, low, mid, high, and max. The mid quality was selected for the patients, considering the short breath-holding duration. Accordingly, the time for one scanning session was 3 s to 11 s (mean 6 s). The number of scanning sessions was 1 to 4 during the early phase, 1 to 2 during the middle phase, and 1 to 4 using the Autosweep 3D function. The data acquired were automatically stored as cineloops in the hard disk of the ultrasound imaging system. Subsequently, we selected the good data obtained in each phase for the image reconstruction.

6. Image reconstruction

3D image reconstruction was performed using the functions with which the LOGIQ 7 ultrasound system was equipped. In the VOI which was presented in an isotropic rectangular coordinate frame, the three orthogonal planes were referred to as plane A,

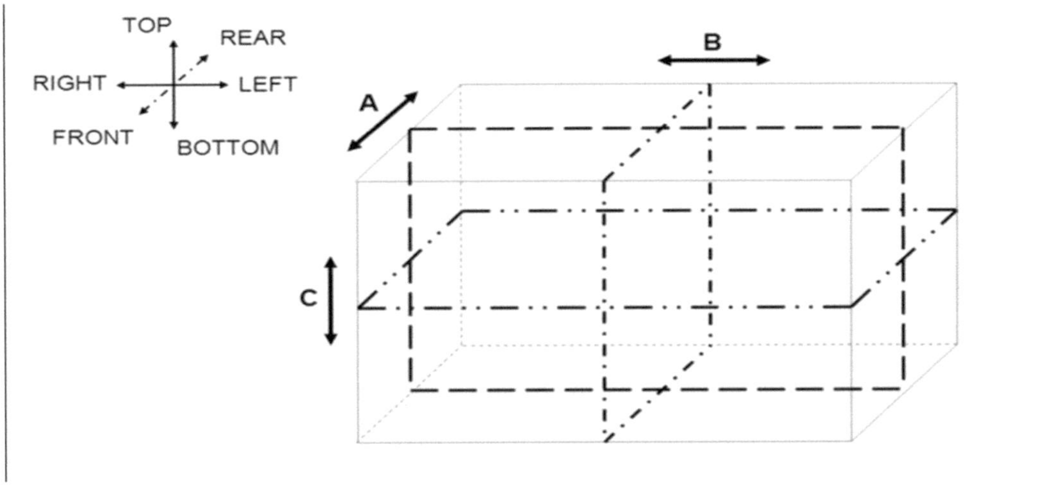

Fig. 1. Illustration of the volume of Interest and three orthogonal planes obtained by automatic 3D acquisition. Plane A moves from the front to the rear, or in the opposite direction, through the volume of interest, whereas plane B moves from the left to the right, or in the opposite direction, and plane C moves from the top to the bottom, or in the opposite direction.

which could migrate from the front to the rear through the VOI, plane B, which moved from the left to the right, and plane C, which moved from the top to the bottom (Fig. 1).
Tomographic ultrasound images (TUI) with presentation of several parallel slices in three orthogonal planes were reconstructed in three phases, while the number of slices that could be selected was 2, 4, or 6 for images obtained using the Autosweep 3D, and 2, 4, or 9 for the Static 3D. In order to show the desired images, the range of distance between two slices in the TUI could be adjusted as required (Figs. 2A-C). The mean time taken for these procedures was about 20 s.
Sonographic angiograms were reconstructed in an angio-like view during the early phase using various rendering modes. When the Autosweep 3D was used, the five rendering modes consisted of the surface mode, texture mode, and maximum intensity projection mode, average intensity mode, and minimum intensity modes, which could be used in any combination (Fig. 2D). The maximum intensity projection mode displaying the maximal gray values in the VOI, combined with the surface mode displaying the gray values on the surfaces of the anatomic structures, was used to visualize the tumor vessels and early tumor enhancement in the early phase. While the average intensity mode displaying the average gray values in the VOI was employed in combination with the surface mode, to define the tumor based on the predominantly unenhanced areas in the early, middle and late phases. The mean time taken for these procedures was about 45 s.
When the Static 3D was used for the reconstruction of the data obtained in the early phase, the transparent maximum mode (as same as the maximum intensity projection mode) combined with the surface smooth mode was selected to depict the tumor vessels and the tumor enhancement distinctly. The transparent X-ray mode (as same as the average intensity mode) combined with the surface smooth mode (as same as the surface mode) was used for detection of the unenhanced areas within the tumors, if these unenhanced portions played an important role in defining the tumors, such as unenhanced portions of metastases

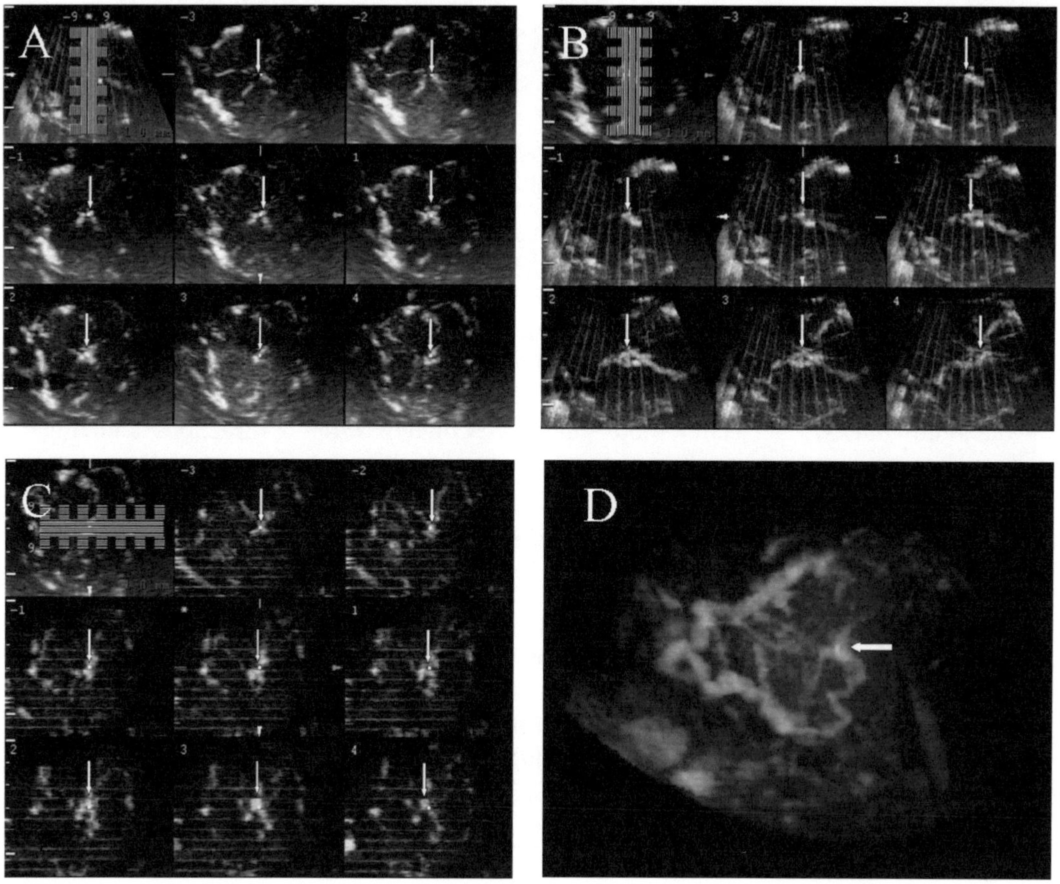

Fig. 2. Early-phase contrast-enhanced three-dimensional ultrasonographic (CE 3D US) images of the liver in a patient with focal nodular hyperplasia (maximum diameter, 50 mm) in the left lobe. A-C: Tomographic ultrasound images (TUI) in plane A, which could be translated from front to back (A), plane B, which could be translated from right to left (B), and plane C, which can be translated from bottom to top. The slice distance is 1.0 mm in each plane. Slight cardiac motion artifacts are seen in planes B and C. Sonographic angiograms acquired by CE 3D US with the Autosweep 3D in the early phase and rendered using the maximum intensity projection mode mixed with the surface mode; the images show the tumor to contain a spoke-wheel artery (D). Arrows indicate the spoke-wheel artery.

with early peripheral ring-like enhancement accounting for large areas of the tumors. In cases of hypervascular tumors, such as typical HCC lesions or focal nodular hyperplasia, the transparent maximum mode (maximum intensity projection mode) alone was selected to simplify the procedure to depict the intratumoral vessels with early tumor enhancement distinctly. Tortuous vessels within the lesion could be clearly visualized (Fig. 3). The mean time taken for these procedures was about 60 s.

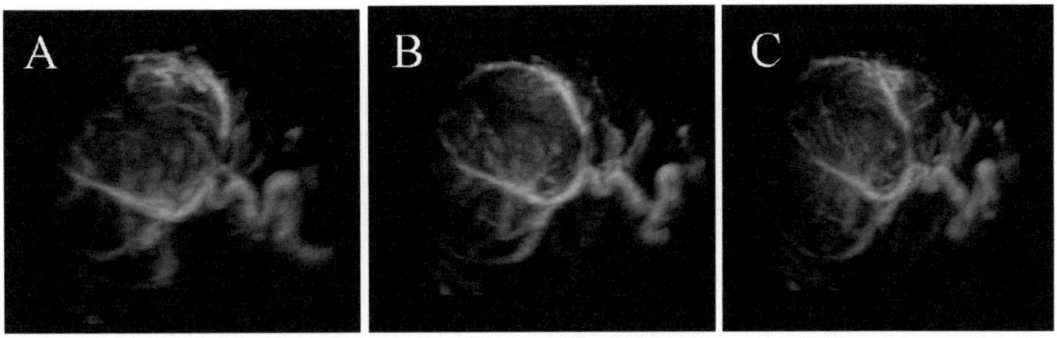

Fig. 3. Early-phase of CE 3D US images of the liver in a patient with a large hepatocellular carcinoma (HCC) (maximum diameter, 75 mm) in the right lobe. A-C: Sonographic angiograms acquired by CE 3D US with the Static 3D in the early phase and rendered using the maximum intensity projection mode alone, presented in different directions, showing the tumor containing the tortuous intratumoral vessels.

7. Characterization of liver lesions by CE 3D US with Sonazoid

Sonazoid-enhanced 3D US also provides important spatial visualization of any part of the VOI. From the early to the late phase, Sonazoid-enhanced 3D US shows tumor vascularity and changes in tumor enhancement patterns in multiplanar images. In our retrospective study of 139 liver lesions, the diagnostic accuracies of Sonazoid-enhanced 3D US and contrast-enhanced 3D CT were assessed for differentiating among liver lesions. The sensitivity of both modalities was 83% or higher, the specificity was 87% or higher for Sonazoid-enhanced 3D US and 92% or higher for contrast-enhanced 3D CT, the positive predictive value was 71% or higher for both modalities, and the area under the receiver operating characteristics curve (*Az*) was 0.89 or more for US and 0.92 or more for CT. The inter-reader agreement was good to excellent ($\kappa \geq 0.76$) for both modalities (Luo et al., 2009c).

8. Features of hypervascular HCCs on CE 3D US with Sonazoid

Typical hypervascular HCCs contain intratumoral vessels and show tumor enhancement in the early phase, show homogeneous or heterogeneous tumor enhancement (slight washout) in the middle phase, and become hypoechoic, showing a distinct boundary with the surrounding liver parenchyma (washout) in the late phase (Figs. 4-6). Most moderately and poorly differentiated HCCs show these enhancement patterns, whereas about half of the hypervascular well-differentiated HCCs appear as isoechogenic areas in the late phase. It must be borne in mind that about half of the hypervascular well-differentiated HCCs are not detected as perfusion defects in the late phase of Sonazoid-enhanced US.

The main rendering mode used for obtaining sonographic angiograms in the early phase for hypervascular HCCs is the maximum intensity projection mode, mixed with some other mode at a different percentage, which enables depiction of the tumor staining and tumor vessels in three dimensions at any visual angles desired. Sonographic angiograms also demonstrate the relationship between the reconstructed tumor staining and the surrounding vessels (Figs. 4C, 5A). The main rendering mode used for obtaining sonographic angiograms in the late phase for typical hypervascular HCCs is the average intensity mode mixed with the surface mode at a different percentage, which enables depiction of the lesions as hypoechogenic (washout) areas.

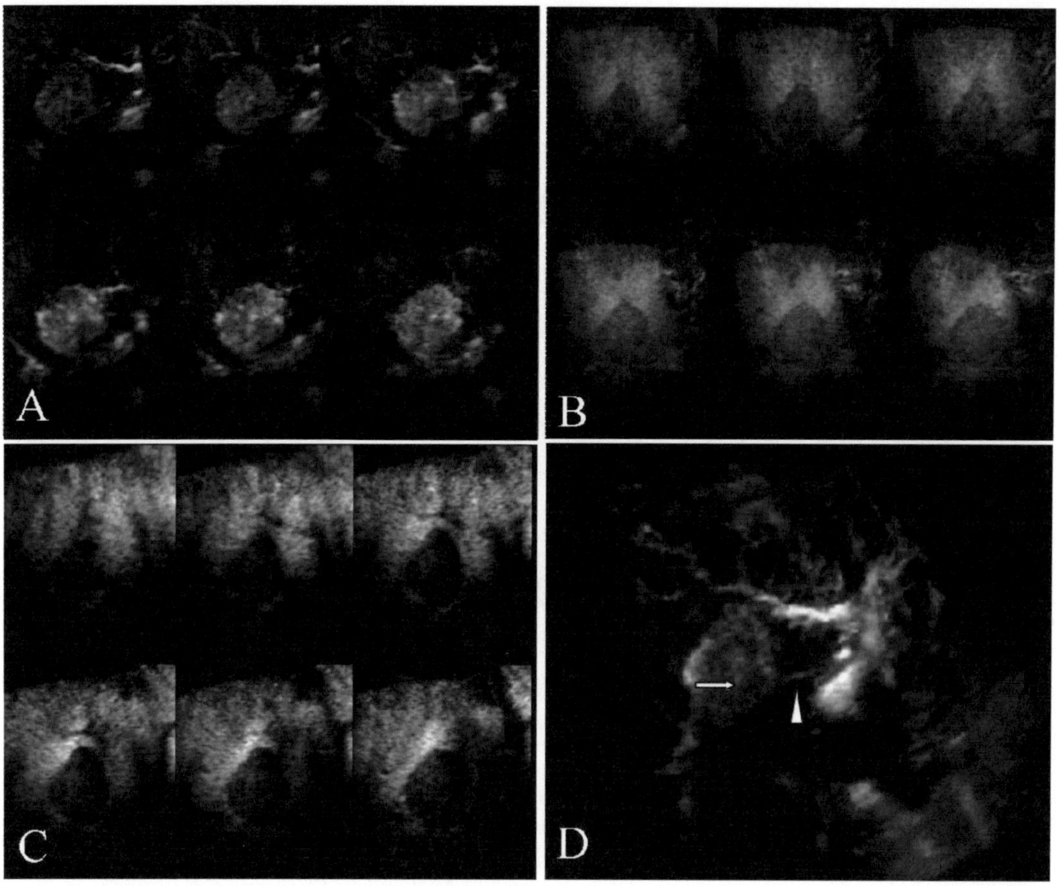

Fig. 4. CE 3D US images of the liver in a patient with HCC (maximum diameter, 40 mm) located adjacent to the left portal vein in segment IV of the left lobe. A-C: TUI in plane A of the early phase (A), middle phase (B), and late phase (C). The slice distance was 3.5 mm in each plane. These images show homogeneous tumor enhancement with intratumoral vessels in the early phase, homogeneous enhancement (slight washout) in the middle phase, and hypoechogenicity (washout) in the late phase. Sonographic angiograms acquired with the Autosweep 3D function in the early phase and rendered using the maximum intensity projection mode mixed with the surface mode showing the feeding artery (arrowhead) and homogeneous tumor enhancement with intratumoral vessels (arrow) (D). The left portal vein is also seen.

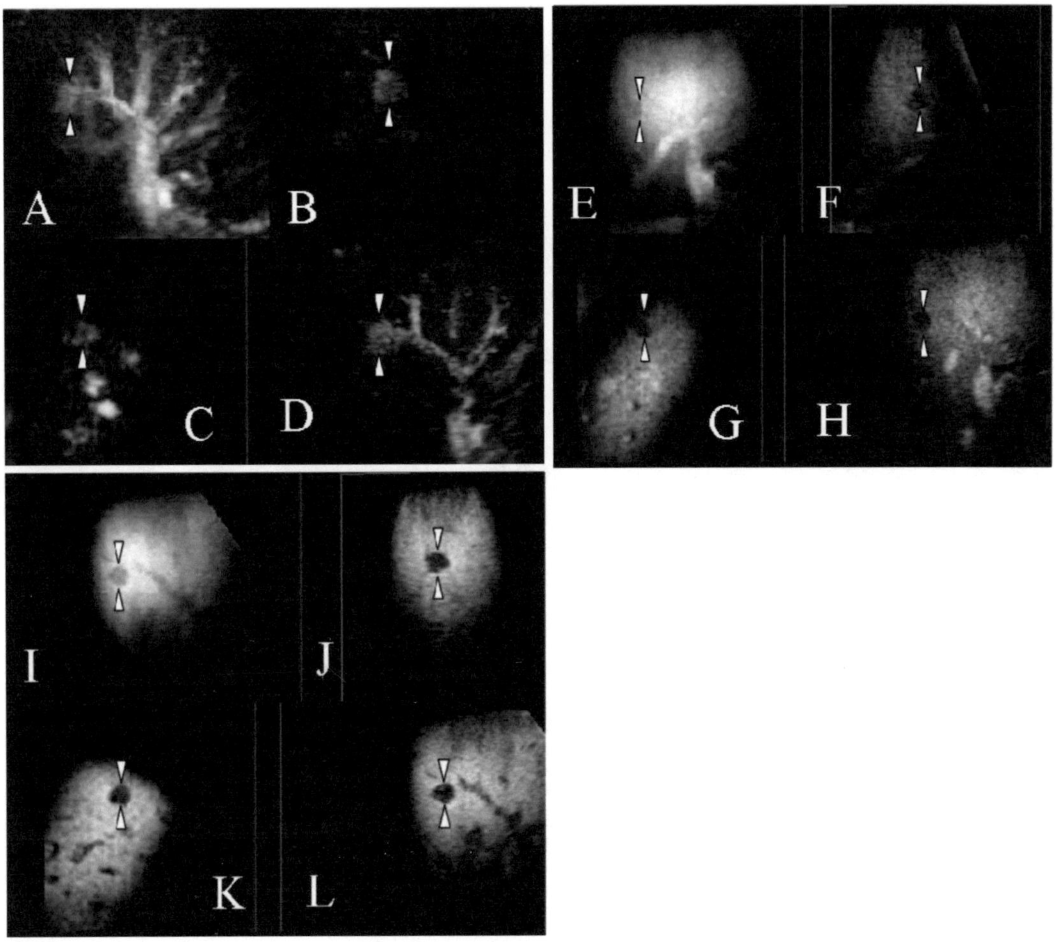

Fig. 5. CE 3D US images of the liver in a patient with a small HCC located adjacent to the right anterior portal vein (maximum diameter, 13 mm) in segment VIII of the right lobe. A-D: Display of a sonographic angiograms acquired with the Autosweep 3D function in the early phase and rendered using the maximum intensity projection mode mixed with the surface mode (A) and 3D plane B, which could be translated from right to left (B), plane C, which could be translated from bottom to top (C), plane A, which could be translated from front to back (D); these images show homogeneous enhancement of the tumor with intratumoral vessels adjacent to the portal vein and hepatic artery. E-H: Display of sonographic angiograms acquired with the Autosweep 3D function in the middle phase and rendered using the average intensity mode mixed with the surface mode (E) and 3D plane B (F), plane C (G), plane A (H); these images exhibit the lesions as perfusion defect. I-L: Display of sonographic angiograms acquired with the Autosweep 3D function in the late phase and rendered using the average intensity mode mixed with the surface mode (I) and 3D plane B (J), plane C (K), plane A (L); these images exhibit the lesion as a hypoechogenic (washout) area. Arrowheads indicate the margin of the tumor. Therefore, this HCC shows homogeneous enhancement with intratumoral vessels in the early phase, appears as a perfusion defect in the middle phase, and as a hypoechogenicity (washout) in the late phase of the CE 3D US.

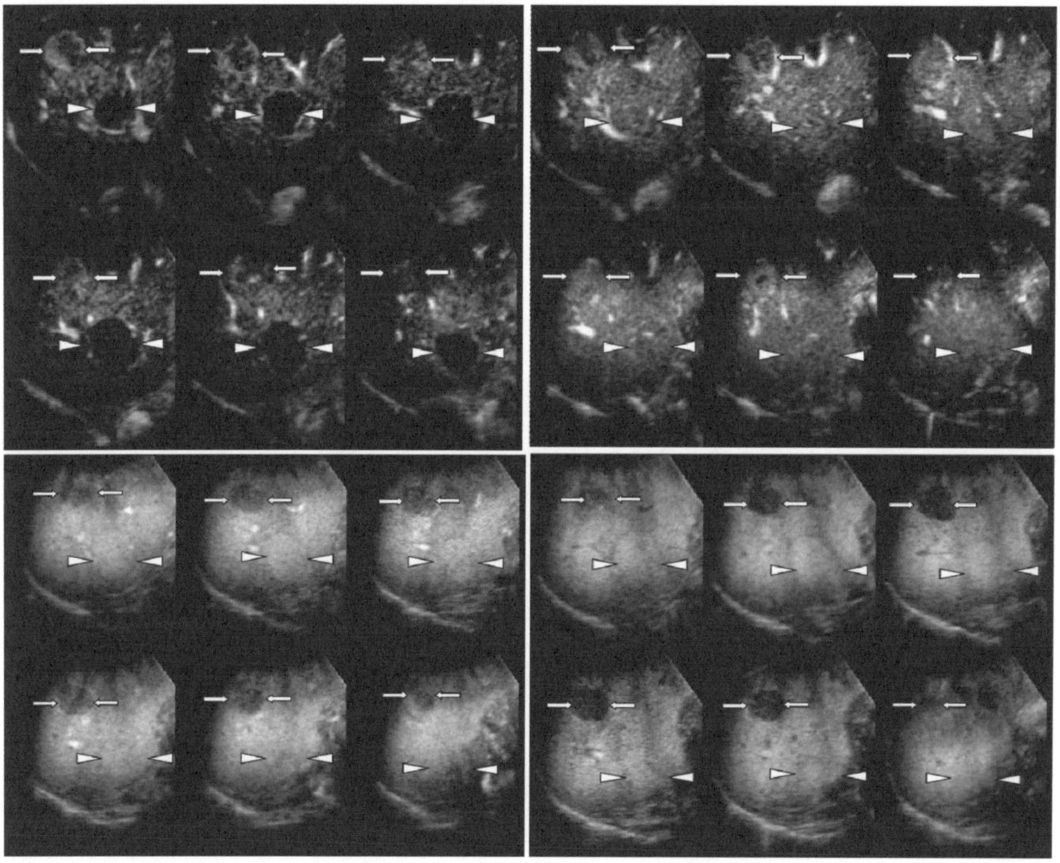

Fig. 6. CE 3D US images of the liver in a patient with a typical hypervascular HCC (maximum diameter, 20 mm) in segment VII (arrows) and a non-hypervascular (atypical) HCC (maximum diameter, 30 mm) in segment VI (arrowheads) in the right lobe. A-D: TUI in plane A obtained at 22 sec (A) and 37 sec (B) (the early phase), 1 min 45 sec (the middle phase) (C), and 6 min 45 sec (the late phase) after injection of Sonazoid (D). The slice distance was 4.4 mm in each plane. As for the HCC located in segment VII (arrows), the tumor shows heterogeneous enhancement with intratumoral vessels in the early phase (A, B), homogeneous enhancement (slight washout) in the middle phase (C), and appears as a hypoechogenic (washout) area in the late phase (D). This HCC was a moderately differentiated HCC. As for the HCC located in segment VI (arrowheads), these images show hypoechogenicity (A), followed by homogeneous tumor enhancement without intratumoral vessels (isoechogenicity) (B) in the early phase, homogeneous enhancement in the middle phase (isoechogenicity) (C), and isoechogenicity (persistence of enhancement) in the late phase (D). This HCC was a well-differentiated HCC.

9. Features of atypical HCCs on CE 3D US with Sonazoid

Most non-hypervascular well-differentiated HCCs (early HCC) are visualized as hypo- to isoechogenic areas without obvious tumor vessels in the early phase, show diffuse enhancement in the middle phase (isoechogenicity), and appear as isoechogenic (persistence

of enhancement) areas in the late phase. Figure 6 shows a TUI showing coexistence of typical hypervascular HCC and early HCC in the right lobe of the liver.
Figure 7 shows a nodule-in-nodule type of HCC. A TUI of this lesion shows heterogeneous enhancement with intratumoral vessels in the early phase, and heterogeneous enhancement in the middle phase. In the late-phase TUI, the lesion exhibits partial hypoechogenicity (washout), corresponding to the enhanced area in the early phase, and isoechogencity (persistence of enhancement) in the remaining area. In general, isoechogenicity in the late phase suggests the diagnosis of well-differentiated HCC and hypoechogenicity in the late phase suggests moderately well-differentiated HCC.

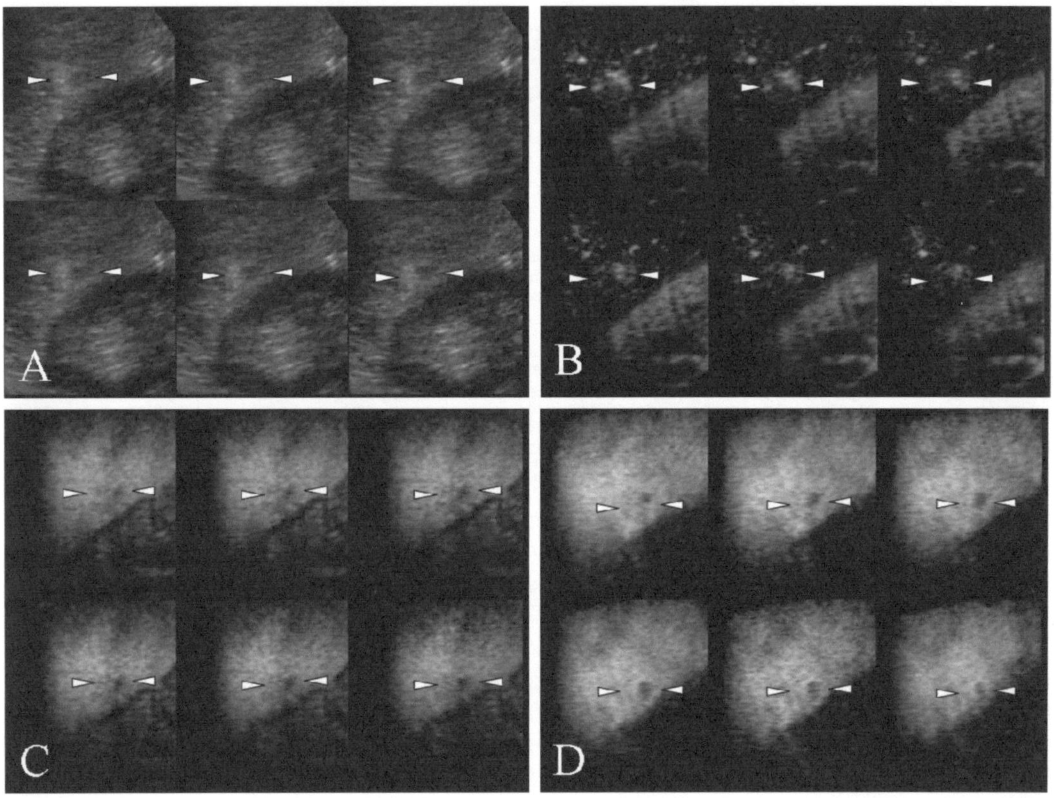

Fig. 7. 3D US and CE 3D US images of the liver in a patient with a nodule-in-nodule type of HCC (maximum diameter, 18 mm) in segment VI of the right lobe. A-D: TUI in plane A of B-mode, early phase (A), middle phase (B), and late phase (C). The slice distance was 0.5 mm in each plane. These images show the nodule-in-nodule lesion in the B-mode (A), heterogeneous enhancement with intratumoral vessels in the early phase (B), and heterogeneous enhancement in the middle phase (C). In the late-phase TUI, the lesion exhibits partial hypoechogenicity (washout), corresponding to the enhanced area in the early-phase image, and isoechogenicity (persistence of enhancement) in the remaining area (D), corresponding to the non-enhanced area in the early-phase image. Arrowheads indicate the margin of the tumor.

10. Features of hepatic metastases on CE 3D US with Sonazoid

The typical enhancement pattern of hepatic metastases consists of peripheral ring-like enhancement with peritumoral vessels (Fig. 8) or intratumoral vessels in the early phase, peripheral ring-like enhancement in the middle phase (wash out), and hypoechogenicity (wash out) in the late phase. As for hypervascular metastases, CE 3D US shows heterogeneous enhancement with intratumoral vessels in the early phase, peripheral ring-like enhancement (wash out) in the middle phase, and hypoechogenicity (wash out) in the late phase (Fig. 9). In this case, the enhancement pattern in the early phase was consistent with that of a hypervascular HCC. However, as compared to a hypervascular HCC, hypervascular metastases have a tendency to show an early washout pattern in the middle phase. This is a valuable finding for differentiating between these two tumors. Hypovascular hepatic metastases show peritumoral vessels without obvious enhancement in the early phase, appear as perfusion defects in the middle phase, and show hypoechogenicity (washout) in the late phase (Fig. 10).

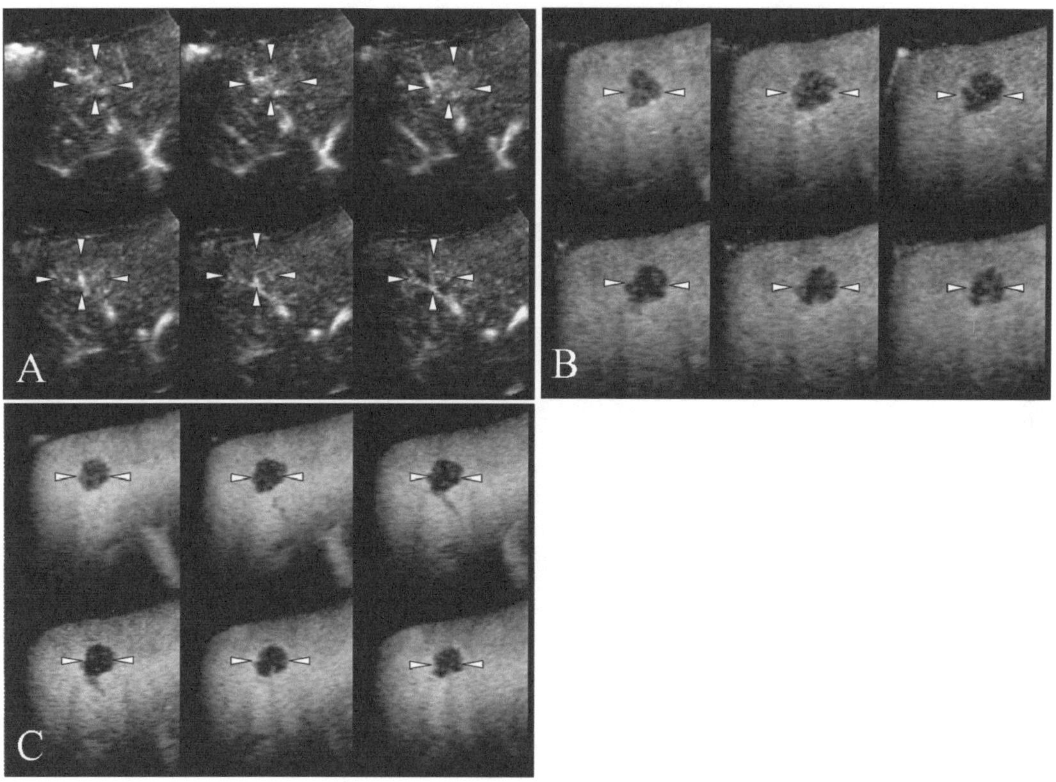

Fig. 8. CE 3D US images of the liver in a patient with metastasis from colon carcinoma (maximum diameter, 16 mm) in segment VIII of the right lobe. A-D: TUI in plane A of the early phase (A), middle phase (B), and late phase (C). The slice distance was 1.5 mm in each plane. These images show peripheral ring-like enhancement with peritumoral vessels in the early phase, peripheral ring-like enhancement in the middle phase (wash out), and hypoechogenicity (wash out) in the late phase. Arowheads indicate the margin of the tumor.

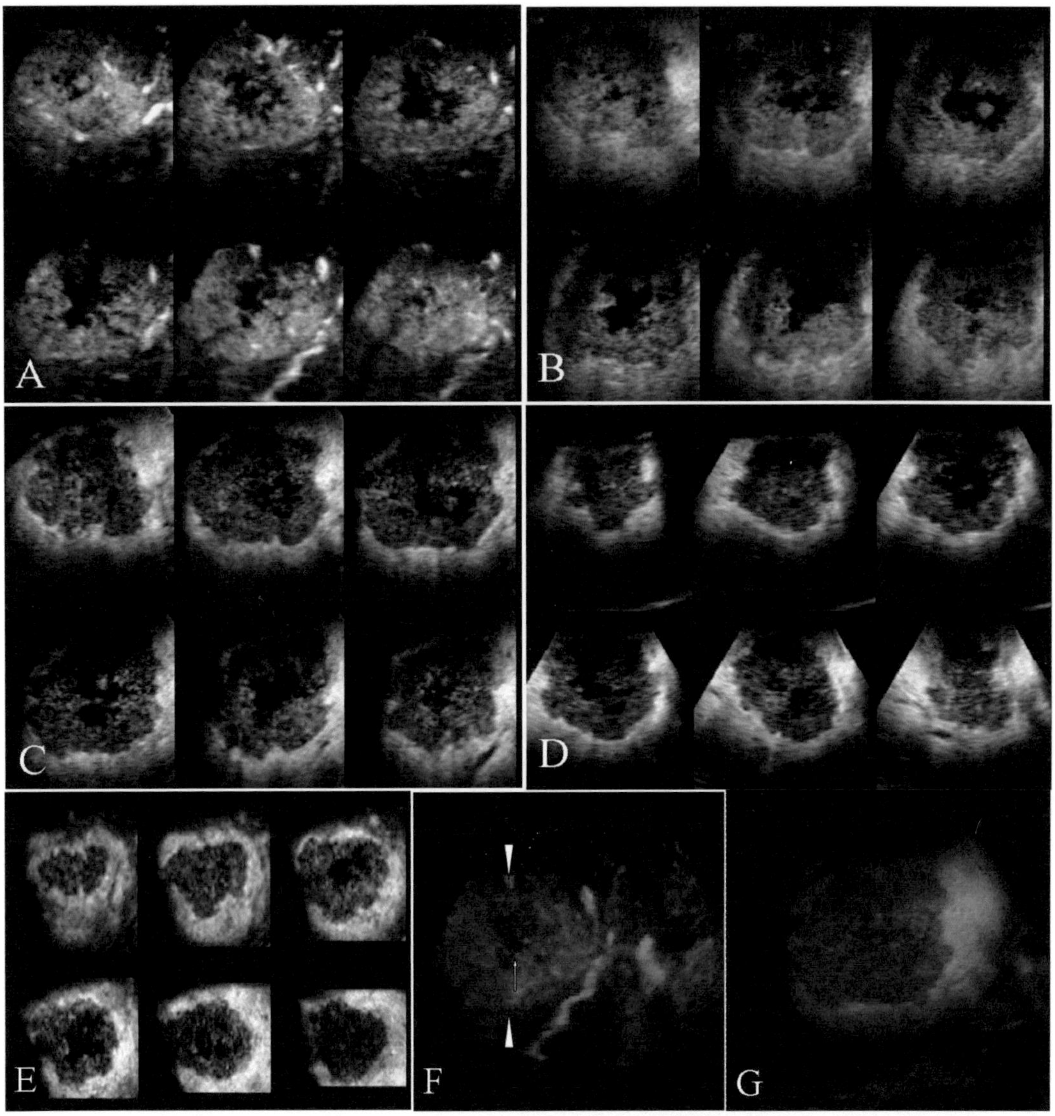

Fig. 9. CE 3D US images of the liver in a patient with metastasis from colon carcinoma (maximum diameter, 65 mm) in the right lobe. A-E: TUI in plane A with a slice distance of 5.4 mm of the early phase (A), middle phase (B), and late phase (C), in plane B with a slice distance of 8.2 mm (D) , and in plane C with a slice distance of 7.0 mm (E) of the late phase. These images show heterogeneous enhancement with intratumoral vessels in the early phase (A), peripheral ring-like enhancement (wash out) in the middle phase (B), and hypoechogenicity (wash out) in the late phase (C-E). A sonographic angiogram acquired with the Autosweep 3D function in the early phase and rendered using the maximum intensity projection mode mixed with the surface mode showing heterogeneous tumor enhancement with intratumoral vessels (arrow) adjacent to the hepatic artery (F). A sonographic angiogram acquired with the Autosweep 3D function in the late phase and rendered using the average intensity mode mixed with the surface mode showing the tumor as a hypoechogenicity (G).

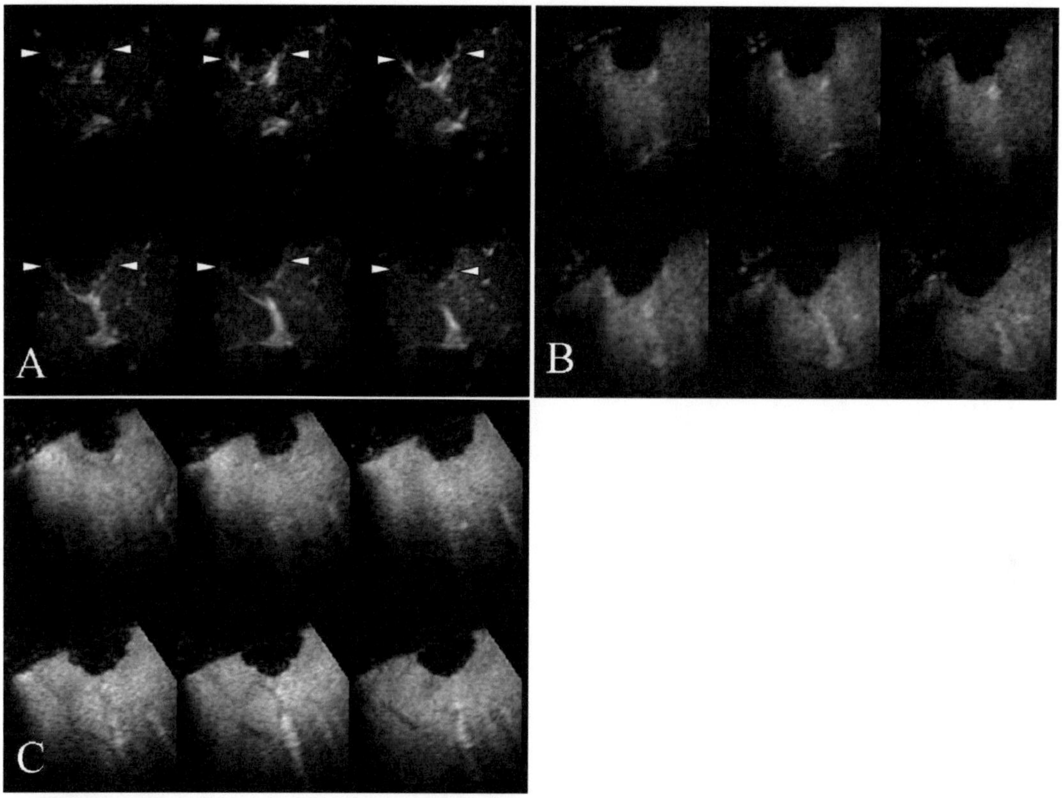

Fig. 10. CE 3D US images of the liver in a patient with metastasis from colon carcinoma (maximum diameter, 25 mm) in segment VIII in the right lobe. A-C: TUI in plane A of the early phase (A), middle phase (B), and late phase (C). The slice distance was 1.8 mm in each plane. These images show peritumoral vessels alone (arrows), without obvious enhancement in the early phase (A), perfusion defect in the middle phase (washout) (B), and hypoechogenicity (washout) in the late phase (C). Arrowheads indicate the margin of the tumor.

The main rendering mode used for obtaining sonographic angiograms in the middle and late phase for metastases is the average intensity mode, mixed with the surface mode at a different percentage, which enables depiction of the lesion as a hypoechogenic (washout) region. According to the vascularity in the early phase, we selected the main rendering mode for obtaining the sonographic angiograms. In cases with hypervascular metastases, the main rendering mode used is the maximum intensity projection mode, and in cases with lesions showing extensive unenhanced areas, we select the average intensity mode as the main rendering mode.

11. Features of hemangiomas on CE 3D US with Sonazoid

The typical enhancement pattern of a hepatic hemangoma consists of peripheral nodular enhancement without tumor vessels in the early phase, peripheral nodular enhancement in the middle phase, and isoechogenicity (persistence of enhancement) in the late phase (Fig. 11). Most hemangiomas appear as isoechogenicities or show incomplete fill-in and

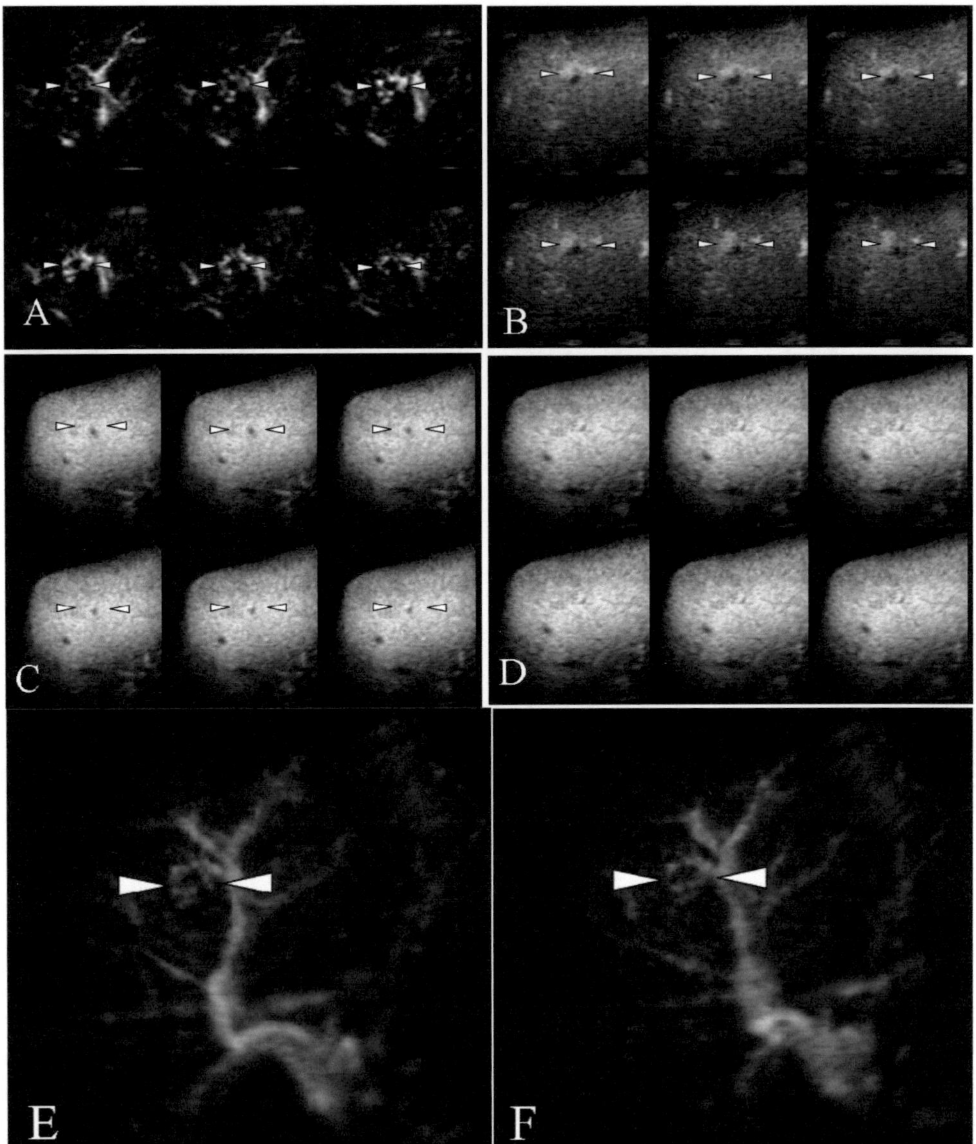

Fig. 11. CE 3D US images of the liver in a patient with a small hemangioma (maximum diameter, 13 mm) in segment VIII of the right lobe. A-D: TUI in plane A obtained at 21 sec (A) and 35 sec (B) (early phase), 1 min 30 sec (middle phase) (C), and 5 min 40 sec (late phase) after the injection of Sonazoid (D). A slice distance is 0.5 mm in each plane. These images show peripheral nodular enhancement without tumor vessels in the early phase (A, B), heterogeneous enhancement in the middle phase (C), and isoechogenicity (persistence of enhancement) in the late phase (D). Arrowheads indicate the margin of the tumor. A sonographic angiogram acquired with the Autosweep 3D function in the early phase and rendered using the average intensity mode mixed with the maximum intensity projection mode, presented in different directions, showing peripheral nodular enhancement without tumor vessels adjacent to the portal vein and the hepatic artery (E, F).

persistence of enhancement in the late phase; however, it must be borne in mind that in some cases, these tumors exhibit slight hypoechogenicity (slight washout) in the late phase (Fig.12). The enhancement pattern of high-flow type hemangiomas consists of homogeneous enhancement immediately after the peripheral nodular enhancement without tumor vessels in the early phase, homogeneous enhancement in the middle phase, and isoechogenicity (persistence of enhancement) in the late phase. Detection of peripheral nodular enhancement without tumor vessels in the early phase is very significant for the diagnosis of hemangioma.

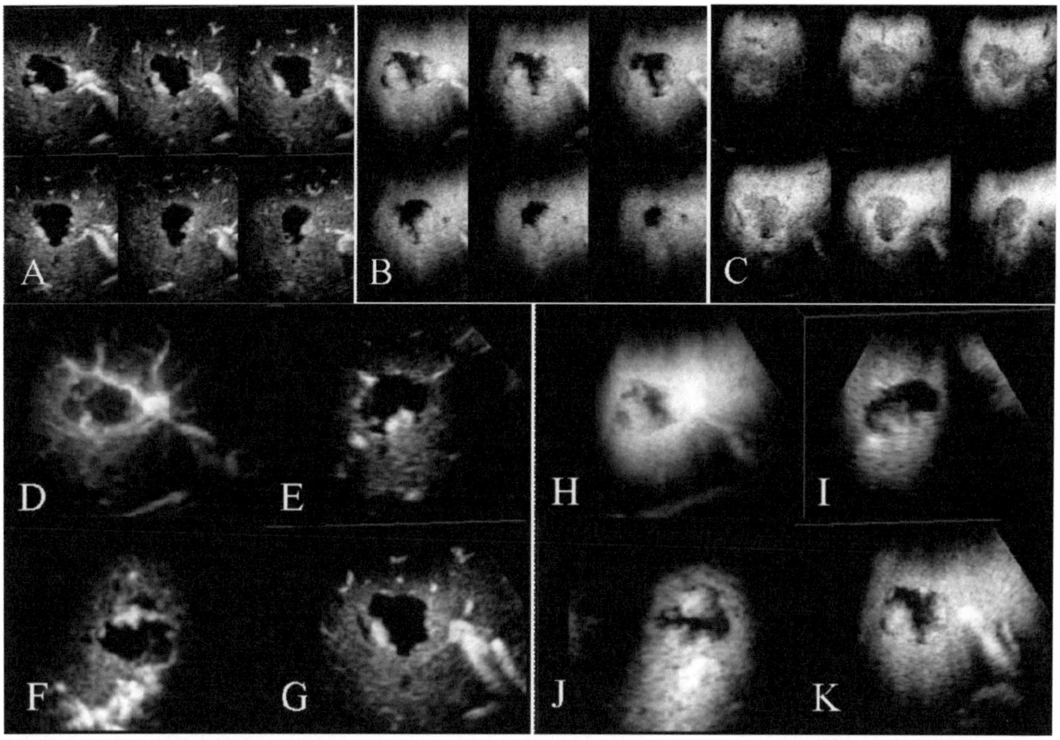

Fig. 12. CE 3D US images of the liver of a patient with hemangioma (maximum diameter, 35 mm) in segment VIII of the right lobe. A-C: TUI in plane A of the early phase (A), middle phase (B), and late phase (C). The slice distance was 3.5 mm in each plane. These images show peripheral nodular enhancement without tumor vessels in the early phase (A), peripheral nodular enhancement in the middle phase (B), and slight hypoechogenicity (slight washout) in the late phase (C). D-G: Display of a sonographic angiogram acquired with the Autosweep 3D function in the early phase and rendered using the average intensity mode mixed with the maximum intensity projection mode (D) and 3D plane B (E), plane C (F), plane A (G). These images show peripheral nodular enhancement without tumor vessels adjacent to the portal vein and the hepatic artery. H-K: Display of a sonographic angiogram acquired with the Autosweep 3D function in the middle phase and rendered using the average intensity mode mixed with the surface mode (H) and 3D plane B (I), plane C (J), plane A (K). These images exhibit the lesions as peripheral nodular enhancement.

The main rendering mode used for obtaining sonographic angiograms in every phase for hemangiomas is the average intensity mode, mixed with some other mode at a different percentage, which enables depiction of the unenhanced areas of the lesion as a hypoechogenic region.

12. Evaluation of the therapeutic efficacy of ablation therapy by CE 3D US with Sonazoid

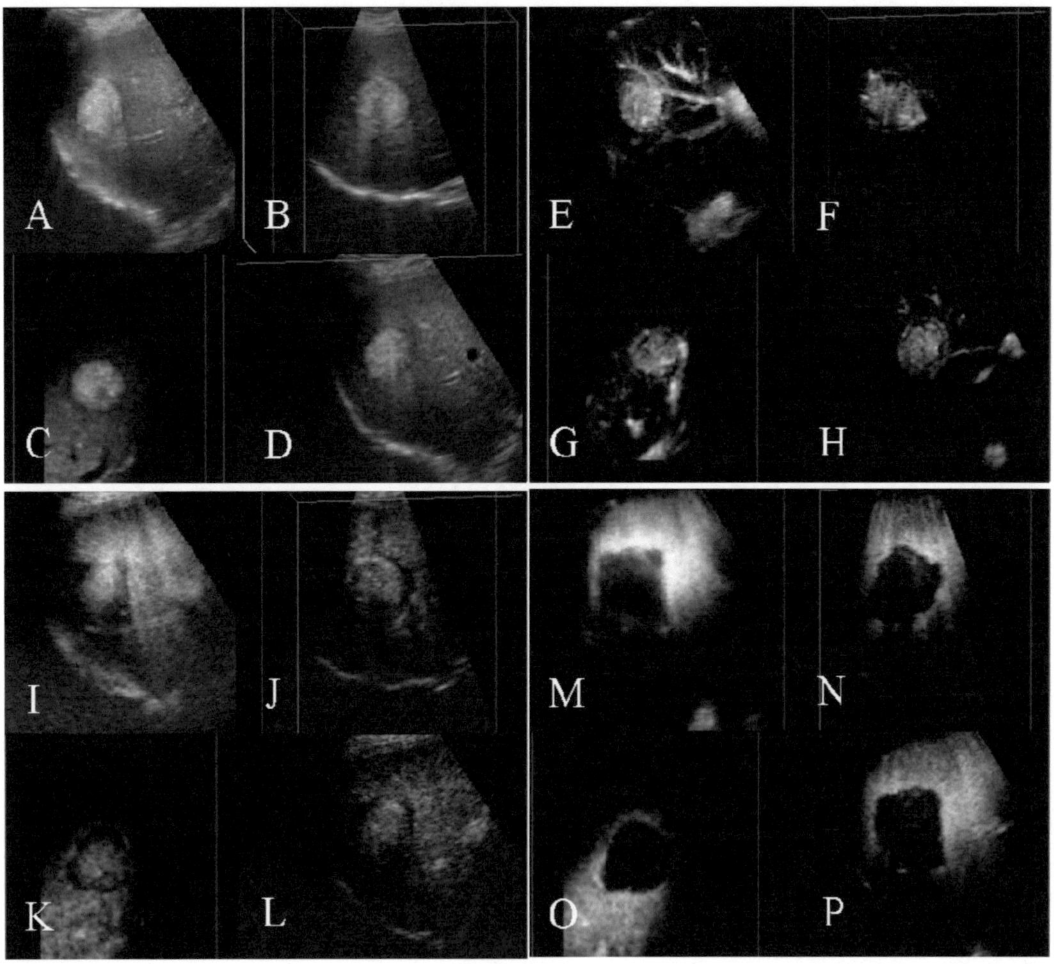

Fig. 13. 3D US and CE 3D US images of the liver in a patient with HCC located adjacent to the right anterior portal vein (maximum diameter, 29 mm), in segment VIII in the right lobe. A-D: Display of sonographic angiograms acquired with the Autosweep 3D function and

rendered using the surface mode (A) and 3D plane B, plane C (C), plane A (D) of the B-mode obtained before RFA showing a hyperechoic tumor.
E-H: Display of sonographic angiograms acquired with the Autosweep 3D function and rendered using the maximum intensity projection mode with the surface mode (E) and 3D plane B (F), plane C (G), plane A (H) of the early-phase images obtained before RFA showing homogeneous enhancement of the tumor with intratumoral vessels.
I-L: Display of sonographic angiograms acquired with the Autosweep 3D function and rendered using the average intensity with the surface mode (I) and 3D plane B (J), plane C (K), plane A (L) of the middle-phase CE 3D US using the CPI mode with a low mechanical index obtained 1 day after RFA showing the tumor itself and the ablated areas. However, the background B-mode appears to interfere with the clear visualization of sufficiently ablated areas.
M-P: Display of a sonographic angiograms acquired with the Autosweep 3D function and rendered using the average intensity with the surface mode (M) and 3D plane B (N), plane C (O), plane A (P) of the middle-phase CE 3D US using the CHA mode with a high mechanical index, which eliminates the background B-mode, obtained 1 day after RFA showing the necrotic areas as clear perfusion defects. This 3D view shows that the ablated area is slightly larger than the original tumor and that the safety of the margin is not sufficient; thus, the patient needed to be monitored closely for tumor recurrence; 22 months after the RFA, local recurrence was detected by dynamic MRI.

CE 3D US imaging with Sonazoid allows 3D visualization for comparison with a high sensitivity of HCC tumors before treatment with the treated areas after ablation. Use of the CHA mode and a high mechanical index eliminates the background B-mode and emphasizes the microbubbles in the vessels, allowing residual tumors to be differentiated from necrotic areas after ablation. Using this method, we recently demonstrated the usefulness of automatically scanned CE 3D US with Sonazoid for early evaluation of the therapeutic efficacy of percutaneous RFA for HCC lesions (Fig. 13) (Luo et al., 2010b).
Sonazoid-enhanced 3D US can also be used to evaluate the immediate therapeutic effects of high-intensity focused ultrasound (HIFU) on small HCC lesions. This modality has the potential to allow detection of residual HCCs after such treatment, thereby enabling additional HIFU ablation to be performed for residual untreated portions (Numata et al., 2010b).

13. Side effects of Sonazoid

Sonazoid is associated with a low incidence of side effects, such as diarrhea 1.6%, albuminuria 1.6%, and neutropenia 1.0%. It is not contraindicated for patients with renal dysfunction or iodine allergy, although one reported contraindication for Sonazoid in patients is a history of egg allergy (Moriyasu & Itoh, 2009).

14. Limitations

First, CE 3D US of focal liver lesions has the shortcoming of potentially including artifacts from the heart and respiratory movements (Figs. 2B, C), rib cage, and interference from abdominal gas, etc. We attempted to minimize the influence of artifacts by requesting the patients to hold their breath during the scanning procedure, selecting the location of the volume transducer, mediating the size and position of the VOI, adjusting the scanning angle, and reconstructing the sonographic angiogram using appropriate rendering modes. Second, when multiple lesions were detected in one VOI, we could scan the lesions simultaneously in the early phase; however, when multiple lesions were located in separate VOI, only one VOI could be evaluated by CE 3D US in the early phase. Third, until recently, Sonazoid was only available in Japan, which might the spread of CE 3D US using this contrast agent.

15. Conclusions

CE 3D US, which is convenient to perform and does not involve radiation exposure, appears to be promising as a novel and useful method for three-dimensional evaluation of the vascular characteristics of liver tumors and for the differential diagnosis of hepatic lesions with good diagnostic capability. These features of CE 3D US are anticipated to be of benefit in the clinical setting. This modality can also be potentially useful for evaluating the effects of RF ablation or HIFU for HCCs, offering unique 3D visualization. We hope that in the near future, a fusion imaging method that would allow fusion and synchronization of CE 3D US images with multiplanar reconstruction CT or MR images on a single screen in real-time will become available in the near future.

16. References

Badea R, Socaciu M, Lupşor M, et al. (2007). Evaluating the liver tumors using three-dimensional ultrasonography: A pictorial essay. *J Gastrointestin Liver Dis*, 16, 1, 85-92.

Benacerraf BR, Shipp TD, Bromley B. (2006). Three-dimensional US of the fetus: volume imaging. *Radiology*, 238, 2, 988-996.

Bosch FX, Ribes J, Díaz M,et al. (2004). Primary liver cancer: worldwide incidence and trends. *Gastroenterology*, 127, 5S1, S5-S16.

Camaggi V, Piscaglia F, Bolondi L. (2007). Recent advances in the imaging of hepatocellular carcinoma. From ultrasound to positron emission tomography scan. *Saudi Med J*, 28, 7, 1007-1014.

Dietrich CF. (2002). 3D real time contrast enhanced ultrasonography, a new technique. *Rofo*, 174, 2, 160-163.

Forsberg F, Goldberg BB, Merritt CR, et al. (2004). Diagnosing breast lesions with contrast-enhanced 3-dimensional power Doppler imaging. *J Ultrasound Med*, 23, 2, 173-182.

Halpern EJ, McCue PA, Aksnes AK, et al. (2002). Contrast-enhanced US of the prostate with Sonazoid: comparison with whole-mount prostatectomy specimens in 12 patients. *Radiology*, 222, 2, 361-366.

Kotsianos-Hermle D, Wirth S, Fischer T, et al. (2009). First clinical use of a standardized three-dimensional ultrasound for breast imaging, *Eur J Radiol*, 71, 1, 102-108.

Krenning BJ, Kirschbaum SW, Soliman OI et al. (2007). Comparison of contrast agent-enhanced versus non-contrast agent-enhanced real-time three-dimensional echocardiography for analysis of left ventricular systolic function. *Am J Cardiol*, 100, 9, 1485-1489.

Kudo M. (2007). New sonographic techniques for the diagnosis and treatment of hepatocellular carcinoma. *Hepatol Res*, 37, S2, S193-S199.

Luo W, Numata K, Morimoto M, et al. (2009a). Clinical utility of contrast-enhanced three-dimensional ultrasound imaging with Sonazoid: findings on hepatocellular carcinoma lesions. *Eur J Radiol*, 72, 3, 425-431.

Luo W, Numata K, Morimoto M, et al. (2009b). Three-dimensional contrast-enhanced sonography of vascular patterns of focal liver tumors: pilot study of visualization methods. *AJR Am J Roentgenol*, 192, 1, 165-173.

Luo W, Numata K, Morimoto M, et al. (2009c). Focal liver tumors: characterization with 3D perflubutane microbubble contrast agent-enhanced US versus 3D contrast-enhanced multidetector CT. *Radiology*, 251, 1, 287-295.

Luo W, Numata K, Morimoto M, et al. (2010a). Differentiation of focal liver lesions using three-dimensional ultrasonography: retrospective and prospective studies. *World J Gastroenterol*, 16, 17, 2109-2119.

Luo W, Numata K, Morimoto M, et al. (2010b). Role of Sonazoid-enhanced three-dimensional ultrasonography in the evaluation of percutaneous radiofrequency ablation of hepatocellular carcinoma. *Eur J Radiol*, 75, 1, 91-97.

Moriyasu F and Itoh K. (2009). Efficacy of perflubutane microbubble-enhanced ultrasound in the characterization and detection of focal liver lesions: phase 3 multicenter clinical trial. *AJR Am. J. Roentgenol*, 193, 1, 86-95.

Numata K, Morimoto M, Ogura T, et al. (2008). Ablation therapy guided by contrast-enhanced sonography with Sonazoid for hepatocellular carcinoma lesions not detected by conventional sonography. *J Ultrasound Med*, 27, 3, 395-406.

Numata K, Luo W, Morimoto M, et al. (2010a).Contrast-enhanced ultrasound of hepatocellular carcinoma. *World J Radiol*. 28, 2, 68-82.

Numata K, Fukuda H, Ohto M, et al. (2010b). Evaluation of the therapeutic efficacy of high-intensity focused ultrasound ablation of hepatocellular carcinoma by three-dimensional sonography with a perflubutane-based contrast agent. *Eur J Radiol*, 75, 2, e67-e75.

Ohto M, Kato H, Tsujii H, Maruyama H, et al. (2005) Vascular flow patterns of hepatic tumors in contrast-enhanced 3-dimensional fusion ultrasonography using plane shift and opacity control modes. *J Ultrasound Med*, 24, 1, 49-57.

Taylor LS, Rubens DJ, Porter BC, et al. (2005). Prostate cancer: three-dimensional sonoelastography for in vitro detection. *Radiology*, 237, 3, 981-985.

Tutschek B, Sahn DJ. (2007). Three-dimensional echocardiography for studies of the fetal heart: present status and future perspectives. *Cardiol Clin*, 25, 2, 341-355.

Wessels T, Bozzato A, Mull M, et al. (2004). Intracranial collateral pathways assessed by contrast-enhanced three-dimensional transcranial color-coded sonography. *Ultrasound Med Biol*, 30, 11, 1435-1440.

Yukisawa S, Ohto M, Masuya Y et al. (2007). Contrast-enhanced three-dimensional fusion sonography of small liver metastases with pathologic correlation. *J Clin Ultrasound,* 35, 1, 1-8.

10

Contrast Enhanced Ultrasonography and Carotid Plaque Imaging: from the Hemodynamic Evaluation to the Detection of Neoangiogenesis - The New Approach to the Identification of the Unstable Plaque: from Morphology to Patophysiology

Maria Fabrizia Giannoni[1], Edoardo Vicenzini[2],
Claudia Monaco[3] and Piergiorgio Cao[4]
[1]Vascular Ultrasound Investigation Unit, Vascular Surgery, Department "P. Stefanini", Sapienza University of Rome,
[2]Department of Neurology and Psychiatry, Sapienza University of Rome,
[3]Kennedy Institute of Rheumatology, Imperial College, London,
[4]Vascular Surgery, Department of Cardioscience, S. Camillo-Forlanini Hospital, Rome,
[1,2,4]Italy
[3]UK

1. Introduction

Ischemic Stroke (IS) represents the third leading cause of death in the Western World and it is particularly relevant because disability is a major frightening issue both for patients' quality of life, as well as for social and therapeutical implications (Engel, 1998).
One of the most frequent causes of Ischemic Strokes and Transient Ischemic Attacks (TIAs) is cerebral embolism that originates from atherosclerotic plaques in the carotid vessels. This "Large artery" (LA) pathogenesis accounts for 25-30% of all IS, i.e. more than 1/4 million per year, worldwide (Diener, 2004). In patients with a previous manifested TIA or IS, LA atherosclerosis is indeed observed in nearly 70% of the cases. Nonetheless, IS is proceeded by a TIA only in half of the patients with carotid atherosclerosis while, in the other half, Stroke may occur without the former manifestation of symptoms (Barnett, 1998).
In regards to preventive surgical strategies for carotid artery diseases, two major fundamental trials represent a "cornerstone" in treatment strategy of the carotid Strokes: these trials clearly and definitively confirmed the relationship between the risk of neurological events and the degree of the internal carotid artery stenosis. According to data collected from European Carotid Surgery Trial (Rothwell, 2004; ECST, 1991; ECST, 1998) and to the North American Symptomatic Carotid Endarterectomy Trial (Barnett, 1998) Stroke risk is correlated to the presence of hemodynamic internal carotid artery stenosis and occurrence of recent cerebrovascular symptoms. A general consensus has been reached on indications for Carotid Endoarterectomy (CEA), that at present has to be performed in

experienced centers in patients with: a) symptomatic severe stenosis (=/>70%); b) symptomatic stenosis (*with soft unstable plaque*) > 50%; c) asymptomatic patients with 70-99% stenosis below 75 years of age (Rothwell, 2004, Goldstein 2010, Hobson 2008, Liapis 2009).
On the other hand, the real benefit of CEA in asymptomatic patients, even though affected by severe hemodynamic degree of stenosis is still nowadays controversial and not clearly defined, as demonstrated by ACAS (ACAS, 1995) and ACST (Halliday, 2004) trials: only carotid stenosis > 70% would benefit from CEA, but only after five years follow-up and only in center where CEA is performed with very low perioperative complication rates (Halliday 2010, Kakkos 2009, Setacci 2009). When stenoses are below this threshold, patients are adressed towards medical therapy, which offers at present good results (Rothwell, 2004; CAPRIE, 1996, Goldberg 2010). Therefore the problem of primary prevention strategy exists for a high number of asymptomatic patients, that may transform into 250.000 new IS per year: in these patients, the surgical approach decided only on the severe degree of internal carotid stenosis may be no more valid.
It is mandatory to ameliorate the balance between risksa nd benefit of CEA in asymptomatic patients: during the last 30 years several potential risk factors have been evaluated to appropriately select subgroups of asymptomatic patients that may really benefit from CEA, but, however, without reaching satisfactory results and clear indications (Abbott, 2007; Nicolaides, 1995). At present, the recent ACES Study performed in asymptomatic patient with severe degree internal carotid artery stenosis (>70%) in order to detect risk factors significantly related with the onset of neurological events concluded that only the microembolism identified at 2 hours Transcranial Doppler monitoring is a true and independent predictor of cerebrovascular events., significantly linked with cerebral ischemia (Markus, 2010). For all the these reasons further studies are mandatory in order to select subgroup populations that really benefit of surgical treatment.
New evaluation methods have to be considered: the detection of the unstable, vulnerable plaques will have to use functional investigations methods, and no longer the morphological investigation alone is sufficient. Advances in carotid plaque imaging could allow functional investigations methods and the detection of vulnerable plaques has to be performed according to these new viewpoints. Due to all the above-mentioned controversial points, the risk-benefit and cost-effectiveness of CEA in asymptomatic patients have to be better characterized, identifying the real subpopulations that would really take advantages from a surgical preventive strategy, in favor of a safe secure benefit and long-term outcome.
In addition, being Stroke an unforeseeable event that occurs in a wide percentage of cases because of carotid embolic lesions, plaque morphology characterization has represented a fundamental step for the selection of patients at risk of cerebrovascular ischemic events. Nonetheless, in recent years, even all information about degree of stenosis and plaque morphology is not yet considered enough to recognize lesions at risk. New further concepts regarding functional activities of carotid plaques represent the future target to be investigated, in order to indentify the so called "vulnerable plaques" and, consequently, to avoid the disabling ischemic event.

1.1 The symptomatic plaque from the histological point of view

Histopathological data collected from carotid specimen of symptomatic patients have clearly identified the different morphological characteristics of the symptomatic plaques (Mauriello, 2010; Fisher, 2005) linked with cerebral ischemia and with the underlying mechanisms of plaque instability.

Beyond the degree of stenosis, the presence of plaques heterogeneity, large areas of intraplaque hemorrhage or a necrotic lipidic core, the presence of surface ulcerations, represent all peculiar characteristics of symptomatic, complicated carotid plaques. All histological studies have then confirmed that the underlying plaque morphology is an important further predictor of stroke risk (Gronholdt, 2001; Stary, 1995). Several studies have shown that plaque morphology have also to be considered an additional independent predictor of cerebral infarction and that carotid plaques at risk for rupture are not always correlated with the severity of stenosis at bifurcation sites. Other morphological characteristics seem to play a more relevant role (Griffin, 2010).
Several histopathological studies have compared the morphological aspects of carotid plaques removed from symptomatic and asymptomatic patients in attempt to better understand the mechanisms underlying plaque destabilization demonstrated that plaque rupture, thin fibrous cap and thrombogenic plaques with relevant inflammatory infiltration and increase of macrophage cells are main features of symptomatic plaques, prone to be responsible of embolic cerebrovascular events (Spagnoli, 2004; Carr, 1996; Fisher, 2005)

1.2 Ultrasonography for plaque characterization

Characterization of plaque morphological aspects seemed an excellent method for risk stratification of neurological events. Over the past twenty years, high-resolution ultrasonography represented a reliable tool for plaque characteristics investigation in vivo and in real-time. Still nowadays Color Duplex Ultrasonography is a reliable, repeatable and noninvasive top-level and first choice investigation method in the evaluation of supraortic vessels.
Historically, in 1983 Reilly and coll. (Reilly, 1983) introduced the first characterization of plaque structure according to data obtained from ultrasound investigations: the concepts of "homogeneous" and "heterogeneous" were introduced in clinical practice to define plaques characteristics related to cerebrovascular risk. Irregular surface and ulcerations has also been identified as morphological features predictors of cerebrovascular events (Dixon, 1982).
In 1985 Johnson and Colleagues (Johnson, 1985) established three different criteria describing plaque composition, including calcified, dense (less hyperechogenic than calcified lesions) or soft plaques (isoechogenic in comparison with blood).
In 1988, Gray-Weale and coworkers (Gray-Weale, 1988) described four different plaque types and proposed a classification of morphological features according to ultrasound imaging: Type 1 (anechoic to echogenic fibrous cap; Type 2 (predominantly, but anechoic areas with echogenic, less than 25% of the plaque); Type 3 (mostly hyperechoic areas with anechoic, less than 25% of the plaque); Type 4 (echogenic and homogeneous plaque).
In 1990, Widder (Widder, 1990) proposed a reverse classification, the most anechogenic plaques being assigned to Type IV and the most echogenic to Type I.
In 1993, Geroulakos (Gerulakos, 1993) introduced a modified version of Gray-Weale's classification including a 5th category of unclassified plaque reflecting calcified plaques which may have zones of acoustic shadowing which obscure the deeper part of the arterial wall as well as the vessel lumen.
Only in the following years the relative risk of plaque related to morphological characteristics according to a numerical quantification was the subject of a consensus meeting (De Bray, 1996) on the characterization of plaques: it was finally decided that the echogenicity of the plaque should have be standardized against 3 reference structures: blood flowing to anechoic, sternocleidomastoid muscle for isoechogenic, next to the transverse

processes of cervical vertebrae for hyperechogenicity Further studies suggested the use of the bright far wall of media-adventitia interface as a reference for hyperechogenicity (Joakimsen, 1997). After these early works many further studies have reported data regarding the successful correlation between the plaque morphology on ultrasound investigation and the histological plaque composition.

To further reduce the possibility of biases due to the subjective evaluation, computerized methods also have been introduced to evaluate echogenicity of carotid plaques. The standardized quantitative computerized assessment of plaque echogenicity by Gray Scale Median (GSM) represents nowadays an objective tool for the definition of the unstable plaques (El-Barghouty, 1995; Biasi, 1999). Data collected from literature have indeed clearly demonstrated that low GSM plaque values identify those lesions that are closely related to the prediction of the risk for embolic events (Biasi, 1999; Mathiesen, 2001).

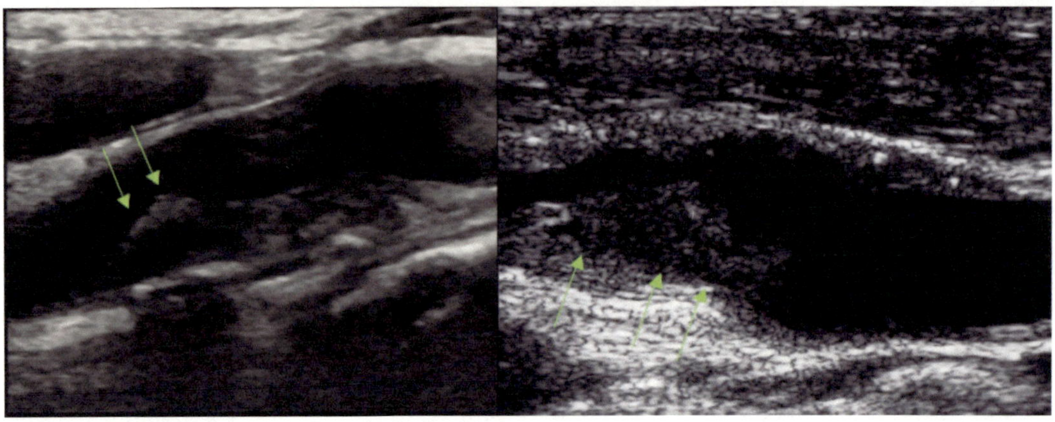

Fig. B-Mode imaging of soft plaques with a clear anechoic part in the distal posterior part of the plaque (green arrows, left) and with a superimposed iso-hypoechoic trhombus (green arrows, right).

1.3 From morphology to patophysiology

There is a general agreement that the identification of carotid artery vulnerable lesions is not possible nowadays only relying on the degree of stenosis and plaque morphological characteristics alone. Even if these features represent the conventional methods used for planning adequate treatment strategies, these methods are not capable of evaluating in vivo inflammation and remodeling of unstable plaques, and consequently to predict the true risk of cerebrovascular events. Surface rupture and luminal thrombus formation related to plaque acute inflammation are nowadays considered the major events related to the development of acute stroke.

Techniques aimed at imaging the biological "functional" status of the plaque are now emerging. Conventional radiological imaging such as Computerized Tomography Angiography with contrast agents (CT), Magnetic Resonance Imaging (MRI) and even Positron Emission Tomography (PET) have been recently applied to image targets of the biological functional pathways of carotid plaques. Nonetheless, up-to-date there is no "in vivo" imaging technique considered as the "gold standard" for the demonstration of the direct temporal correlation between inflammation and morphological features of carotid vulnerable plaques responsible of neurological events (Warburton, 2006). Moreover, being not widely available and being expensive and radiation risk techniques, these tools cannot be used in the current ordinary follow-up. Despite the excellent results obtained on the validation and accuracy of ultrasonography, the true mechanism able to convert an asymptomatic plaque to a symptomatic one failed to be clearly identified and even if Duplex evaluation represented a further step in the knowledge, it seemed inadequate. Preoperative ultrasound carotid imaging can be used to detect the histological characteristics of plaque with the possibility of post-operative validation. Since recent clinicopathological studies have indicated the role of intraplaque hemorrhage and ulceration in symptomatic carotid disease, identification of these features is of high value in choosing therapy, especially for the asymptomatic patient.

From clinical studies a new concept has emerged: plaque 'vulnerability' i.e. the inner stability and risk for rupture other than morphology and degree of stenosis may be more adequate (Reilly, 1983; Hennerici 2004). Thus, a functional diagnostic test (instead of a pure anatomical imaging) would be preferable as current clinical anatomical investigations have a poor ability to predict which plaques become symptomatic in the immediate future.

2. Plaque angiogenesis

The clinical complications of atherosclerosis are caused by local thrombus formation, which results from the rupture and fissuration of surface of an unstable atherosclerotic plaque. The formation of microvessels (angiogenesis) in an atherosclerotic plaque contributes to the development of plaques, increasing the risk of plaque rupture.

Only recently has the in vivo evaluation of angiogenesis received attention for its possible role in assessing the vulnerability of the atheroma. The presence of microvessels in atherosclerotic plaques was firstly described by Paterson in 1936-38 and Geiringer (1951) as well as their lack in the non atherosclerotic - normal, non pathological - arterial wall: these were simply pure observational studies, very far to connect with a patophysiological mechanism. From histological reports it is well known that angiogenesis is linked with the vulnerable, unstable plaque characteristics. Moreover, although the detailed pathophysiological mechanisms of plaque formation and rupture are still under debate, there seems to be reasonable evidence that smooth muscle cell hypertrophy, proliferation and migration through the basal membrane, macrophage infiltration, LDL deposition and intimal neoangiogenesis are crucial steps finally leading to plaque vulnerability and rupture. Histological studies have indeed shown that microvessels are not usually present in the normal human intimal layers and that intima becomes vascularized only with the development of the atherosclerotic process and when its layer grows in thickness (Geiringer, 1951).

Only in the last 20 years the presence of the adventitial vasa vasorum and the occurrence of plaque neovascularization was recognized and identified as a significant marker of plaque instability and confirmed in histological studies, as predictors of unstable atheromasic lesions in cerebro and cardiovascular patients (McCarthy, 1999; Mofidi, 2001).

3. Ultrasound contrast agents for functional plaque imaging

In the last few years, Contrast Enhanced Ultrasonography (CEUS) performed with 2nd generation contrast agents and new dedicated software represent a useful tool that improved not only the diagnostic accuracy of ultrasonography, but allowed the detection of

vascularization and tissue perfusion in real-time and with excellent spatial resolution in many fields.
CEUS is a safety (Piscaglia 2006, Abdelmoneim 2009), emerging tool that allows to obtain more reliable information in daily practice (Claudon, 2008). As a matter of fact, regarding the evaluation of carotid atherosclerosis, CEUS provides an enhanced assessment of the arterial lumen and plaque morphology, an improved resolution of carotid intima-media thickness, and they even allow the direct visualization of adventitial vasa vasorum and plaque neovascularization (Purushothman, 2006; Feinstein, 2004). Feinstein et al reported in 2006 first experiences identifying carotid plaque neovascularization with CEUS in a patient with a significant and symptomatic carotid stenosis, confirmed by the histological findings after endarterectomy. They also observed the neovascularization regression after 8 months of statins therapy in a plaque of a diabetic patient. In a recent paper from our group (Vicenzini, 2007), we also observed that plaque vascularization can be easily detected with contrast ultrasound imaging in the the fibrous and fibro-fatty tissue and not observed in the calcific nor in the necrotic and haemorrhagic areas, as expression of plaque remodeling. More evidences are now confirming the reliability of this technique (Shah, 2007; Huang, 2008, Staub, 2010; Coll 2010).
In our research, we focus on the possibility to detect neoangiogenesis in carotid plaques with ultrasound and second-generation ultrasound contrast agents. In order to detect possible differences between atherosclerotic lesions correlated with clinical symptomatology, we studied patients to be submitted to carotid endarterectomy for severe, hemodynamic internal carotid artery stenosis, both asymptomatic as well as acute/recent symptomatic cerebrovascular patients. Data obtained were also confronted with post-operative histological findings. Moreover, asymptomatic patients with moderate internal carotid artery stenosis suitable for medical treatment and sonographic surveillance were investigated. Aim of our study was to evaluate the characteristics of carotid plaque vascularization detected with contrast ultrasound investigation according clinical findings, and to correlate contrast ultrasound investigation with histology and immunohisto-chemichal (VEGF, MMP3,CD 31-34).

3.1 Methods of CEUS investigation

Carotid duplex scanning was performed with an Acuson/Siemens Sequoia 512 and Siemens S2000 scanners, equipped with the software "Cadence Contrast Pulse Sequencing technology" (Cadence CPS). Linear phased array probes (6, 8 and 15 Mhz for the Sequoia, 9, 14, 18 MHz for the S2000). General Electric (GE Logiq9) and Philips IUD 22 scanner were also used. The same presets were maintained for all patients, in order to reduce pitfalls reproducibility.
Internal carotid artery plaques were digitally documented in B-Mode, Color and Power modes on both longitudinal and transversal scans, to obtain the best visualization of the atherosclerotic lesions. Angle corrected blood flow velocities were obtained with Pulsed Wave Doppler at the maximum site of stenosis. Plaque echographic morphology has been described according to criteria already well-established in literature (Gray-Weale, 1988; El Bargouthy, 1995): plaque structure according to the echogenicity, and considered as hyperechoic with acoustic shadow, hyperechoic, isoechoic, hypoechoic, and consequently as calcific, fibrous, fibro-calcific, fibro-fatty/haemorrhagic. Plaque surface as regular, irregular and ulcerated, when a surface irregularity > 2 mm was detected. Echogenicity was also quantified with Gray Scale Median (GSM) computerized analysis (Biasi, 1999) in order to

better define the plaque risk. The degree of stenosis was evaluated according to European Carotid Surgery Trial criteria (ECST, 1995), as percentage of the difference between the original and the residual lumen at the maximum site of stenosis and to the relative increase of blood flow velocities (Sabeti, 2004).

Contrast ultrasound investigation was performed, as already described (Vicenzini, 2007), after small repeated bolus injections of SonoVue (Bracco Altana Pharma, Konstanz, Germany) in an antecubital vein (20 Gauge Venflon), followed by saline flushes. After identifying the plaque on longitudinal and transverse scans, and after having obtained the baseline B-mode, Color and Power images of the plaque, the 15 Mhz linear array probe with a mechanical index varying from 0.4 to 1.4 with CPS continuous real-time recording software was used to achieve the best visualization of plaque morphology and vascularization, in the same longitudinal view. Freezed images and clips were stored throughout the investigation, in order to compare the basal images with the same images obtained after contrast administration. The "Contrast Agent only" software feature, in which the image is derived only from the signals originating from the microbubbles, has been used. All the investigations were digitally stored onto an external hard-disk for the off-line review analysis, performed by two different sonographers.

Carotid endarterectomies have been carefully performed in order to obtain the whole plaque with minimal trauma. The removed plaques were immediately placed in formalin and subsequently probed with hematossilin-eosin coloration, to have a general view of plaque cellularity, and immunostained with antibodies for Vascular Endotelial Growth Factors (VEGF) and Matrix MetalloProteinases 3 (MMP3) (DAKO, Glostrup Denmark). After the complete observation of the lesion, the regions of interest observed at ultrasound images were identified and discussed with the sonographers.

4. Contrast ultrasound findings

Ultrasound contrast agent microbubbles are visualized few seconds after the injection as a hyperechoic dynamic flow in the carotid vessel lumen, providing an enhanced visualization of the carotid intima-media complex and a better identification of the plaque surface. They may be of help in better defining plaque surface and to indentify plaque ulceration, especially when B-Mode imaging and Color imaging are blurry or have a low definition.

Mainly during the diastolic cardiac phase, probably due to the reduced local pressure, the distribution of UCA inside the plaque allowed the visualization of vascularization. Microvesseles were detected through the visualization of microbubbles penetrating in the iso-hyperechoic fibrous and fibro-fatty tissue, as a little vessel perpendicular to the carotid lumen, regardless the severity of stenosis.

Further, a different pattern of plaque vascularization was observed in the acute symptomatic patients, represented by a major and more diffuse contrast enhancement, completely different from the pattern of the majority of the asymptomatic plaques. These data have been confirmed by other Authors (Xiong, 2009; Staub, 2010, Chowdhury ,2010, Cosgrove, 2009).

Histological specimens with immunostaining obtained from CEA confirmed a relevant angiogenesis in symptomatic plaques when compared to asymptomatic ones. From our experience (Vicenzini, 2007, 2009; Giannoni, 2009 a, 2009 b), we observed that microbubbles diffuse easily in the fibrous tissue of carotid plaques and that histologically correspond to the newly generated vessels, so confirming that plaques angiogenesis could be related to

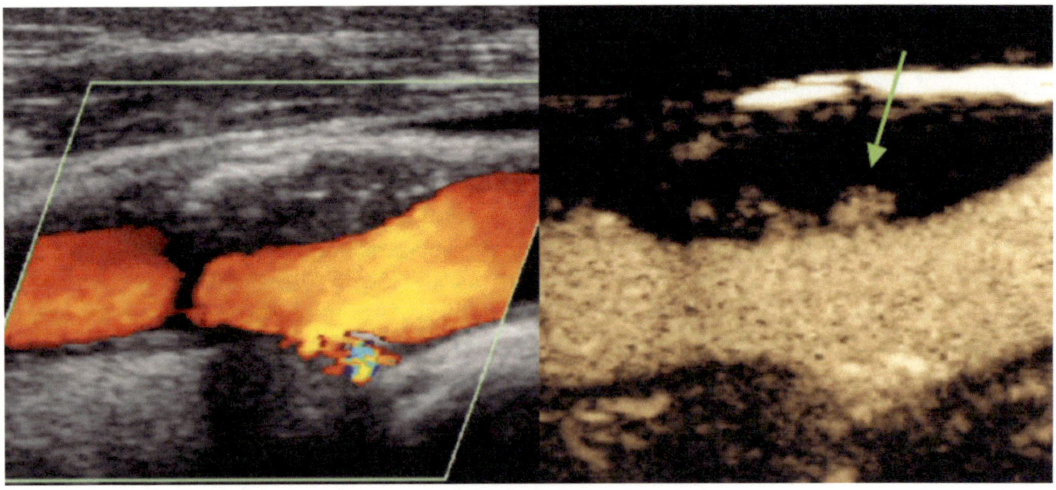

Fig. 1. Contrast carotid ultrasound of a ulcerated plaque. Ultrasound contrast agents better identify plaque surface and ulceration (green arrow).

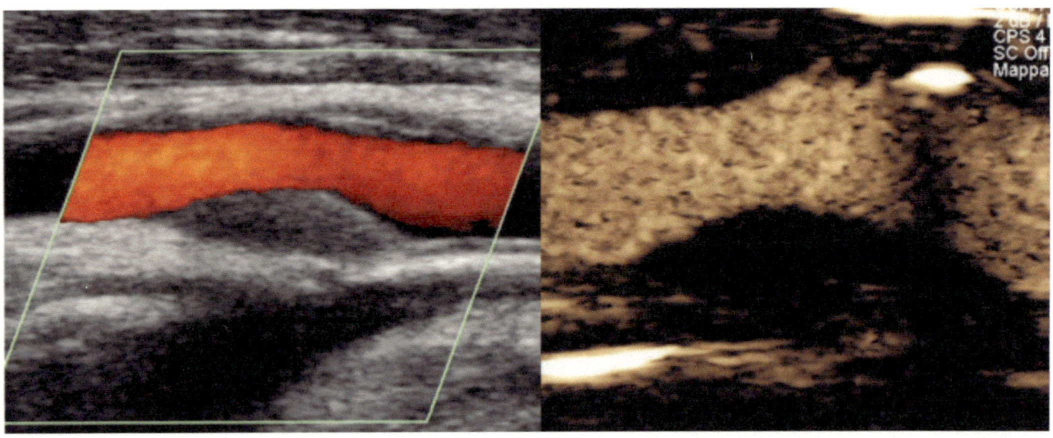

Fig. Isoechoic, fibrous plaque with regular surface determining moderate internal carotid artery stenosis in an asymptomatic patient. No vascularization observed at contrast ultrasound.

progression and remodeling. In these regards, several Authors reported the strong histological correlation between the density of the new vessels in the intima and the incidence of luminal stenosis, the extent of chronic inflammatory infiltrates, the evidence of granulation tissue, thus confirming that symptomatic coronary and carotid artery plaques are characterized by a high vascularized pattern (McCarthy, 1999; Mofidi, 2001; Fleiner, 2004; Spagnoli, 2004; Dunmore, 2007).

The relevance of angiogenesis in atherosclerosis is driving efforts to develop accurate and reliable imaging modalities able to quantify plaque neovessels in-vivo. The ideal non-invasive technique should have a high resolution and be widely available and reproducible. In cardiology, angiogenesis and microvessels observed in coronary atheromas in histological studies have proven to be strongly associated with unstable angina and myocardial infarction. These observations lead then to the concept that the coronary atherosclerotic plaque, when in a late phase of development, becomes richly vascularized, unstable and responsible of the coronary artery occlusion and/or distal embolization, with consequent myocardial ischemic damage (Fryer, 1987; El Barghouty, 1995; Mofidi, 2001; Spagnoli, 2004). Morevoer, in our experience, contrast ultrasound shows vasa-vasorum and plaque newly-formed microvessels with an outward-inward direction, probably witnessing the patophysiological mechanism responsible of intraplaque microvessels rupture resulting in plaque increase of volume and surface rupture, trombotically active. The immunohistochemical sampling confirmed the relevant neoangiogenesis in these areas. On the other hand, the vascularization pattern was quite different in asymptomatic plaques, that showed less contrast enhancement with histological demonstration of more mature microvessels of higher caliber, rarely distributed in the plaque context. These contrast ultrasonographic findings are confirming histological data showing that every plaque has its own vascularization and that neoangiogensis is relevant in the unstable and symptomatic carotid plaque, as in the coronary arteries (Barger, 1984). New vessels formed within an atherosclerotic lesion have to be considered a "locus minoris resistentiae", because they are particularly prone to rupture, thus causing intra-plaque haemorrhage, increased plaque volume and instability. Several factors have been identified as contributors to the neovascular response of the atherosclerotic plaque: hypoxia and ischemia occurs when the intima and media undergoes thickening, inducing the production of angiogenic factors such as vascular endothelial grow-factor (VEGF), in particular in the diabetic patient (Williamson 1993). With the rupture of these microvessels, intraplaque haemorrhage stimulates the inflammatory response of macrophages and T cells to produce angiogenic factors, further promoting angiogenesis and increase of plaque volume.

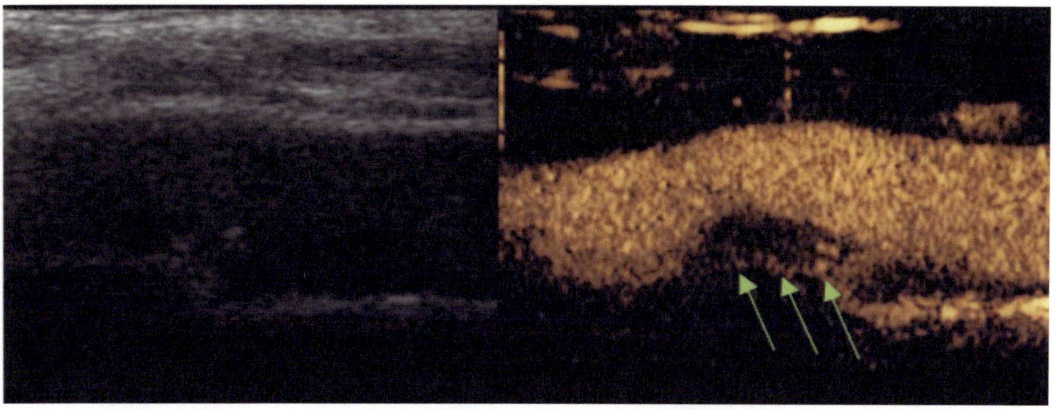

Fig. Acute symptomatic vascularized plaque. Green arrows show microbubbles in the plaque texture.

5. Role of inflammation and intraplaque angiogenesis

The patophysiological mechanisms responsible for progression and change towards carotid plaque instability remain incompletely defined. Consequently, there is an important need to identify if other elements play a key role in the progression and embolism from carotid plaques. Nowadays, the importance of inflammation and inflammatory markers has been claimed as a fundamental factor involved in the development and progression of the atherosclerotic plaques; furthermore, the association between inflammation, atherosclerosis progression and cardiovascular events have been well established for coronary and carotid artery diseases (Libby, 2002; Ridker, 2003, Monaco 2009, Monaco 2010, Shalhoub 2009, Shalhoub 2010.). Histological studies have observed that stable plaques are indeed characterized by a chronic inflammatory infiltrate, whereas vulnerable and ruptured plaques are characterized by an active inflammation and "plaque activity" processes involved in the thinning of the fibrous cap, predisposing to plaque rupture (de Nooijer, 1996; Spagnoli, 2004; Spagnoli, 2007). Nonetheless, the occurrence of high plaque neovascularization originating from the external layers and the increased number of adventitial vasa-vasorum have been considered, and confirmed in histological studies, as other important predictors of unstable achromatic lesions in symptomatic and asymptomatic carotid artery plaques (Mofidi, 2001; Dunmore, 2007), through different mechanisms that may be connected with plaque inflammation. Angiogenesis occurs indeed regularly within atherosclerotic plaques and plaque vulnerability and symptomatic carotid disease have been associated with an increased number of microvessels (Fleiner, 2004). It is indeed believed that the absence of pericytes in new vessels causes the "leak" of potentially noxious and inflammatory plasma components into the extracellular matrix of the media/intima, increasing the plaque volume, gradually reducing vessel wall oxygen diffusion, enhancing further angiogenesis. In the final phase, the plaque is enveloped in adventitial vasa vasorum and rich network of small caliber microvessels, a hallmark of symptomatic atherosclerosis (Carlier, 2005). The processes that lead to intramural haemorrhage and plaque ulcerations are other important issues that have been extensively studied. Some theories claims the hypothesis that atherosclerosis progression is due to an "outside-in" process and, effectively, intimal vessels originating from the adventitial layers have been observed much more frequently that those originating from the luminal side, resembling microvessels that grow within tumors (Kumamoto, 1995; Mofidi, 2001; Dunmore, 2007). This datum was also confirmed in our patients, in which the microbubbles diffusion seems to be oriented from the external adventitial layers towards the internal intimal lumen and, constantly, through a little vessel present under the plaque ulcerations.

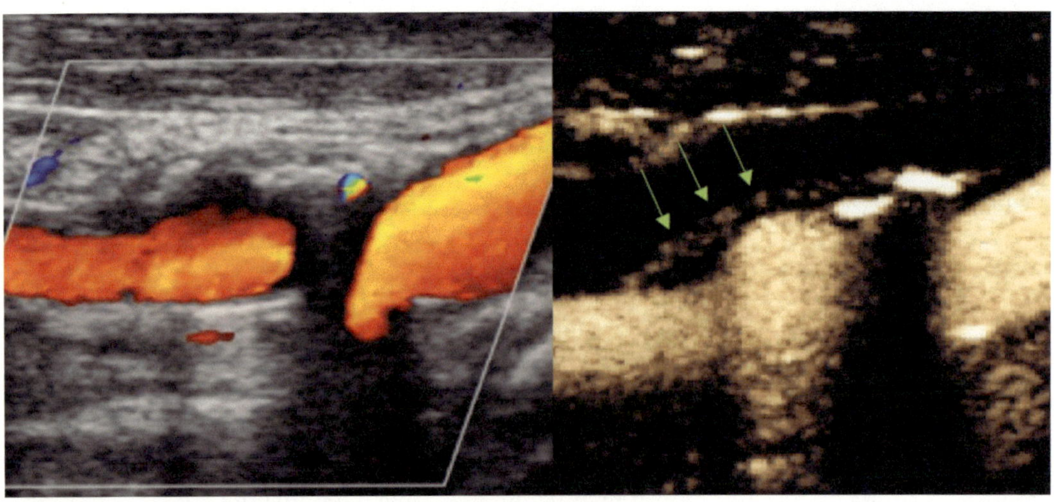

Fig. Plaque vascularization in the area below ulcerations

This latter observation further supports the theory that intraplaque hemorrhage and ulcerations can be related to the rupture of newly formed intraplaque microvessels, that, being immature and with a thin wall, are submitted to local triggering factors such as mechanical forces and shear stress. The histological observation that intraplaque hemorrhages are common in every atherosclerotic lesion, usually deep and not connected with the vessel lumen, is another indicator that the bleeding originates locally (Bornstein, 1990; Milei, 1998).

6. What is new and good, what is not good

The most relevant information that can be obtained with CEUS is that plaque angiogenesis is possible to be demonstrated in vivo and in "real time". A limitation of this approach is the modality of the evaluation of these patterns of vascularization: at present, a method of a real numerical objective quantification is indeed not available for carotid plaques. Differently from the evaluation of myocardium, in which tissue perfusion is the expression of a normal condition, and differently from small coronary plaques, in which there is a different ratio due to the size of the vessel, this pattern may interest limited regions of the carotid plaque and the quantitative analysis of the mean signal enhancement deriving from the whole plaque cannot be easily applicable. The semi-quantitative evaluation, being arbitrary, may not be considered as really representative of plaque vascularization, also because evaluated in bi-dimensional images on user-defined region of interest. The identification of these patterns requires then a very careful visual and morphological observation. Moreover, at present, conventional CEUS imaging is provided through a bidimensional plane, that is not able to give complete information regarding the whole plaque angiogenesis, also considering that plaques can be either or not vascularized with avascular areas, due to necrosis, hemorrhage or calcifications.

7. Future research

Standard ultrasound carotid duplex is one of the most diffuse and available technique to assess plaque morphology and to identify the "plaque at risk". With Ultrasound Contrast Agents, more information on carotid atherosclerosis can be identified in routine clinical practice: as a matter of fact, an enhanced assessment of the arterial lumen and plaque morphology and an improved resolution of carotid intima-media thickness can be obtained. Consistent data also report that the direct visualization of adventitial vasa vasorum and plaque neovascularization is now possible with this technique, with the main advantage of being simple, low cost, minimally invasive and "in vivo". These data could open future perspectives to study unstable carotid plaques with contrast ultrasound to evaluate plaque progression and the possible efficacy of medical therapies. In these regards, the efficacy of statins in cardiovascular prevention has been established (Mizuguchi, 2008). Several papers suggested that the pleiotrophic effects of statins may contribute to plaque stabilization reducing inflammation (Yamagami 2008; Kadoglou, 2008) and, potentially, all these features could be evaluated with contrast ultrasound. The innovative aspect of this study is that data obtained from histological specimens are detectable "in vivo", with minimal invasiveness, by contrast ultrasound investigation.

8. References

A randomised, blinded, trial of clopidogrel versus aspirin in patients at risk of ischaemic events (CAPRIE). CAPRIE Steering Committee. Lancet (1996); 348: 1329-1339

Abbott AL, Bladin CF, Levi CR, Chambers BR What should we do with asymptomatic carotid stenosis? Int J Stroke (2007); 2: 27-39

Abdelmoneim SS, Bernier M, Scott CG, Dhoble A, Ness SA, Hagen ME, Moir S, McCully RB, Pellikka PA, Mulvagh SL. Safety of contrast agent use during stress echocardiography: a 4-year experience from a single-center cohort study of 26,774 patients. JACC Cardiovasc Imaging. (2009); 2: 1048-1056.

Asymptomatic Carotid Atherosclerosis Study Group. Carotid endarterectomy for patients with asymptomatic internal carotid artery stenosis. JAMA (1995); 273: 1421–1428

Barger AC, Beeuwkes R, Lainey LL, Silverman KJ. Hypothesis: vasa vasorum and neovascularization of human coronary arteries. A possible role in the pathophysiology of atherosclerosis. NEJM (1984); 310: 175-177

Barnett HJ, Taylor DW, Eliasziw M, Fox AJ, Ferguson GG, Haynes RB, Rankin RN, Clagett GP, Hachinski VC, Sackett DL, Thorpe KE, Meldrum HE, Spence JD Benefit of carotid endarterectomy in patients with symptomatic moderate or severe stenosis. North American Symptomatic Carotid Endarterectomy Trial Collaborators. N Engl J Med (1998); 339: 1415-1425.

Biasi GM, Sampaolo A, Mingazzini P, De Amicis P, El-Barghouty N, Nicolaides AN: Computer analysis of ultrasonic plaque echolucency in identifying high risk carotid bifurcation lesions. Eur J Vasc Endovasc Surg (1999); 17: 476–479

Bornstein NM, Krajewski A, Lewis AJ, Norris JW. Clinical significance of carotid plaque hemorrhage. Arch Neurol (1990); 47: 958-959

Carlier S, Kakadiaris IA, Dib N, Vavuranakis M, O'Malley SM, Gul K, et al. Vasa vasorum imaging: a new window to the clinical detection of vulnerable atherosclerotic plaques. Curr Atheroscler Rep (2005); 7: 164-169

Carr S, Farb A, Pearce WH, Virmani R, Yao JS. Atherosclerotic plaque rupture in symptomatic carotid artery stenosis. J Vasc Surg (1996); 23: 755–765

Chowdhury M, Ghosh J, Slevin M, et al A comparative study of carotid atherosclerotic plaque microvessel density and angiogenic growth factor expression in symptomatic versus asymptomatic patients Eur J Vasc Endovasc Surg. 2010 ; 39:388-395.

Claudon M, Cosgrove D, Albrecht T, Bolondi L, Bosio M, Calliada F, Correas JM, Darge K, Dietrich C, D'Onofrio M, Evans DH, Filice C, Greiner L, Jäger K, Jong N, Leen E, Lencioni R, Lindsell D, Martegani A, Meairs S, Nolsøe C, Piscaglia F, Ricci P, Seidel G, Skjoldbye B, Solbiati L, Thorelius L, Tranquart F, Weskott HP, Whittingham T. Guidelines and good clinical practice recommendations for contrast enhanced ultrasound (CEUS) - update 2008. Ultraschall Med. (2008); 29: 28-44.

Cole JE, Mitra AT, Monaco C. Treating atherosclerosis: the potential of Toll-like receptors as therapeutic targets. Expert Rev Cardiovasc Ther. (2010); 8: 1619-1635.

Cole JE, Georgiou E, Monaco C.The expression and functions of toll-like receptors in atherosclerosis. Mediators Inflamm. (2010)3 93946. Epub 2010 Jun 24. Review

Coll B, Nambi V, Feinstein SB. New advances in noninvasive imaging of the carotid artery: CIMT, contrast-enhanced ultrasound, and vasa vasorum. Curr Cardiol Rep. (2010); 12: 497-502.

De Bray JM, Baud JM, Dauzat M. Consensus concerning the morphology and the risk of carotid plaques. Cerebrovasc Dis (1996);7:289–296

de Nooijer R, Verkleij CJ, von der Thüsen JH, Jukema JW, van der Wall EE, van Berkel TJ, et al. Lesional over expression of matrix metalloproteinase-9 promotes intraplaque hemorrhage in advanced lesions but not at earlier stages of atherogenesis. Arterioscler Thromb Vasc Biol (2006); 26: 340-346

Diener HC, Bogousslavsky J, Brass LM, Cimminiello C, Csiba L, Kaste M, Leys D, Matias-Guiu J, Rupprecht HJ; MATCH investigators. Aspirin and clopidogrel compared with clopidogrel alone after recent ischaemic stroke or transient ischaemic attack in high-risk patients (MATCH): randomised, double-blind, placebo-controlled trial. Lancet. (2004) ;364: 331-337

Dixon S, Pais SO, Raviola C.: Natural history of non stenotic ulcerative lesions of the carotid artery. Arch Surg (1982); 117: 1493-1498

Dunmore BJ, McCarthy MJ, Naylor AR, Brindle NP. Carotid plaque instability and ischemic symptoms are linked to immaturity of microvessels within plaques. J Vasc Surg (2007); 45: 155-159

El-Barghouty N, Gerulakos G, NicolaidesAN, Androulakos A, Bahn V: Computer assisted carotid plaque characterization. Eur JVasc Endov Surg (1995); 9: 389–393

Engel-Nitz NM, Sander SD, Harley C, Rey GG, Shah H. Costs and outcomes of noncardioembolic ischemic stroke in a managed care population. Vascular Health and Risk Management .6 : 905 - 913, 2010)European Carotid Surgery Trialists' Collaborative Group. Randomised trial of endarterectomy for recently symptomatic carotid stenosis: final results in the MRC European carotid surgery trial (ECST). Lancet (1998); 351: 1379–1387

European Carotid Surgery Trialists' Collaborative Group. MRC European Carotid Surgery Trial: interim results for symptomatic patients with severe (70–99%) or with mild (0–29%) carotid stenosis. Lancet. (1991); 337: 1235–1243

Executive Committee for the Asymptomatic Carotid Atherosclerosis Study. Endarterectomy for asymptomatic carotid artery stenosis. JAMA. (1995); 273:1421–1428

Feinstein SB. Contrast ultrasound imaging of the carotid artery vasa vasorum and atherosclerotic plaque neovascularization. J Am Coll Cardiol (2006); 48: 236-243

Feinstein SB. The powerful microbubble: from bench to bedside, from intravascular indicator to therapeutic delivery system, and beyond. Am J Physiol Heart Circ Physiol (2004); 287: H450-457.

Fisher M, Paganini-Hill A, Martin A, et al. Carotid plaque pathology: thrombosis,ulceration, and stroke pathogenesis. Stroke (2005); 36:253–257

Fleiner M, Kummer M, Mirlacher M, Sauter G, Cathomas G, Krapf R, Biedermann BC. Arterial neovascularization and inflammation in vulnerable patients: early and late signs of symptomatic atherosclerosis. Circulation. (2004); 110: 2843-2850

Fryer J.A, Myers PC, Appleberg M Carotid intraplaque hemorrhage: the significance of neovascularity. J Vasc Surg (1987); 6: 341-349

Geiringer E: Intimal vascularisation and atherosclerosis. Histologic characteristics of carotid atherosclerotid plaque. J Pathol Bacteriol (1951); 63: 201–211

Geroulakos G, Ramaswami G, Nicolaides A. Characterisation of symptomatic and asymptomatic carotid plaques using high resolution real time ultrasound. Br J Surg (1993); 80:1274–1277

Giannoni MF, Vicenzini E, Citone M, Ricciardi MC, Irace L, Laurito A, Scucchi LF, Di Piero V, Gossetti B, Mauriello A, Spagnoli LG, Lenzi GL, Valentini FB. Contrast carotid ultrasound for the detection of unstable plaques with neoangiogenesis: a pilot study. Eur J Vasc Endovasc Surg. (2009); 37: 722-727

Giannoni MF, Vicenzini E. Focus on the "unstable" carotid plaque: detection of intraplaque angiogenesis with contrast ultrasound. Present state and future perspectives. Curr Vasc Pharmacol. (2009); 7: 180-184 a

Goldstein LB, Bushnell CD, Adams RJ, Appel LJ, Braun LT, Chaturvedi S, Creager MA, Culebras A, Eckel RH, Hart RG, Hinchey JA, Howard VJ, Jauch EC, Levine SR, Meschia JF, Moore WS, Nixon JV, Pearson TA; on behalf of the American Heart Association Stroke Council, Council on Cardiovascular Nursing, Council on Epidemiology and Prevention, Council for High Blood Pressure Research, Council on Peripheral Vascular Disease, and Interdisciplinary Council on Quali. Guidelines for the Primary Prevention of Stroke. A Guideline for Healthcare Professionals From the American Heart Association/American Stroke Association. Stroke. 2010 Dec 6.

Gray-Weale AC, Graham JC, Burnett JR, Byrne K, Lusby RJ.Carotid artery atheroma: Comparison of B-mode ultrasound appearance with preoperative pathology carotid endarterectomy sample J Cardiovasc Surg (1988); 29: 676-681

Griffin MB, Kyriacou E, Pattichis C, Bond D, Kakkos SK, Sabetai M, Geroulakos G, Georgiou N, Doré CJ, Nicolaides A. Juxtaluminal hypoechoic area in ultrasonic images of carotid plaques and hemispheric symptoms. J Vasc Surg. (2010) ; 52: 69-76

Grønholdt ML, Nordestgaard BG, Schroeder TV, Vorstrup S, Sillesen H. Ultrasonic echolucent carotid plaques predict future strokes. Circulation (2001); 104:68–73

Halliday A, Mansfield A, Marro J, MRC Asymptomatic Carotid Surgery Trial (ACST) Collaborative Group. Prevention of disabling and fatal strokes by successful carotid endarterectomy in patients without recent neurological symptoms: randomised controlled trial. Lancet (2004); 363:1491–1502

Halliday A, Harrison M, Hayter E, Kong X, Mansfield A, Marro J, Pan H, Peto R, Potter J, Rahimi K, Rau A, Robertson S, Streifler J, Thomas D; Asymptomatic Carotid Surgery Trial (ACST) Collaborative GroupResults: 1 to 20 of 33 1.10-year stroke prevention after successful carotid endarterectomy for asymptomatic stenosis (ACST-1): a multicentre randomised trial. Lancet. (2010);37:1074-1084

Hennerici MG. The unstable plaque. Cerebrovasc Dis. 2004; 17 Suppl 3: 17-22.

Hobson RW 2nd, Mackey WC, Ascher E, Murad MH, Calligaro KD, Comerota AJ, Montori VM, Eskandari MK, Massop DW, Bush RL, Lal BK, Perler BA; Society for Vascular Surgery Management of atherosclerotic carotid artery disease: clinical practice guidelines of the Society for Vascular Surgery. J Vasc Surg. (2008);48: 480-486

Huang PT, Huang FG, Zou CP, Sun HY, Tian XQ, Yang Y, et al. Contrast-enhanced sonographic characteristics of neovascularization in carotid atherosclerotic plaques. J Clin Ultrasound. (2008); 36: 346-351

Huang P, Huang F, Cosgrove D. Analysis of Neovascularization within Carotid Plaques in Patients with Ischemic Stroke using Contrast-Enhanced Ultrasound . 12th World congress of Ultrasound in Medicine and Biology, Sydney sept 2009. Ultrasound in Medicine and Biology 2009; 35, (8S), S4.

Joakimsen O, Bonaa KH, Stensland-Bugge E. Reproducibility of ultrasound assessment of carotid plaque occurrence, thickness,and morphology. The Tromso Study. Stroke (1997);28: 2201–2207

Johnson JM, Kennely M, Decesale D, Morgan S, Sparrow S. Natural history of asymptomatic plaque. Arch Surg (1985); 120: 1010–1012

Kadoglou NP, Gerasimidis T, Moumtzouoglou A, Kapelouzou A, Sailer N, Fotiadis G, Vitta I, Katinios A, Kougias P, Bandios S, Voliotis K, Karayannacos PE, Liapis CD.Intensive lipid-lowering therapy ameliorates novel calcification markers and GSM score in patients with carotid stenosis.Eur J Vasc Endovasc Surg. (2008); 35: 661-668

Kakkos SK, Sabetai M, Tegos T, Stevens J, Thomas D, Griffin M, Geroulakos G, Nicolaides AN; Asymptomatic Carotid Stenosis and Risk of Stroke (ACSRS) Study Group. Silent embolic infarcts on computed tomography brain scans and risk of ipsilateral hemispheric events in patients with asymptomatic internal carotid artery stenosis. J Vasc Surg. (2009); 49:902-909

Kumamoto M, Nakashima Y, Sueishi K Intimal neovascularization in human coronary atherosclerosis: its origin and pathophysiological significance, Hum Pathol (1995); 26: 450-456

Liapis CD, Bell PR, Mikhailidis D, Sivenius J, Nicolaides A, Fernandes e Fernandes J, Biasi G, Norgren L; ESVS Guidelines Collaborators . ESVS guidelines. Invasive treatment for carotid stenosis: indications, techniques. Eur J Vasc Endovasc Surg. (2009) 37: 1-19

Libby P, Ridker P, Maseri A. Inflammation and atherosclerosis. Circulation (2002); 105: 1135-1143

Lindner JR, Coggins MP, Kaul S, Klibanov AL, Brandenburger GH, Ley K. Microbubble persistence in the microcirculation during ischemia/reperfusion and inflammation is caused by integrin- and complement-mediated adherence to activated leukocytes. Circulation (2000); 101: 668-675

Markus H S, King A, Shipley M, Topakian R, Cullinane M, Reihill S, Bornstein N, , Schaafsma A. ACES A prospective observational study. Lancet Neurol (2010); 9: 663-671

Mathiesen EB, Bønaa KH, Joakimsen O. Echolucent plaques are associated with high risk of ischemic cerebrovascular events in carotid stenosis: the TROMSO study. Circulation. 2001; 103: 2171-2175

Mauriello A, Sangiorgi GM, Virmani R, Trimarchi S, Holmes DR Jr, Kolodgie FD, Piepgras DG, Piperno G, Liotti D, Narula J, Righini P, Ippoliti A, Spagnoli LG. A pathobiologic link between risk factors profile and morphological markers of carotid instability. Atherosclerosis. 2010; 208: 572-580

McCarthy MJ, Loftus IM, Thompson MM Angiogenesis and the atherosclerotic carotid plaque: an association between symptomatology and plaque morphology. J Vasc Surg (1999); 30: 261-268

Milei J, Parodi JC, Alonso GF, Barone A, Grana D, Matturri L. Carotid rupture and intraplaque hemorrhage: immunophenotype and role of cells involved. Am Heart J 1998; 136: 1096-1105

Mizuguchi Y, Oishi Y, Miyoshi H, Iuchi A, Nagase N, Oki T.Impact of statin therapy on left ventricular function and carotid arterial stiffness in patients with hypercholesterolemia.Circ J. (2008); 72: 538-544

Mofidi R, Crotty TB, McCarthy P, Sheehan SJ, Mehigan D, Keaveny TV Association between plaque instability, angiogenesis and symptomatic carotid occlusive disease, Br J Surg (2001); 88: 945-950

Monaco C. Innate immunity meets arteriogenesis: The versatility of toll-like receptors. J Mol Cell Cardiol. 2010 Oct 21.

Monaco C, Gregan SM, Navin TJ, Foxwell BM, Davies AH, Feldmann M Toll-like receptor-2 mediates inflammation and matrix degradation in human atherosclerosis. Circulation. (2009); 120: 2462-2469

Nicolaides AN. Asymptomatic carotid stenosis and risk of stroke. Identification of a high-risk group. Int Angiol (1995); 14: 21–23

Paterson JC. Vascularization and hemorrhage of the intima of the atherosclerotic coronary arteries. Arch Pathol. (1936); 22: 313-324

Paterson JC: Capillary rupture with intimal haemorrhage as the causative factor in coronary thrombosis. Arch Pathol (1938); 25: 474–487

Piscaglia F, Bolondi L; Italian Society for Ultrasound in Medicine and Biology (SIUMB) Study Group on Ultrasound Contrast Agents. The safety of Sonovue in abdominal applications: retrospective analysis of 23188 investigations. Ultrasound Med Biol. (2006) ; 32: 1369-1375

Purushothaman KR, Sanz J, Zias E, Fuster V, Moreno PR. Atherosclerosis neovascularization and imaging. Curr Mol Med (2006); 6: 549-556

Randomised trial of endarterectomy for recently symptomatic carotid stenosis: final results of the MRC European Carotid Surgery Trial (ECST) Lancet. (1998); 351: 1379-1387

Reilly LM, Lusby RJ, Hugues L, Ferrell LD, Stoney RJ, Ehrenfeld WK. Carotid plaque histology using real-time ultrasonography: clinical and therapeutic implications. Am. J. Surg. (1983); 146: 188-193

Ridker PM, Buring JE, Cook NR, Rifai N. C-reactive protein, the metabolic syndrome, and risk of incident cardiovascular events: an 8-year follow-up of 14719 initially healthy American women. Circulation (2003); 107: 391-399

Rothwell PM, Eliasziw M., Carotid Endarterectomy Trialists Collaboration.et al. Endarterectomy for symptomatic carotid stenosis in relation to clinical subgroups and timing of surgery. Lancet (2004); 363: 915–24

Sabeti S, Schillinger M, Mlekusch W, Willfort A, Haumer M, Nachtmann T, et al. Quantification of internal carotid artery stenosis with duplex US: comparative analysis of different flow velocity criteria. Radiology (2004); 232: 431-439

Shalhoub J, Owen D, Gauthier T, Monaco C, Leen E, Davies A H. The use of contrast enhanced ultrasound in carotid arterial disease. EJVES (2010); 39:381-387

Shalhoub J, Owen DR, Gauthier T, Monaco C, Leen EL, Davies AH. The use of contrast enhanced ultrasound in carotid arterial disease. Eur J Vasc Endovasc Surg. (2010); 39: 381-387

Shah F, Balan P, Weinberg M, Reddy V, Neems R, Feinstein M, et al. Contrast-enhanced ultrasound imaging of atherosclerotic carotid plaque neovascularization: a new surrogate marker of atherosclerosis? Vasc Med (2007); 12: 291-297

Setacci C, Lanza G, Ricci S, Cao PG, Castelli P, Cremonesi A, Inzitari D, Novali C, Pratesi C, Speziale F, Mangiafico S, Zaninelli A, Gensini GF; Stroke Prevention and Educational Awareness Diffusion (SPREAD). SPREAD Italian Guidelines for stroke. Indications for carotid endarterectomy and stenting J Cardiovasc Surg (Torino). 2009;50:171-182.

Spagnoli LG, Mauriello A, Sangiorgi G, et al. Extracranial thrombotically active carotid plaque as a risk factor for ischemic stroke. JAMA (2004); 292:1845–1852

Stary HC, Chandler AB, Dinsmore RE, Fuster V, Glagov S, Insull W Jr, Rosenfeld ME, Schwartz CJ, Wagner WD, Wissler RW. A definition of advanced types of atherosclerotic lesions and a histological classification of atherosclerosis. A report from the Committee on Vascular Lesions of the Council on Arteriosclerosis, American Heart Association. Circulation (1995); 92: 1355–1374

Staub D, Schinkel AF, Coll B, Coli S, van der Steen AF, Reed JD, Krueger C, Thomenius KE, Adam D, Sijbrands EJ, ten Cate FJ, Feinstein SB. Contrast-enhanced ultrasound imaging of the vasa vasorum: from early atherosclerosis to the identification of unstable plaques. JACC Cardiovasc Imaging. (2010); 3: 761-771

Staub D, Patel MB, Tibrewala A et al Vasa vasorum and plaque neovascularization on contrast-enhanced carotid ultrasound imaging correlates with cardiovascular disease and past cardiovascular events. Stroke. 2010

Vicenzini E, Giannoni MF, Benedetti-Valentini F, Lenzi GL. Imaging of carotid plaque angiogenesis. Cerebrovasc Dis. (2009); 27 Suppl 2: 48-54

Vicenzini E, Giannoni MF, Puccinelli F, Ricciardi MC, Altieri M, Di Piero V, Gossetti B, Valentini FB, Lenzi GL. Detection of carotid adventitial vasa vasorum and plaque vascularization with ultrasound cadence contrast pulse sequencing technique and echo-contrast agent. Stroke. (2007); 38: 2841-2843

Warburton L, Gillard J. Functional imaging of carotid atheromatous plaques. J Neuroimaging. (2006); 16: 293-301

Widder B, Paulat K, Hachspacher J. Morphological characterization of carotid artery stenoses by ultrasound duplex scanning.Ultrasound Med Biol (1990); 16: 349–354

Williamson JR, Chang K, Frangos M, Hasan KS, Ido Y, Kawamura T, et al. Hyperglycemic pseudohypoxia and diabetic complications. Diabetes (1993); 42: 801-813

Xiong L, Deng YB, Zhu Y, Liu YN, Bi XJ. Correlation of carotid plaque neovascularization detected by using contrast-enhanced US with clinical symptoms. Radiology (2009); 251:583-589

Yamagami H, Sakaguchi M, Furukado S, Hoshi T, Abe Y, Hougaku H, Hori M, Kitagawa K. Statin Therapy Increases Carotid Plaque Echogenicity in Hypercholesterolemic Patients. Ultrasound Med Biol. (2008); 34: 1353-1359

11

Ultrasound Imaging for Pediatric Anesthesia: A Review

Santhanam Suresh MD, Lauren J. Taylor BA and Amar S. Minhas
Department of Pediatric Anesthesiology, Children's Memorial Hospital, Northwestern University Feinberg School of Medicine, Chicago, IL USA

1. Introduction

There has been a recent increase in the use of regional anesthesia in pediatric patients (Lacroix, 2008). This explosive growth, particularly in the use of truncal blocks, can be attributed in part to the refinement of anatomically based ultrasound imaging to facilitate nerve localization. Historically, pediatric regional anesthesia has posed a significant challenge due to the close proximity of nerves to critical structures and the need for limiting the local anesthetic volume below toxic levels in children. Ultrasound guidance, however, allows the visualization of important anatomy and can help overcome many of these traditional obstacles.

This chapter will review a variety of common peripheral nerve and central neuraxial blocks that can be performed using ultrasound guidance in children. This aspect of regional anesthesia has the potential for significant contributions to evidence-based medicine. Because ultrasound guidance is a relative newcomer to the field of regional anesthesia, most of the current literature is not evidence based. As a result, much of the data comes from case reports and case series. This chapter is based on an extensive review of the literature using MEDLINE and EMBASE from 1980 to May 28, 2009. Our goal is to provide the pediatric anesthesiologist with a comprehensive summary of the relevant sonoanatomy, techniques, and outcomes of ultrasound guidance for peripheral nerve blocks of the extremities and trunk as well as neuraxial blocks in pediatric patients based on currently available literature.

2. Peripheral nerve blocks

2.1 Upper extremity blocks

Peripheral regional anesthesia is of great utility in children undergoing surgery on the upper extremities. Although many approaches to the brachial plexus have been described, the axillary block using conventional methods is still the most commonly performed and reported brachial plexus blockade in children. This may be due to the fact that other block sites are situated near critical structures such as the cervical pleura (supraclavicular and infraclavicular) and the spinal cord (interscalene). Although there is a paucity of related literature, the introduction of ultrasound imaging will likely greatly increase the performance of brachial plexus blocks in infants and children at locations besides the commonly described axillary approach by allowing for real-time visualization of anatomical structures.

2.1.1 Axillary block

2.1.1.1 Sonoanatomy

The axillary approach blocks the radial, median and ulnar nerves. A probe placed perpendicular to the anterior axillary fold provides a short-axis view of the neurovascular bundle with the biceps brachii and coracobrachialis muscles lateral and the triceps brachii medial and deep to the biceps. The axillary artery is a useful ultrasound landmark and appears as a circular anechoic structure adjacent to the biceps and coracobrachialis muscles. Terminal nerves surround the artery with the radial nerve located deep and along the midline of the artery. The median and ulnar nerves are both superficial to the artery, with median nerve visible between the artery and biceps muscle while the ulnar nerve is found more medial (Figure 1). It is important to be aware of anatomic variation, particularly in the location of the median nerve. The musculocutaneous nerve is located between the coracobrachialis and biceps muscles, but it is difficult to detect in children (Rapp & Grau, 2004). In contrast to the textbook anatomical description, in an ultrasound image the radial, median, and ulnar nerves often appear the same size as the axillary artery (Rapp & Grau, 2004).

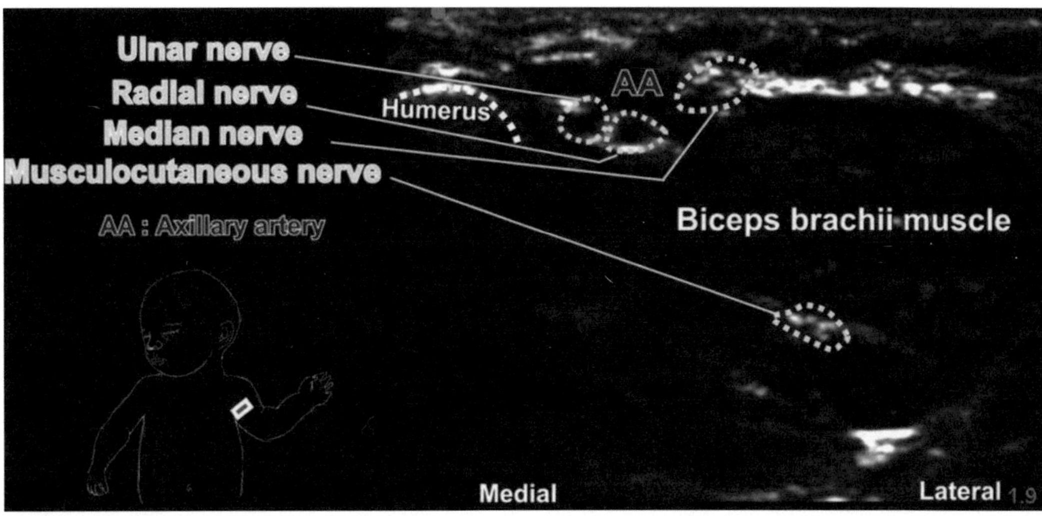

Fig. 1. Sonoanatomy of the axillary block location using a linear hockey stick probe (SLA 6-13 MHz, 25-mm footprint) placed transversely to the humerus.

2.1.1.2 Technique

An axillary block may be used for procedures on the elbow, forearm, or hand. The use of ultrasound guidance for this block in children, however, is not well described in the literature; a recent search produced no original reports (Fleischmann et al., 2003). This block may be performed in children using techniques borrowed from adult patients. With a hockey stick or linear small footprint probe placed proximally in the axilla and transverse to the humerus, an in-plane technique may be used. It is best to use multiple injections with needle redirections to ensure that the local anesthetic surrounds all the terminal nerves of the plexus. Due to the close proximity of the axillary vein and artery, multiple punctures may be necessary to avoid intravascular injection.

2.1.1.3 Outcome and discussion

In children, the axillary block is one of the most popular approaches to the brachial plexus (Cregg et al., 1996). Due to the abundance of vessels in the axillary region, caution must be taken when performing this block to avoid intravascular injection. This is particularly important when multiple punctures are required to achieve the desired circumferential local anesthetic spread. The use of ultrasound for real-time visualization may reduce this risk. Color Doppler is also a helpful tool to identify the axillary vasculature. Due to the superficial location of the plexus, ultrasound guidance may help the anesthesiologist guide the needle advancement (Tsui & Suresh, 2010a).

2.1.2 Interscalene block

2.1.2.1 Sonoanatomy

Ultrasound imaging allows visualization of the C5, C6, and C7 nerve roots between the anterior and middle scalene muscles (Figure 2). In a transverse oblique plane at the level of the cricoid cartilage and at the posteriolateral aspect of the sternocleidomastoid muscle, the muscle appears as a triangular shaped structure overlying the internal jugular vein and common carotid artery. The scalene muscles serve as useful landmarks; the anterior scalene lies deep to the sternocleidomastoid and lateral to the subclavian artery, while the middle and posterior scalenes are located more posterolaterally. The neurovascular (interscalene) sheath appears as a hyperechoic structure within the interscalene groove. The trunks and/or roots of the brachial plexus may be visible as round or oval-shaped hypoechoic structures.

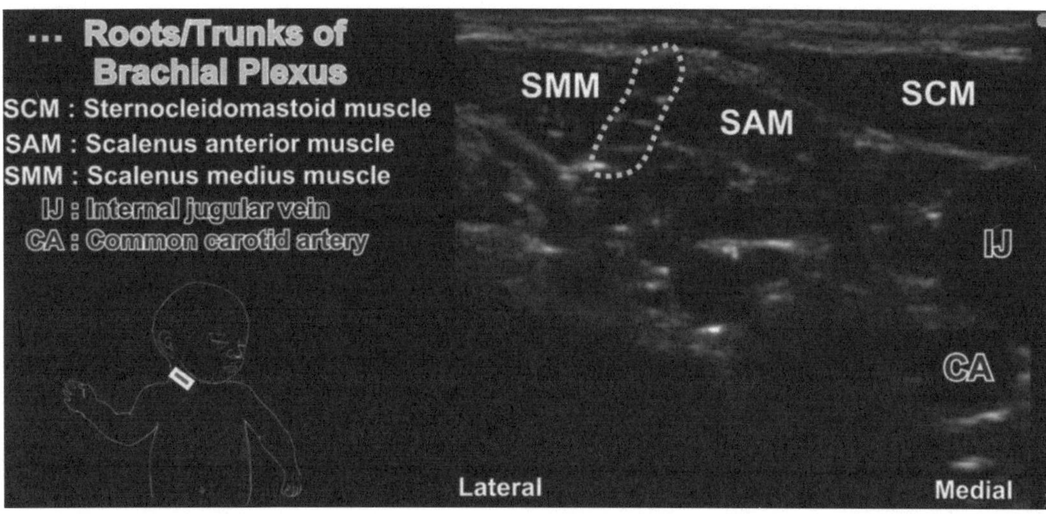

Fig. 2. Sonoanatomy at the interscalene groove using a linear hockey stick probe (SLA, 6-13 MHz, 25-mm footprint).

2.1.2.2 Technique

For optimal imaging, the probe is placed in a transverse oblique plane at the level of the cricoid cartilage. A combined ultrasound-guided nerve stimulating technique may facilitate nerve localization. Using an in-plane approach and slight redirections to advance the needle close to the brachial plexus, local anesthetic spread around the nerve roots or trunks may be visualized. Precise needle placement may limit the dose of local anesthetic required (Tsui & Suresh, 2010a). This combined ultrasound guided-nerve stimulation technique has also been described in the literature using an out-of plane approach and displacement of the middle scalene muscle tissue as a means of tracking the needle tip (Fredrickson, 2007).

2.1.2.3 Outcome and discussion

An interscalene approach is a means of providing analgesia for patients undergoing surgery of the shoulder or proximal arm that can last 6-12 hours. This block may also be used for catheter placement for continuous analgesia (Marhofer et al, 2005). While it may be advantageous to use nerve stimulation in conjunction with ultrasound to confirm the identity of the localized nerve root, a report documenting the performance of an interscalene block in a 7-year-old child with femur fibula ulna syndrome suggests that ultrasound guidance may be of special value for patients in whom the use of nerve stimulation is impossible (Van Geffen et al., 2006).

Due to potential adverse effects including pneumothorax, vertebral artery injection, and intrathecal injection, the intrascalene block is not common in pediatrics. Palpation of the interscalene grove often proves challenging in children under general anesthesia and as a result a recent report states that this block is not recommended for any heavily sedated or anesthetized patient (Bernards et al., 2008). However, the improvements in nerve localization made possible due to ultrasound guidance have the potential to increase the use of this block in children.

2.1.3 Supraclavicular Block

2.1.3.1 Sonoanatomy

At the level of a supraclavicular approach, the trunks and divisions of the brachial plexus are superiolateral to the subclavian artery and above the first rib. This relationship is most clearly visualized with the probe in a coronal oblique plane. The subclavian artery may be used as a primary ultrasound landmark and appears as an anechoic, hypodense, pulsatile structure. Color Doppler may be useful to confirm vascular identification. The trunks and divisions of the plexus appear as three hypoechoic grape-like clusters around the artery while a hyperechoic line with dorsal shadowing indicates the first rib (Figure 3).

2.1.3.2 Technique

Literature describing the supraclavicular technique in children is limited (Suresh et al., 2009). A recent report describes an approach similar to that used in adult patients (De Jose Maria et al, 2008). With a high frequency probe in the coronal oblique plane, the plexus divisions and/or roots are visible lateral to the subclavian artery. Using an in-plane approach, directing the needle from lateral to medial avoids vascular structures in contact with the plexus. An out-of plane approach may also be successful.

2.1.3.3 Outcome and discussion

The supraclavicular block may be performed for patients undergoing most procedures of the upper extremities. However, when compared to other brachial plexus blocks there is an increased risk of pneumothorax due to the proximity of the lung parenchyma at the level of this block. By using an in-plane approach, ultrasound guidance may reduce this risk by providing clear visibility of the needle shaft and tip, making the supraclavicular approach one of the most reliable and effective blocks of the brachial plexus (Tsui & Suresh, 2010a).

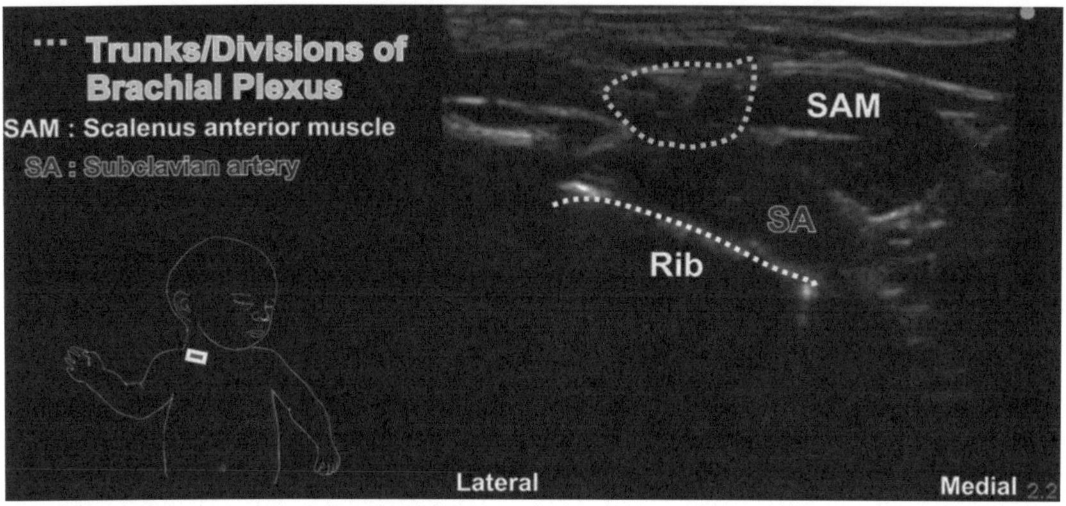

Fig. 3. Sonoanatomy at the supraclavicular block location using a linear hockey stick probe (SLA, 6-13 MHz, 25-mm footprint) placed in the coronal oblique plane.

2.1.4 Infraclavicular block

2.1.4.1 Sonoanatomy

In the infraclavicular approach to the brachial plexus, the cords are located inferior and medial to the coracoid process. Both the axillary artery and vein serve as useful ultrasound landmarks for the infraclavicular approach. These vessels are located deep and medial to the cords, with the vein positioned medial and caudal to the artery (Figure 4). Although all the cords surround the artery, they are not visualized with equal clarity. The lateral cord is most

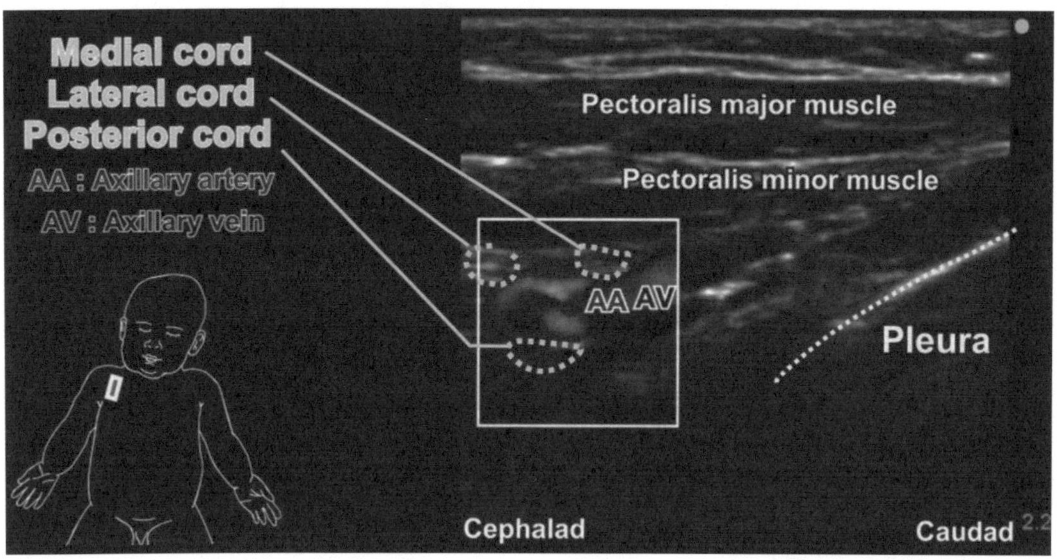

Fig. 4. Sonoanatomy at the infraclavicular block location using a linear hockey stick probe (SLA, 6-13 MHz, 25-mm footprint) placed below the clavicle in a parasagittal plane.

easily viewed and appears as a hyperechoic oval structure. In contrast, the posterior and medial cords may be difficult to visualize, in part because the view may be obstructed by the axillary vasculature; the medial cord lies between the artery and vein while the posterior cord is deep to the artery. The pectoralis major and minor muscles lie superficial to the neurovascular bundle and are separated by a hyperechoic lining (perimysium).

2.1.4.2 Technique

While the plexus lies quite deep in adults, the structure is much more superficial in children, making a higher frequency probe optimal. Marhofer *et al.* described a lateral approach to this block in which the probe was placed transversely below the clavicle with the patient in the supine position (Marhofer et al, 2004). The authors achieved sufficient visualization of the plexus in all 40 patients studied. With the needle inserted using an out-of-plane approach 1 cm inferior to the probe, the local anesthetic dispersion was also clearly visualized.

A recent report by De Jose Maria *et al* described a different technique in which the probe was placed either parallel or in a slightly parasagittal plane to the clavicle (De Jose Maria et al., 2008). The authors recommended using a medium frequency probe to maximize visibility of deeper structures in older children. The needle was inserted cephalad to the probe and redirected when necessary to ensure optimal spread of the local anesthetic around the cords.

2.1.4.3 Outcome and discussion

The infraclavicular block is commonly used for patients undergoing surgery of the upper arm and elbow. It may also be a useful approach for placing a catheter in the posterior cord during more extensive procedures. The risks of this block are similar to the supraclavicular approach, with the danger of pneumothorax being most serious. Just as with the supraclavicular block, an in-plane needle insertion under ultrasound guidance may minimize the risk by allowing clear visualization of the needle tip and shaft (Chin et al., 2008). In addition, due to the closer proximity of the cervical pleura to the plexus cords medially, a lateral puncture site is recommended (Greher et al., 2002). Ultrasound imaging may also be advantageous in avoiding multiple puncture sites and visualizing underdeveloped structures like the coracoid process that may be difficult to palpate in children using "blind" techniques (Marhofer et al., 2004; de Jose Maria & Tielens, 2004).

The first controlled study by Marhofer *et al* in 2004 compared ultrasound guidance to traditional nerve stimulation technique for performance of the infraclavicular block in children. The authors reported ultrasound guidance to be associated with superior visual analog scores during block puncture, better sensory onset times (mean times of onset were 9 vs. 15 mins), longer duration of sensory block, and better sensory and motor block scores 10 mins after the block was performed. The authors explained the faster onset and longer duration of the blocks by the more accurate deposition of local anesthetic possible under ultrasound guidance (Marhofer et al, 2004). Although this study was a prospective, randomized controlled blinded study, the authors did not comment on the power necessary to determine statistical significance.

2.2 Lower extremity blocks

Multiple regional anesthesia techniques may be used for children undergoing surgery of the lower extremities, including lumbar plexus, femoral, and sciatic nerve blockades. These procedures can be performed successfully with the aid of ultrasound, which allows clearer localization of structures as well as visual confirmation of the local anesthetic spread.

2.2.1 Lumbar plexus block

2.2.1.1 Sonoanatomy

Lumbar plexus blocks provide analgesia to the major branches of the lumbar plexus, including the femoral, genitofemoral, lateral femoral cutaneous, and obturator nerves and are therefore indicated for surgical procedures involving the hip, knee, or foot. In infants, a transverse (axial) view using a linear probe reveals several bony structures including spinous processes, laminae, and transverse processes, as well as musculature such as the erector spinae and quadratus lumborum. The plexus is located deep to these structures and is embedded in the psoas muscle (Figure 5). In a transverse scan, the spinous processes appear hypoechoic (likely due to dorsal shadowing effect) and extend superficially, whereas the transverse processes are hyperechoic masses or lines at the lateral edge of each vertebra. In the longitudinal scan, the lateral edges of the transverse processes can be identified at the most lateral point near multiple hyperechoic nodules (Tsui & Suresh, 2010a). In this view the plexus lies between and just deep to the lateral tips of the processes.

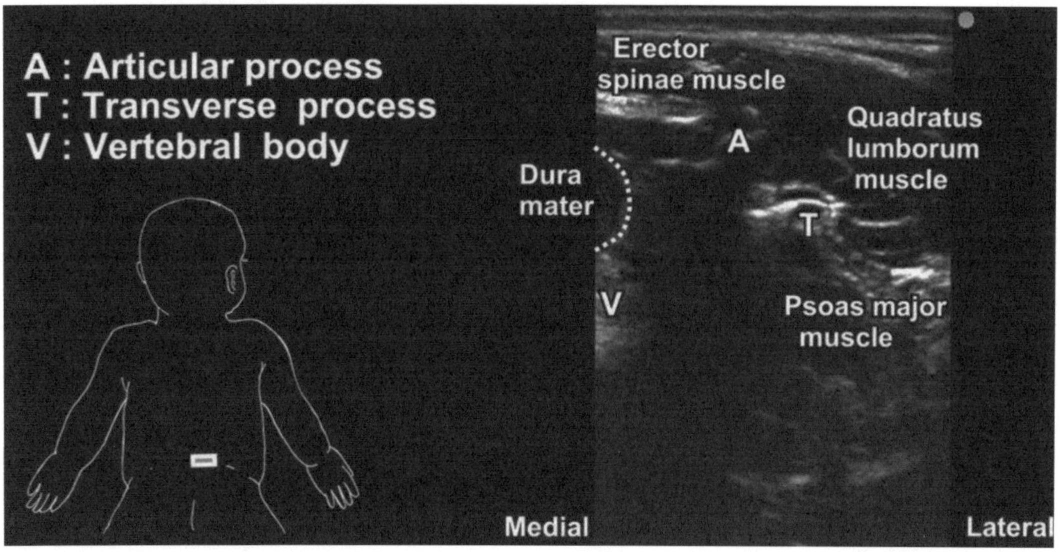

Fig. 5. Sonoanatomy at the lumbar plexus block location using a linear probe (HFL38, 6-13 MHz, 38-mm footprint) placed transversely at L4/5.

2.2.1.2 Technique

With the patient in the lateral decubitus position, ultrasound guidance may be used to identify the transverse processes of L4 or L5 and visualize the psoas major muscle and the plexus in relation to the paravertebral musculature. To locate the bony landmarks, it is important to alternate between transverse and longitudinal planes to survey the region of between the processes. Because of the depth and the similar echogenicity of the plexus to psoas major, however, ultrasound visualization of the nerves may not be possible in older children. In these patients, instead of real-time guidance the block is usually ultrasound *aided*, meaning that location and depth of the transverse processes are determined using ultrasound but the actual needle placement is not imaged. In younger children the plexus is easier to identify because the muscle tissue appears relatively more hypoechoic than the nerve structures, which contain hyperechoic connective tissue layers (Kirchmair et al., 2004). It is best to insert the needle in a cephalad or caudad direction rather than medially towards the spinal canal.

2.2.1.3 Outcome and discussion

Visualization of the lumbar paravertebral region using sonographic imaging has been described in the literature, with the authors reporting successful intra and postoperative analgesia (Johr, 2005). Although ultrasound may enable visualization of the transverse processes or the plexus itself, use of a nerve stimulator, maintaining a needle puncture relatively lateral and cranial (Schuepfer & Johr, 2005), and performing a regular aspiration during injection are recommended to increase safety of the block. Without clear tracking of the needle tip and it may be difficult to achieve an adequate view of the local anesthetic spread, especially if the needle is inserted in a relatively medial and caudal location (Tsui & Suresh, 2010a). Therefore, a risk-benefit analysis is necessary before performing this block.

There is a lack of data in the pediatric literature describing the use of ultrasound imaging for other blocks of the nerves of the lumbar plexus, notably the fascia iliaca block, 3-in-1 block, or individual blocks of the lateral femoral cutaneous or obturator nerves. However, these blocks could all benefit from the advantages offered by ultrasound guidance. In particular, visualization of local anesthetic spread will likely reduce reliance on injecting larger than necessary volumes of local anesthetic in an attempt to block all of the related nerves (Simion & Suresh, 2007).

2.2.2 Femoral nerve block

2.2.2.1 Sonoanatomy

The femoral nerve originates from nerve roots L2, L3, and L4 and when blocked provides surgical anesthesia and analgesia for the anterior thigh extending to the knee. The femoral artery is easily visualized and serves as the principle ultrasound landmark (Figure 6). With the probe placed perpendicular to the nerve axis (*i.e.*, coronal oblique) at the level of and parallel to the inguinal crease, the nerve appears lateral to the large, circular, and anechoic femoral artery. Color Doppler may be helpful to identify the femoral vasculature. The nerve typically assumes a triangular shape but may be of variable size. The fascia lata (most superficial) and iliaca (separating the nerve from the artery) are visible superficial to the femoral nerve and most often appear as bright and longitudinally angled echogenic signals (Tsui & Suresh, 2010a).

2.2.2.2 Technique

A femoral nerve block may be used for surgical procedures on the anterior thigh and knee, including anterior thigh biopsy and knee arthroscopy. With the patient supine, the femoral artery, vein, and nerve can all be visualized with a linear probe placed along the inguinal-femoral crease. When inserted using an in-plane approach, the needle tip can be visualized as it enters the fascia iliaca. It is important that the needle be placed inside the fascia iliaca compartment. In a study comparing ultrasound guidance to nerve stimulator technique, the nerve was visible in all children studied when the probe was placed parallel and inferior to the inguinal ligament and lateral to the femoral artery. Ultrasound was also used effectively to visualize the needle tip and facilitate needle redirections (Oberndorger et al., 2007).

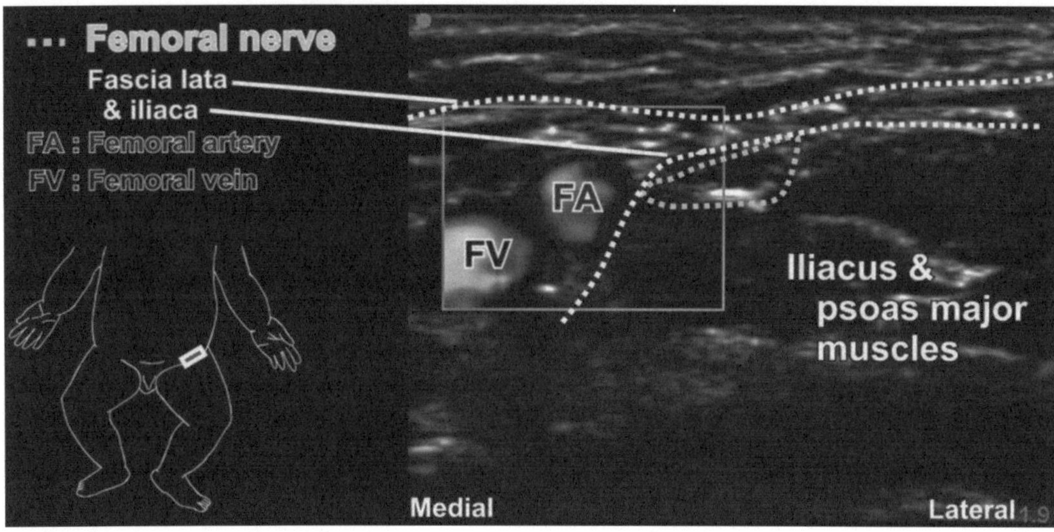

Fig. 6. Sonoanatomy at the femoral nerve block location using a linear hockey stick probe (SLA, 6-36 MHz, 25-mm footprint) placed parallel and inferior to the inguinal ligament.

2.2.2.3 Outcome and discussion

The proximity of the femoral nerve to major vasculature increases the potential for inadvertent vessel puncture and hematoma formation. Although there is no direct evidence to prove that ultrasound could reduce this risk, it is the authors' experience that fewer adverse events occurred when this block was performed under ultrasound guidance. In addition, precise ultrasound imaging of the local anesthetic spread may reduce the need for larger volumes used when injecting blindly.

2.2.3 Sciatic nerve block

2.2.3.1 Sonoanatomy

The sciatic nerve is formed by nerve roots L4 to S3 and innervates the posterior thigh and leg below the knee, with the exception of the medial portion. As it leaves the pelvis through the greater sciatic foramen, the sciatic nerve can be found inferior to the gluteus maximus muscle. The nerve lies between the ischial tuberosity and the greater trochanter, however typically only the greater trochanter can be seen when using a small foot print linear probe (Figure 7). Curved probes (curvilinear) with moderate-low frequency (*e.g.*2-5MHz) allow deeper ultrasound beam penetration and are often necessary in older children. Although the greater trochanter and ischial tuberosity serve as the principle bony landmarks for the subgluteal approach, they must be palpated with great care as these structures do not reach adult morphology until puberty (Scheuer et al., 2000). Thus, since the size of the greater trochanter is dependent on the age of the child, it is only highly recognizable at 6 to 8 years of age (Scheuer, 2000). While the medial aspect of the greater trochanter appears largely hypoechoic, the sciatic nerve is predominantly hyperechoic and is typically elliptical in a short-axis view.

The pathway of the sciatic nerve continues through the posterior popliteal fossa before bifurcating to form the common peroneal and tibial nerves. A linear probe transversely oriented in the popliteal crease captures both the tibial and common peroneal nerves located

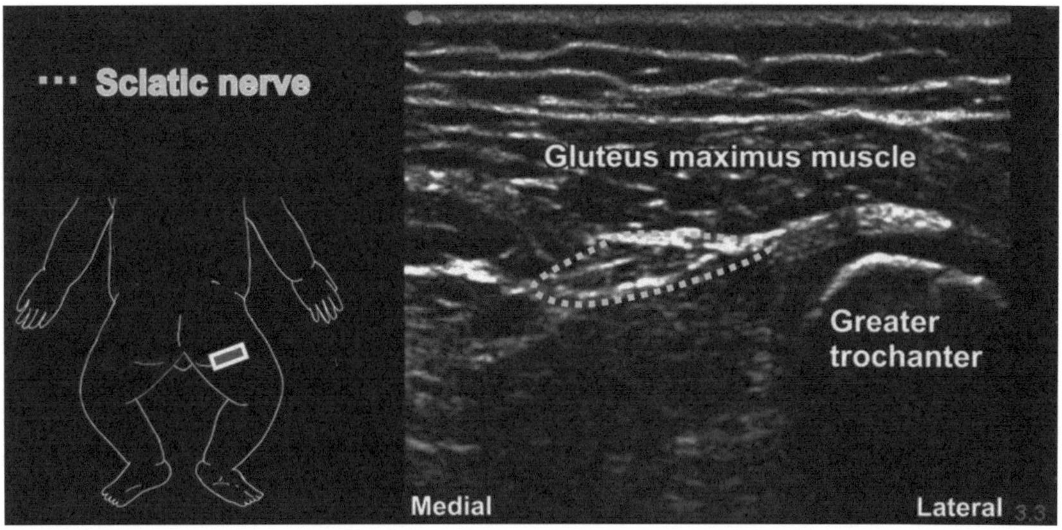

Fig. 7. Sonoanatomy at the subgluteal location using a linear probe (HFL38, 6-13 MHz, 38mm footprint). Image shows where the sciatic nerve lies at the midpoint between the ischial tuberosity and the greater trochanter of the femur.

medially and laterally, respectively, to the popliteal vessels (Figure 8). This vasculature, particularly the popliteal artery, serves as useful ultrasound landmarks (color Doppler may be useful). At the popliteal crease, the tibial nerve is found more superficial and most adjacent to the artery. However, as the probe is moved cephalad, the artery becomes deeper and more distant as the tibial nerve moves laterally to join the common peroneal nerve. At and cephalad to the bifurcation, the sciatic nerve appears as a large round to flat-oval hyperechoic structure. The biceps femoris muscle lies superficial to the bifurcating nerves and appears as a large oval shaped structure with less internal punctuate areas (hyperechoic spots) than the nerves.

2.2.3.2 Technique

A sciatic block is commonly used for surgical procedures of the foot and ankle, as well as in combination with a femoral nerve block for patients undergoing knee surgery (De Jose Maria et al., 2008). In children, subgluteal and popliteal approaches are most commonly employed. For the subgluteal approach, the child should be in the Sim's position with the hip and knee flexed (van Geffen & Gielen, 2006). To visualize the sciatic nerve in cross section, the probe should be oriented transversely at the mid point of the ischial tuberosity and the greater trochanter. The nerve can be seen deep to and at the junction where the gluteus maximus muscle meets the biceps femoris-semitendinosus muscle complex. Both in- and out-of-plane approaches have been described with success.

For a more distal block of the sciatic nerve at the popliteal fossa, it is best to place the patient in the prone position with the probe above the popliteal crease. The probe is moved cephalad until the nerves merge together. Using an in-plane approach, the needle is placed in close proximity to the sciatic nerve and the local anesthetic spread surrounds the nerve.

To achieve an ideal image, a probe appropriate to the size of the child must be used. Deeper structures in older children require lower frequency probes for sufficient visualization. Such a low frequency probe might be necessary for the subgluteal approach as there is considerable variation in the depth of the sciatic nerve in older children. In contrast, high-frequency linear probes are more advantageous for popliteal blocks.

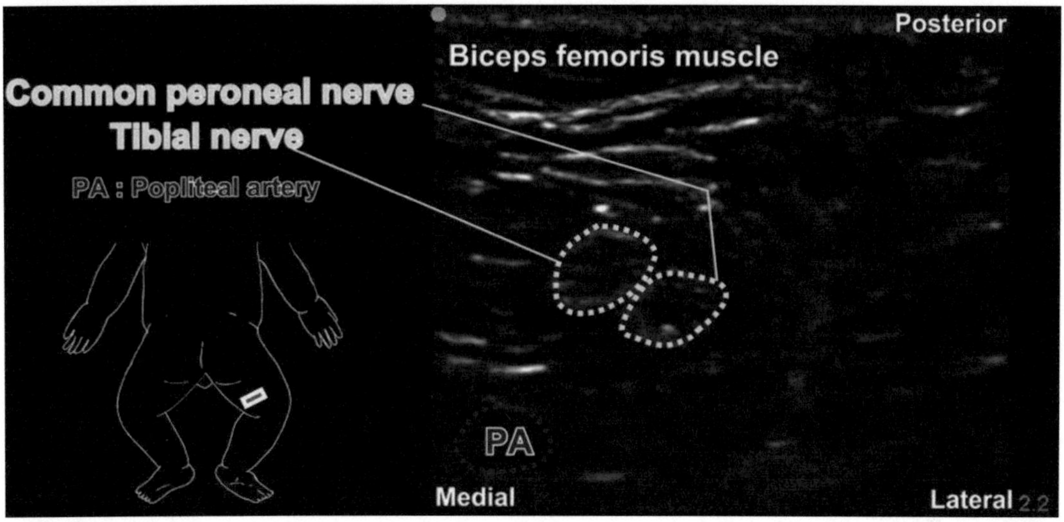

Fig. 8. Sonoanatomy in the popliteal fossa just distal to bifurcation of the sciatic nerve using a linear hockey stick probe (SLA, 6-13, 25-mm footprint).

2.2.3.3 Outcome and discussion

Ultrasound imaging can be particularly beneficial when using blind catheter insertion to confirm the spread of local anesthetic around the nerve. In addition, ultrasound guidance can be advantageous in instances in which a blind technique is likely to fail. An example of this was described for patients with venous malformations. The use of ultrasound in these patients helped the anesthesiologist avoid vascular puncture during needle placement (van Geffen et al., 2007). Due to the high degree of variability in the division of the sciatic nerve, ultrasound also offers considerable advantages in nerve localization when using the popliteal approach (Schwemmer et al., 2004).

2.3 Truncal blocks

Truncal blocks are becoming a more popular means of providing analgesia for procedures in the umbilical or epigastric regions. The ability to visualize relevant musculature and fascial layers with ultrasound offers an advantage over the more subjective conventional technique of detecting "pops" or "clicks" upon penetration into fascial compartments. This is particularly beneficial in children due to the close proximity of nerve and critical abdominal structures. In addition, visualization of the local anesthetic spread made possible with ultrasonography has the potential to improve success rates and allow for administration of minimal volumes of local anesthetic (Willschke et al., 2005, Willschke et al., 2006).

2.3.1 Ilioinguinal-iliohypogastric block

2.3.1.1 Sonoanatomy

The ilioinguinal and iliohypogastric nerves supply the groin area and are derived from the L1 nerve root of the thoracolumbar plexus. Both nerves are seen as hypoechoic structures between the internal oblique and transversus abdominis muscles. A short-axis view of the ilioinguinal nerve running in the transversus abdominis plane (TAP) can be viewed using a probe placed medial to the superior aspect of the anterior superior iliac spine (ASIS) (Figure 9). The ASIS appears nodular in shape and hypoechoic due to the dorsal shadowing beyond the highly reflective periosteum. The lateral abdominal muscles appear with numerous hyperechoic dots within a hypoechoic background (a "starry night" appearance). Any hyperechoic divisions between the muscles represent fascial compartments.

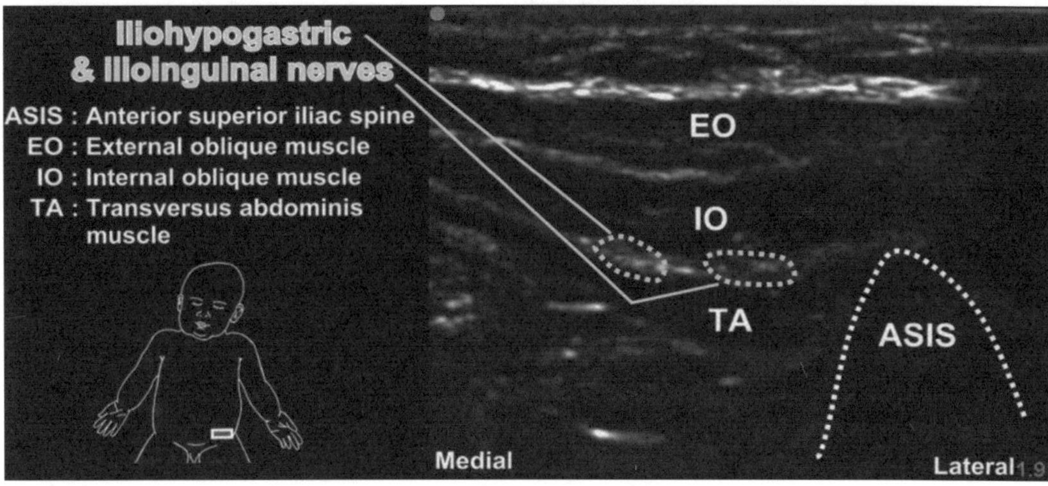

Fig. 9. Sonoanatomy of the ilioinguinal-iliohypogastric nerve block location medial to the ASIS using a linear hockey stick probe (SLA, 6-13 MHz, 25-mm footprint).

2.3.1.2 Technique

This block is commonly used for patients undergoing surgery involving the inguinal region, including hernia repair, orchiopexy, or groin surgery. When performed successfully, these blocks can be as effective as caudal blocks and may be used when a caudal block is contraindicated (Markham et al., 1986). When using a linear probe, it should be placed at the highest point of the iliac crest with the axis facing the umbilicus. This orientation provides a clear view of the relevant muscle layers and nerves as they run in the TAP. Using an in-plane approach, a needle is inserted toward the ilioinguinal and iliohypogastric nerves. After a small test injection of dextrose (1-2ml) to confirm the spread between the muscles and close to the nerves, local anesthetic can be injected into the space.

2.3.1.3 Outcome and discussion

The use of conventional techniques for the ilioinguinal nerve block based on the observance of clicks to determine penetration of the abdominal muscles as a reported success rate of approximately 70% (Lim et al., 2002). Part of the block failure may be attributed to inaccurate nerve localization using traditional landmark-based needle insertion sites and the fascial click method to determine injection. A study by Wientraud et al, used ultrasonography to determine the actual location of local anesthetic distribution when it was injected using traditional methods. The local anesthetic surrounded the nerves in only 14% of blocks (Wientraud et al, 2008). Thus, the use of ultrasound guidance to visualize the plane of nerve localization, needle trajectory, and local anesthetic dispersion offers significant opportunity for improvement.

Pharmacodynamic studies have demonstrated the efficacy of lower doses of local anesthetics for managing postoperative pain in children who received these blocks under ultrasound guidance. The authors also believe using lower volumes could reduce the risk of local anesthetic toxicity (Willschke et al., 2006). The use of lower volumes of local anesthetic is also supported by a recent pharmacokinetic study that found higher plasma levels of ropivacaine using ultrasound guidance when compared to a single pop technique (Weintraud et al., 2009).

2.3.2 Transversus Abdominis Plane (TAP) block

2.3.2.1 Sonoanatomy

The TAP is a potential space located between the internal oblique and the transversus abdominis muscles. The thoracolumbar nerve roots, T8-L1, run in the TAP. The 3 muscle layers: external oblique, internal oblique, and transversus abdominis, serve as easily identified landmarks in an ultrasound image (Figure 10). However, there may not be a clear distinction between the individual muscles. The external oblique is most superficial and lies above the internal oblique, followed by the transversus abdominis. Deep to the muscles, the peritoneum appears as a hypoechoic region. The nerves for this block have similar echogenicity when compared to the muscles and travel tangentially to the ultrasound beam axis. As a result, the nerves will not be visualized.

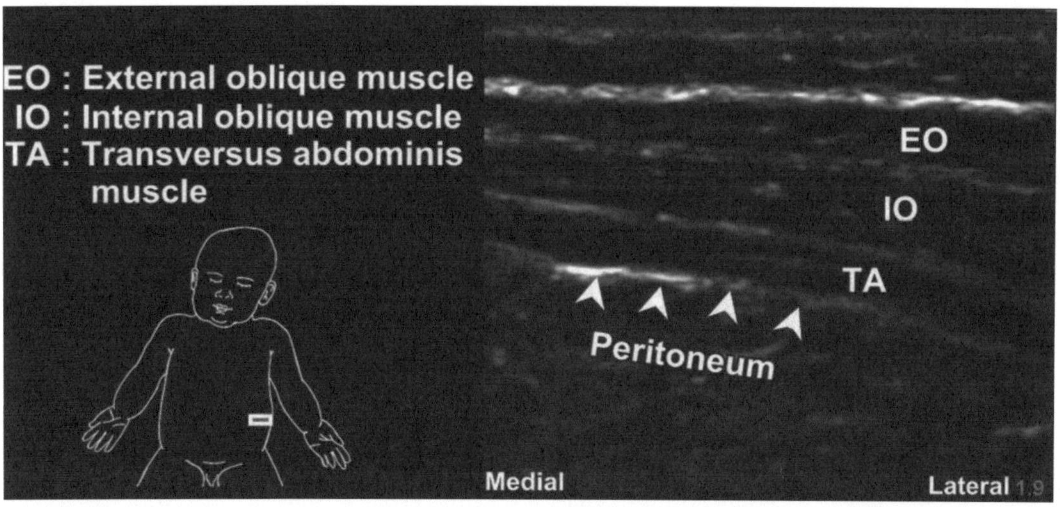

Fig. 10. Sonoanatomy at the TAP using a linear hockey stick probe (SLA, 6-13 MHz, 25-mm footprint).

2.3.2.2 Technique

TAP blocks may be used to provide analgesia for a variety of abdominal procedures as well as chronic neuropathic abdominal wall pain (McDonnell et al., 2007). This block is particularly useful when a central neuraxial blockade is contraindicated. Performing a TAP block in pediatric patients under ultrasound guidance has been described using a step-by-step approach (Pak et al., 2009). A high-frequency linear probe or hockey stick probe is placed on the abdomen lateral to the umbilicus. The probe can be shifted laterally to identify the three layers of the abdominal wall. Next, a needle is placed at or slightly posterior to the midaxillary line using an in-plane approach. The needle should be inserted into the plane between the internal oblique and the transversus abdominis muscles and the local anesthetic is injected into this potential space. The local anesthetic dispersion will appear as an elliptical opening of the potential space. If this spread is not observed, it is important to hydrodissect with small injections of local anesthetic solution or saline until the exact plane of injection is recognized.

2.3.2.3 Outcome and discussion

In adults, the anesthesiologist may rely on palpating the lumbar triangle of Petit to find the internal oblique muscle that lies at its base (Rafi, 2001). However, this triangle is not easily palpable in children, making ultrasound a valuable tool for determining needle placement. Because it includes blockade of the first lumbar nerve root, a TAP block may be used instead of an ilioinguinal/iliohypogastric block when images from the region anterior and medial to the ASIS are not ideal (Fredrickson et al., 2008).

3. Neuraxial blocks

Performing central neuraxial blocks in pediatric patients can be challenging, due in part to the narrow safety margin for needle placement in the spinal canal and tight positioning of anatomical structures. While the use of ultrasound in neuraxial anesthesia in adults is somewhat limited because of poor beam penetration through the ossified bony vertebral column, it could be of much greater value in pediatric patients. In contrast to adults, children have limited ossification, thus allowing good visual resolution of the anatomy and block-related equipment or solutions (Tsui & Suresh, 2010b). Despite an increasing amount of literature supporting the use of ultrasound guided neuraxial blocks, the benefit of ultrasound has not yet been established for block performance or outcome in all patients.

3.1 Epidural Analgesia

3.1.1 Sonoanatomy

Visualization is typically easier in younger children because of the largely cartilaginous composition of their vertebral columns. To capture an overview of neuraxial structures, the probe should be placed both in transverse and longitudinal planes. In a transverse view, the central vertebral body in the region of L3/L4 appears as a hyperechoic "V" in contrast to the more hypoechoic paravertebral muscles. Bony structures such as the spinous processes are useful in identifying the midline (Figure 11). The *ligamentum flavum* and *dura mater* may be visualized as hyperechoic lines in the transverse view, although the *dura mater* becomes more difficult to see in children older than 6 months (Tsui & Suresh, 2010b). Deep to the *dura*, fibers of the cauda equina appear as hyperechoic dots in an anechoic space filled with cerebrospinal fluid.

Using a paramedial longitudinal view at the level of the thoracic vertebrae, the spinous processes and laminae are easy to identify as slanted hyperechoic lines. Deep to the *ligamentum flavum* and *dura mater*, the spinal cord appears as a hypoechoic structure with two distinguishing features: a central line of hyperechogenicity representing the median sulcus, and a bright outer covering of the pia mater (Figure 12).

3.1.2 Technique

A report by Rapp *et al.* examined the use of ultrasound preoperatively to visualize the sacral, lumbar, and thoracic regions (Rapp et al., 2005). The authors used ultrasound to measure the skin to *ligamentum flavum* distance to determine the depth of loss of resistance. An assistant is recommended during catheter placement if real time imaging is desired. In this study a separate individual positioned the probe in the paramedial longitudinal plane at the level of insertion while the anesthesiologist performed the epidural puncture. Ultrasound images were used to monitor the loss of resistance, seen as a ventral displacement of the *dura mater* and widening of the epidural space.

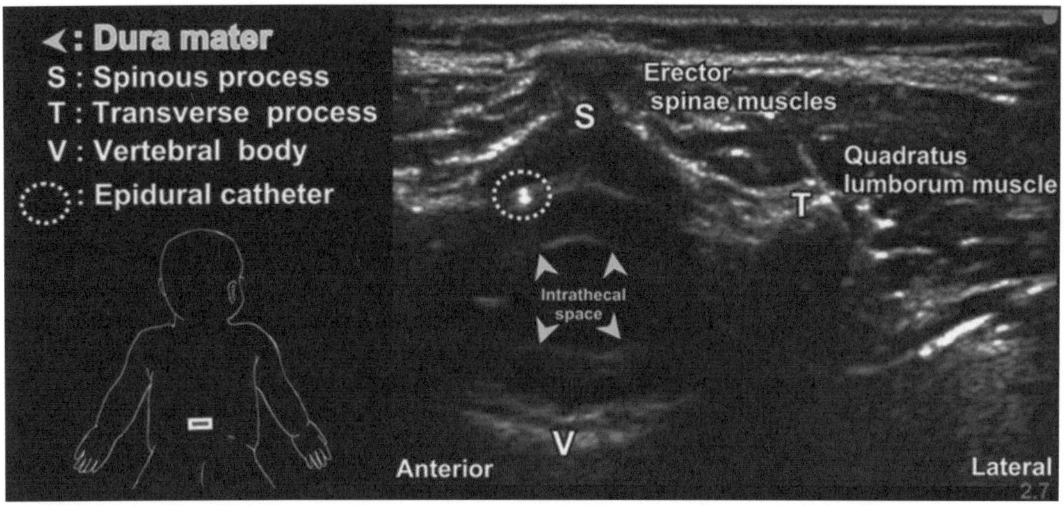

Fig. 11. Sonoanatomy of the spinal column and canal in a transverse axis at the L3/L4 level using a linear probe (HFL38, 6-13 MHz, 38 mm footprint).

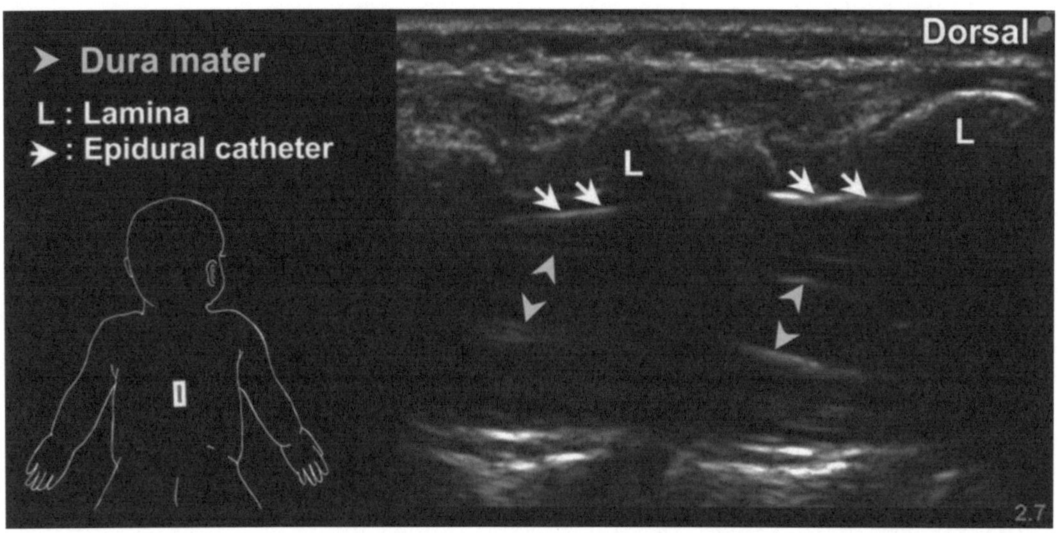

Fig. 12. Sonoanatomy of the spinal column and canal in a paramedian longitudinal view at the midthoracic level using a linear probe (HFL38, 6-13 MHz, 38 mm footprint).

A randomized controlled trial by Willschke et al. also studied the use of ultrasound guidance for determining loss of resistance (Willschke et al., 2006). The procedure was performed with the child in the lateral position with knees flexed. Similar to the technique described by Rapp et al, an assistant operated the probe in a paramedial longitudinal plane while the anesthesiologist performed a midline puncture. The needle was inserted after visualization of the *dura mater* and the needle was followed on its course through the *ligamentum flavum* into the epidural space. Ultrasound imaging was also used to confirm the tip of the catheter and local anesthetic spread.

3.1.3 Outcome and discussion

Ultrasound imaging for epidural analgesia may be beneficial either preprocedurally (before puncture) or during (in real time) block performance to estimate the depth to the epidural space as well as the spread of the local anesthetic. When identifying the epidural space, studies have found that the *dura mater* is typically more clearly visible than the *ligamentum flavum* (Marhofer et al., 2005; Kil et al., 2007). The benefits of preprocedural ultrasound may be more substantial in obese children in whom the landmarks are difficult to palpate (Kawaguchi et al., 2007). A randomized study compared ultrasound guidance with loss of resistance technique for the placement of both lumbar and thoracic level epidural catheters (Willschke et al., 2006). Although the authors found ultrasound guidance to be superior in terms of the number of bone contacts and speed of execution, at this time ultrasound guidance does not obviate continuous testing for loss of resistance.

There is also evidence to suggest that ultrasound may enable visualization of static structures like catheters (Chawathe et al., 2003). This is possible by one of two methods: monitoring the movement of the local anesthetic as the catheter moves through the solution, or noting the ventral movement of the *dura mater.*

3.2 Caudal block

3.1.1 Sonoanatomy

Preprocedural imaging in both the transverse and longitudinal planes is important to identify the sacrococcygeal ligament, dural sac, and cauda equina. With the probe placed in the transverse plane at the level of the coccyx, the sacral hiatus is visible between two hyperechoic lines: the superior line represents the sacrococcygeal ligament while the inferior represents the dorsum of the pelvic surface of the sacrum (Figure 13). When the probe is placed in a longitudinal plane between the sacral cornua, the dorsal surface of the sacrum, dorsal aspect of the pelvic surface of the sacrum, as well as the sacroccygeal ligament are viewed. The ligament can be identified as a thick, linear, hyperechoic band that slopes caudally. When ossification has occurred at the midline, as is the case in older children, the paramedial longitudinal view is optimal because it allows the ultrasound beam to penetrate the spaces lateral to the spinous processes (Roberts & Galvez, 2005).

3.2.2 Technique

Current research supports the use of ultrasound imaging in both the transverse (Raghunathan et al., 2008; Schwartz et al., 2008) and longitudinal (Roberts & Galvez, 2005; Park et al., 2006) planes to guide needle placement during a caudal block. For the transverse technique, the probe was placed just cephalad to the point of injection. Ultrasound imaging allowed visualization of local anesthetic injection within the caudal epidural space, made evident by the presence of localized turbulence and a swelling of the caudal space (Schwartz et al., 2008).

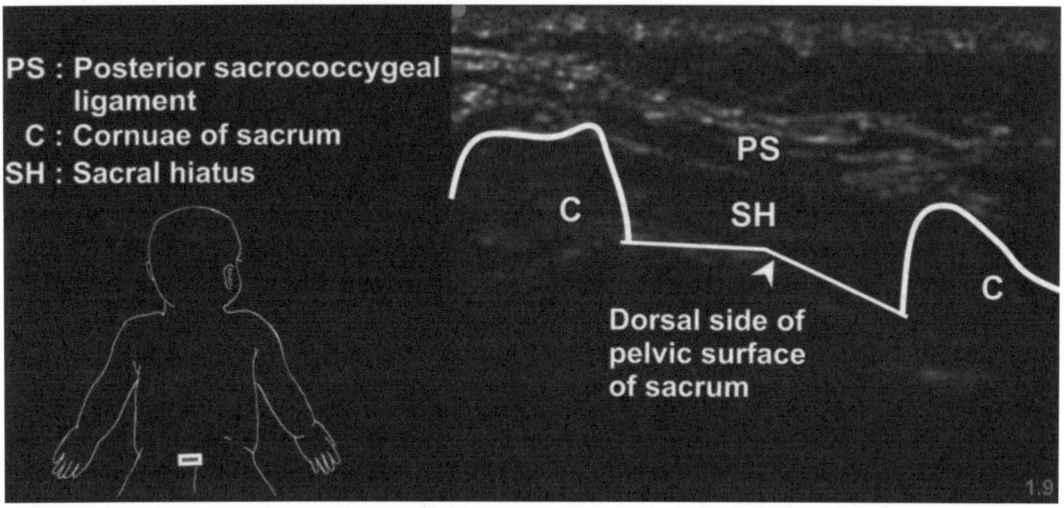

Fig. 13. Sonoanatomy of the caudal epidural space at the level of the sacral hiatus using a linear hockey stick probe (SLA, 6-13 MHz, 25 mm footprint) placed in the transverse plane.

The longitudinal technique allows a long axis view of the needle as is penetrates the sacrococcygeal ligament and thus is particularly valuable in determining accurate angle and depth of the needle. Park et al. used ultrasound in children age 2-84 months to determine the optimal angle of needle entry (Park et al., 2006). The authors found a needle angle of 21 degrees to the skin surface to be successful in 92.3% of patients studied. A similar technique has been found to be successful for catheter insertion into the caudal space. The position of the catheter is possible with ultrasound imaging (Roberts & Galvez, 2005).

3.2.3 Outcome and discussion

Caudal blocks for lower extremity and perineal perioperative analgesia are one of the most commonly practiced regional anesthesia techniques in children. However, they can be associated with higher rates of complications than peripheral blocks, notably bloody punctures and intravascular injections (Giaufre et al., 1996; Lacroix, 2008). To reduce these risks, it is important to have correct needle placement when performing the block. The use of epidural electrical simulation may be used in conjunction with ultrasound guidance to ensure proper needle placement within the caudal epidural space. When compared to the swoosh test for confirming caudal epidural placement, investigators found real time ultrasonography to have significantly higher sensitivity and negative predictive value (Raghunathan et al., 2008). The low negative predictive value may be explained in part by the older age of the patients (5-8 yrs).

Similar to that described in the adult literature, it may be beneficial to use both transverse and longitudinal planes; the longitudinal plane to view the needle puncture followed by a transverse plane to ensure local anesthetic dispersion (Chen et al., 2004). Although there is an increasing amount of literature illustrating the advantages of clearer visualization of anatomical structures as well as the needle, more evidence is needed to clearly define the benefits of ultrasound imaging in neuraxial blocks. For the caudal block in particular, ultrasound guidance may be considered cumbersome for the standard patient, however it may be a useful tool in obese patients in whom poorly palpable landmarks make the blind approach more difficult.

Block	Indications	Ultrasound Landmark
Axillary	Surgery of the elbow, forearm, or hand	Axillary artery
Interscalene	Surgery of the shoulder or proximal arm, catheter placement for postoperative pain control	Scalene muscles and subclavian artery
Supraclavicular	Most surgical procedures of the upper extremity distal to the midhumerus	Subclavian artery
Infraclavicular	Surgery of the arm and elbow, catheter placement for major reconstructive procedures	Subclavian artery and vein
Lumbar plexus	Surgery of the hip or knee	Transverse processes
Femoral nerve	Surgical procedures of the anterior knee and thigh	Femoral artery
Sciatic nerve	Most surgical procedures of the foot and ankle, may be used in conjunction with a femoral block for knee surgery	Subgluteal: greater trochanter and ischial tuberosity Popliteal: popliteal artery
Ilioinguinal-iliohypogastric	Hernia repair or groin surgery	Two to three muscle layers (external oblique and aponeurosis) and the anterior superior iliac spine
Transversus abdominis plane	Major abdominal procedures, chronic neuropathic abdominal wall pain	Three muscle layers: external oblique, internal oblique, transversus abdominis
Epidural analgesia (lumbar)	Surgery of the lower extremity or abdomen	*Ligamentum flavum, dura mater,* and bony structures (midline spinous processes in transverse plane, laminae in paramedial longitudinal plane)
Caudal	Perineal surgery	Dorsum of pelvic surface of the sacrum and hyperechoic sacrococcygeal membranes on the two coruna

Table 1. Common peripheral and neuraxial nerve blocks in children

3.3 Spinal anesthesia

Although ultrasound imaging has the potential to facilitate needle guidance and determination of the depth of the subarachnoid space, to the authors' knowledge there is no published literature available at this time that has studied this aspect of pediatric spinal anesthesia.

4. References

Bernards, CM.; Hadzic, A.; Suresh, S. & Neal, JM. (2008). Regional anesthesia in anesthetized or heavily sedated patients. *Reg Anesth Pain Med,* Vol. 33, 189-93

Chawathe, MS.; Jones, RM. ; Gildersieve, CD. ; Harrison, SK. ; Morris, SJ. & Eickmann, C. (2003). Detection of epidural cathéters with ultrasound in children. *Pediatr Anesth,* Vol. 13, 681-4

Chen, CP. ; Tang, SF. ; Hsu, TC. ; Tsai, WC. ; Liu, HP. ; Chen, MJ, Date, E. & Lew, HL. (2004). Ultrasound guidance in caudal épidural needle placement. *Anesthesiology,* Vol. 101, 181-4

Chin, KJ. ; Chan VW. & van Geffen, GJ. (2008). Ultrasound-guided infraclavicular block : The in-plane versus out-of-plane approach. *Paediatr Anaesth,* Vol. 18, 1279-80

Cregg, N. ; Conway, F. & Casey, W. (1996). Analgesia after otoplasty : regional nerve blockade vs local anaesthetic infiltration of the ear. *Can J Anesth,* Vol. 43, No. 2, 141-7

De Jose Maria, B. & Tielens, LK. (2004). Vertical infraclavicular brachial plexus block in children : A preliminary study. *Paediatr Anaesth,* Vol. 14, 931-5

De Jose Maria, B. ; Banus, E. ; Navarro, EM. ; Serrano, S. ; Perello, M. & Marbok, M. (2008). Ultrasound-guided supraclaicular vs infraclavicular brachial plexus blocks in children. *Pediatr Anesth,* Vol. 18, 838-44

Fleischmann, E. ; Marhofer, P. ; Greher, M. ; Waltl, B. ; Sitzwohl, C. & Kapral, S. (2003). Brachial plexus anesthésia in children : latéral infraclavicular vs axillary approach. *Pediatr Anaesth,* Vol. 13, No. 2, 103-8

Fredrickson, MJ. (2007). Ultrasound-assisted interscalene catheter placement in a child. *Anesth Intensive Care,* Vol. 35, 807-8

Fredrickson, M. ; Seal, P. & Houghton, J. (2008). Early expérience with the transversus abdominis plane block in children. *Paediatr Anaesth,* Vol. 18, 891-2

Giaufre, E. ; Dalens, B. & Gombert, A. (1996). Epidemiology and morbidity of régional anesthesia in children : A one year prospective Survey of the French-Language Society of Pediatric Anesthesiologists. *Anesth Analg,* Vol. 83, 904-12

Greher, M. ; Retzl, G. ; Niel, P. ; Kamolz, L. ; Marhofer, P. & Kapral, S. (2002). Ultrasonographic assessment of topographic anatomy in volunteers suggests a modification of the infraclavicular vertical brachial plexus block. *Br J Anaesth,* Vol. 88, 632-6

Johr, M. (2005). The right thing in the right place : Lumbar plexus block in children. *Anesthesiology,* Vol. 101, 445-50

Kawaguchi, R. ; Yamauch, M. ; Sugino, S. ; Tsukigase, N. ; Omote, K. & Namiki, A. (2007). Two cases of epidural anesthesia using ultrasound Imaging. *Masui,* Vol. 56, 702-5

Kil, HK. ; Cho, JE. ; Kim, WO. ; Koo, BN. ; Han, SW. & Kim, JY. (2007). Prepuncture ultrasound-measured distance : An accurate reflection of épidural depth in infants and small children. *Reg Anesth Pain Med,* Vol. 32, 102-6

Kirchmair, L. ; Enna, B. ; Mitterschiffthaler, G. ; Moriggl, B. ; Greher, M. ; Marhofer, P. ; Kapral, S. & Grassner, I. (2004). Lumbar plexus in children. A sonographic study and its relevance to pediatric regional anesthesia. *Anesthesiology,* Vol. 101, 445-50

Lacroix, F. (2008). Epidemiology and morbidity of regional anesthesia in children. *Curr Opin Anesthesiol,* Vol. 21, 345-9

Lim, SL. ; Ng, SA. & Tan, GM. (2002). Ilioinguinal and iliohypogastric nerve block revisited : Single shot versus double shot technique for hernia repair in children. *Paediatr Anesth,* Vol 12, 255-60

McDonnell, JG. ; O'Donnell, B. ; Curley, G. ; Heffernan, A. ; Power, C. & Laffey, JG. (2007). The analgesic efficacy of transversus abdominis plane block after abdominal surgery : a prospective randomized controlled trial. *Anesth Analg,* Vol. 104, 193-197

Marhofer, P. ; Bosenber, A. ; Sitzwohol, C. ; Willschke, H. ; Wanzel, O. & Kapral, S. (2005). Pilot study of neuraxial Imaging by ultrasound in infants and children. *Pediatr Anesth,* Vol. 32, 102-6

Marhofer, P. ; Greher, M. & Kapral, S. (2005). Ultrasound guidance in regional anaesthesia. *Br J Anaesth,* Vol. 94, No. 1, 7-17

Marhofer, P. ; Sitzwohl, C. ; Greher, M. & Kapral, S. (2004). Ultrasound guidance for infraclavicular brachial plexus anaesthesia in children. *Anesthesia,* Vol. 59, 642-6

Markham, SJ. ; Tomlinson, J. & Hain, WR. (1986). A comparison with caudal block for intra and postoperative analgesia. *Anesthesia,* Vol. 41, 1098-103

Oberndorfer, U. ; Marhofer, P. ; Bosenberg, A. ; Wilschke, H. ; Felfernig, M. ; Weintraud, M. ; Kapral, S. & Kettner, SC. (2007). Ultrasonographic guidance for sciatic and femoral nerve blocks in children. *Br J Anaesth,* Vol. 98, 797-801

Park, JH. ; Koo, BN. ; Kim, JY. ; Cho, JE. ; Kim, WO. & Kil, HK. (2006). Determination of the optimal angle for needle insertion during caudal block in children using ultrasound Imaging. *Anesthesia,* Vol. 61, 946-9

Pak, T. ; Mickelson, J. ; Yerkes, E. & Suresh, S. (2009). Transverse abdominis plane block : a new approach to the management of secondary hyperalgesia following major abdominal surgery. *Paediatr Anaesth,* Vol. 19, No. 1, 54-56

Rafi, AN. (2001). Abdominal field block : A new approach via the lumbar triangle. *Anesthesia,* Vol. 56, 1024-6

Raghunathan, K. ; Schwartz, D. & Connelly, NR. (2008). Determining the accuracy of caudal needle placement in children : A comparison of the swoosh test and ultrasonography. *Pediatr Anesth,* Vol. 18, 606-12

Rapp, HJ. ; Folger, A. & Grau, T. (2005). Ultrasound-guided epidural catheter insertion in children. *Anesth Analg,* Vol. 101, 333-9

Rapp, H. & Grau, T. (2004). Ultrasound-guided regional anesthesia in pediatric patients. *Techn Reg Anesth Pain Manag,* Vol. 8, 179-98

Roberts, SA. & Galvez, I. (2005). Ultrasound assessment of caudal cathéter position in infants. *Pediatr Anesth,* Vol. 15, 429-32

Scheuer, L. (2000). The lower extremity, in Scheuer, L. (ed), *Developmental Juvenile Osteology,* Academic Press, London, pp. 374-467

Scheuer, L. ; Black, S. & Christie, A. (2000). The pelvic girdle in Scheuer, L. (ed.),. *Developmental Juvenile Osteology,* Academic Press, London, pp. 342-73

Schuepfer, G. & Johr, M. (2005). Psoas compartment block in children : Part I- Description of the technique. *Paediatr Anaesth,* Vol. 15, 461-4

Schwartz, D. ; Raghunanathan, K. ; Dunn, S. & Connelly, NR. (2008). Ultrasonography and pediatric caudals. *Anesth Analg,* Vol. 106, 97-9

Simion, C. & Suresh, S. (2007). Lower extremity peripheral nerve blocks in children. *Tech Reg Anesth Pain Manag,* Vol. 11, 222-8

Suresh, S. ; Barcelona, SL. ; Young, NM. ; Seligman, I. ; Heffner, CL. & Cote, CJ. (2009). Postoperative pain relief in children undergoing tympanomastoid surgery : is a regional block better than opioids ? *Anesth Analg,* Vol. 94, No. 4, 859-62

Schwemmer, U. ; Markus, CK. ; Greim, CA. ; Brederlau, J. ; Trautner, H. & Roewer, N. (2004). Sonographic Imaging of the sciatic nerve and its division in the popliteal fossa in children. *Pediatr Anesth,* Vol. 14, 1005-8

Tsui, BC. & Suresh, S. (2010a). Ultrasound imaging for regional anesthesia in infants, children, and adolescents : a review of current literature and its application in the practice of extremity and trunk blocks. *Anesthesiology,* Vol. 112, No. 2, 473-92

Tsui, BC. & Suresh, S. (2010b). Ultrasound Imaging for régional anesthesia in infants, children and adolescents : A review of current littérature and its application in the practice of neuraxial blockade. *Anesthesiology,* Vol. 112, 719-28

Van Geffen, GJ & Gielen, M. (2006). Ultrasound-guided subluteal sicatic nerve blocks with stimulating catheters in children : A descriptive study. *Anesth Analg,* Vol 103, 328-337

Van Geffen, GJ. ; McCartney, CJ. ; Gielen, M. & Chan, VW. (2007). Ultrasound as the only nerve localization technique for peripheral nerve block. *J Clin Anesth,* Vol 19, 381-5

Van Geffen, GJ. ; Tielens, L . & Gielen, M. (2006). Ultrasound-guided interscalene brachial plexus block in a child with femur fibula ulna syndrome. *Pediatr Anesth,* Vol. 16, 330-2

Weintraud, M. ; Lundblad, M. ; Kettner, SC. ; Wilschke, H. ; Kapral, S. ; Lonnqvist, PA. ; Koppatz, K. ; Turnheim, K. ; Bsenberg, A. & Marhofer, P. (2009). Ultrasound versus Landmark-based technique for ilioinguinal-iliohypogastric nerve blockade in children : The implications on plasma levels of ropivacaine. *Anesth Analg,* Vol. 108, 1488-92

Weintraud, M. ; Marhofer, P. ; Bosenberg, A. ; Kapral, S. ; Sillschke, H. ; Felfernig, M. & Kettner, S. (2008). Ilioinguinal/iliohypogastric blocks in children : Where do we administer the local anesthetic without direct visualization ? *Anesth Analg,* Vol. 18, 89-93

Willschke, H. ; Bosenberg, A. ; Marhofer, P. ; Johnston, S. ; Kettner, S. ; Eichenberger, U. ; Wanzel, O. & Kapral, S. (2006). Ultrasonographic-guided ilioinguinal/ iliohypogastric nerve block in pediatric anesthesia : What is the optimal volume ? Anesth Analg, Vol. 102, 1680-4

Willschke, H. ; Marhofer, P. ; Bosenberg, A. ; Johnston, S. ; Wanzel, O. ; Cox, SG. ; Sitzwohl, C. & Kapral, S. (2005). Ultrasonography for ilioinguinal/iliohypogastric nerve blocks in children. *Br J Anaesth,* Vol. 95, 226-30

Willschke, H. ; Marhofer, P. ; Bosenberg, A. ; Johnston, S. ; Wanzel, O. ; Sitzwohl, C. ; Kettner, S. & Kapral, S. (2006). Comparing a novel approach using ultrasound guidance and a standard loss-of-resistance technique. *Br J Anaesth,* Vol. 97, 200-7